Self-Assessment Questions for the MRCP Part 2

Volume 2

Self-Assessment Questions for the MRCP Part 2

Volume 2

Dr Bilal Iqbal

Consultant Interventional Cardiologist, Royal Jubilee Hospital, Victoria, British Columbia, Canada
Professor of Medicine, University of Victoria Faculty of Medicine, University of British Columbia, Canada
Honorary Consultant Interventional Cardiologist, Royal Brompton and Harefield Hospitals, Middlesex, UK

Dr Amin Oomatia

Specialist Registrar in Nephrology, Royal Free Hospital, London, UK

Dr John Waters

Consultant in Acute Medicine and Nephrology, Addenbrooke's Hospital, Cambridge, UK

Dr Gautam Mehta

Associate Professor of Hepatology, University College London, London, UK

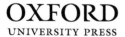
OXFORD
UNIVERSITY PRESS

OXFORD
UNIVERSITY PRESS

Great Clarendon Street, Oxford, OX2 6DP,
United Kingdom

Oxford University Press is a department of the University of Oxford.
It furthers the University's objective of excellence in research, scholarship,
and education by publishing worldwide. Oxford is a registered trade mark of
Oxford University Press in the UK and in certain other countries

Published in the United States of America by Oxford University Press
198 Madison Avenue, New York, NY 10016, United States of America

British Library Cataloguing in Publication Data

Data available

Library of Congress Control Number: 2020946615

Set ISBN 978–0–19–879178–2
Volume 1 978–0–19–879179–9
Volume 2 978–0–19–879180–5

Printed and bound by
CPI Group (UK) Ltd, Croydon, CR0 4YY

DEDICATION AND ACKNOWLEDGEMENTS

I would like to thank my co-authors Gautam, John, and Amin for all their hard work, time, and patience without which this work would have never been completed. I am also grateful to all the contributors and reviewers for their knowledge, expertise, and valuable input. I cannot thank Fiona, from Oxford University Press, enough for her patience from outset with the idea and conception of the books to the completion of what once felt like a never-ending project.

These books have come together with years of hard work involving busy schedules, jobs, and not to mention the move and relocation from UK to Canada. I cannot be grateful enough to my wife, Nabila, and children, Adam, Anna, and Amelia, for their everlasting love, support, resilience, and patience at home, without which I would never had been able to complete this work.

Finally, I would like to dedicate these books to my wife and children, Nabila, Adam, Anna, and Amelia.

Bilal Iqbal

I would like to thank Gautam for involving me in this project, which has been a real privilege. Not only have I learnt a great deal of medicine from writing, editing, and re-drafting the countless versions of the manuscript, but it has reminded me how fascinating medicine actually is. We are truly lucky to be physicians in a day and age when not only do we know more than we ever have before about diseases, but we are also able to provide cutting edge treatment to our patients. I hope that after reading this book, our readers feel the same. A big thank you to Fiona Sutherland from Oxford University Press for being patient with us authors (especially when it came to missed deadlines) and being meticulous and thorough during the synthesis of this book.

Lastly, I'd like to dedicate my contribution in this book to my parents. To my mother, Masuma: thank you for always being patient and supportive, especially when I've been stressed and irritable. To my dad, Asgarali: without your hard work—which included studying for medical school under streetlights in 1960s India—I would not have been granted so many amazing opportunities in my life and I certainly wouldn't have been inspired to go to medical school. Thank you both.

Amin Oomatia

I dedicate these books to my wife for her patience, my mother for her love, and to my late father for his lifelong dedication to his family.

John Waters

This book is dedicated to my parents, for their love and unfailing support in everything I do.

Gautam Mehta

CONTENTS

ABBREVIATIONS

ACE	angiotensin-converting enzyme
ACR	American College of Rheumatology
ADEM	acute disseminated encephalomyelitis
ADM	abductor digiti minimi
ADPKD	autosomal dominant polycystic kidney disease
AIN	acute interstitial nephritis
AION	anterior ischaemic optic neuropathy
AKI	acute kidney injury
AMD	age-related macular degeneration
AML	acute myeloid leukaemia
ANA	antinuclear antibody
ANCA	anti-neutrophil cytoplasm antibodies
anti-U1-RNP	anti-ribonucleoprotein antibodies
APB	abductor pollicis brevis
APTT	activated partial thromboplastin time
AQ4	aquaporin 4
AQP2	aquaporin 2
ARB	angiotensin II receptor blocker
ARDS	acute respiratory distress syndrome
AS	ankylosing spondylitis
AT	antithrombin
ATIN	acute tubulointerstitial nephritis
ATN	acute tubular necrosis
BEP	bleomycin, etoposide, cisplatin
BPAD	bipolar affective disorder
BTS	British Thoracic Society
CAPS	cryopyrin-associated periodic syndromes
CBT	cognitive behavioural therapy
CFH	complement factor H
CHOP chemotherapy	cyclophosphamide, doxorubicin, vincristine, prednisone
CK	creatinine kinase

CKD	chronic kidney disease
CKD-MBD	chronic kidney disease—mineral bone disorder
CMV	cytomegalovirus
CNI	calcineurin inhibitors
COX-2	cyclo-oxygenase 2
CPP	calcium pyrophosphate
CPPD	calcium pyrophosphate disease
CREST	calcinosis cutis, Raynaud's phenomenon, oesophageal dysmotility, sclerodactyly, and telangiectasia
CRC	colorectal cancer
CRP	C-reactive protein
CRPS	complex regional pain syndrome
CRVO	central retinal vein occlusion
CSF	cerebrospinal fluid
CTPA	CT pulmonary angiography
CVAD	central venous access devices
DAS	disease activity scale
DAT	dopamine transporter
DAVF	dural arteriovenous fistula
DAWS	dopamine agonist withdrawal syndrome
DBT	dialectic behaviour therapy
dcSSc	diffuse cutaneous systemic sclerosis
DDS	dialysis disequilibrium syndrome
D+ HUS	diarrhoea-positive haemolytic uraemic syndrome
D- HUS	drug-induced haemolytic uraemic syndrome
DIC	disseminated intravascular coagulopathy
DLBCL	diffuse large B cell lymphoma
DM	dermatomyositis
DMARD	disease-modifying anti-rheumatic drugs
DMO	diabetic macular oedema
DRPLA	dentatorubral-pallidoluysian atrophy
DSA	donor-specific antibody
dsDNA	double stranded DNA
DYT5	dopa-responsive dystonia
EBV	Epstein-Barr virus
EGFR	epidermal growth factor receptor
EGPA	eosinophilic granulomatosis with polyangiitis
ENA	extractable nuclear antigens
ERCP	endoscopic retrograde cholangio-pancreatography

ESR	erythrocyte sedimentation rate
FDIO	first dorsal interosseus
FDP	flexor digitorum profundus
FES	fat embolism syndrome
FFA	fundus fluorescence angiography
FFP	fresh frozen plasma
FGF 23	fibroblast growth factor 23
FIGO	International Federation of Gynaecology and Obstetrics
FMF	familial Mediterranean fever
FPL	flexor pollicis longus
FSGS	focal segmental glomerular sclerosis
FTD	frontotemporal dementia
GAVE	gastric antral vascular ectasia
GBM	glomerular basement membranes
GBS	Guillain-Barré syndrome
GCA	giant cell arteritis
GCH1	GTP cyclohydrolase 1
GDNF	glial cell-derived neurotrophic factor
GPA	granulomatosis with polyangiitis
HAART	highly active anti-retroviral therapy
HADS	Hospital Anxiety and Depression Scale
HD	Huntington's disease
HELLP	haemolysis (H), elevated liver enzymes (EL) and low platelet count (LP)
HHT	hereditary haemorrhagic telangiectasia
HLA	human leukocyte antigen
HNPCC	hereditary non-polyposis colorectal cancer
HPV	human papillomavirus
HUS	haemolytic uraemic syndrome
IBM	inclusion body myositis
IGE	idiopathic generalized epilepsy
IP	intraperitoneal
ISN	International Society of Nephrology
IVC	inferior vena cava
IVU	intravenous urography
JIA	juvenile idiopathic arthritis
JME	juvenile myoclonic epilepsy
KCO	transfer coefficient
KDIGO	Kidney Disease: Improving Global Outcomes
LAM	lymphangioleiomyomatosis

LBD	Lewy body dementia
lcSSc	limited cutaneous systemic sclerosis
LD	legionnaires disease
LEMS	Lambert-Eaton myasthenic syndrome
LETM	longitudinally extensive transverse myelitis
LMWH	low molecular weight heparin
LTOT	long-term oxygen therapy
MAHA	microangiopathic haemolytic anaemia
MGRS	monoclonal gammopathy of renal significance
MGUS	monoclonal gammopathy of undetermined significance
MPGN	membranoproliferative glomerulonephritis
MPO	myeloperoxidase
MRC	Medical Research Council
MS	multiple sclerosis
MSK	medullary sponge kidney
MUGA	multi-gate acquisition
MWS	Muckle-Wells syndrome
NAC	N-acetylcysteine
NAPQI	N-acetyl-p-benzoquinoneimine
NIV	non-invasive ventilation
NMDA	N-methyl-D-aspartate
NMO	neuromyelitis optica
NMS	neuroleptic malignant syndrome
NOAC	novel oral anticoagulant
NSAIDS	non-steroidal anti-inflammatory drugs
NSCLC	non-small cell lung cancer
OCD	obsessive compulsive disorder
OCT	optical coherence tomography
OCTA	optical coherence tomography angiography
OMM	oculomasticatory myorhythmia
PAS	Periodic acid-Schiff
PAVM	pulmonary arteriovenous malformation
PCNSL	primary central nervous system lymphoma
PCOM	posterior communicating
PD	Parkinson's dementia
PD	peritoneal dialysis
PE	pulmonary embolism
PET	positron emission tomography
PICC	peripherally inserted central catheter

PLA2R	phospholipase A2 receptor
PM	polymyositis
PML	progressive multifocal leukoencephalopathy
PMR	polymyalgia rheumatica
POEMS	polyneuropathy, organomegaly, endocrinopathy, M-band, and skin changes
PPD	purified protein derivative
PPI	proton-pump inhibitor
PPMS	primary progressive multiple sclerosis
PRA	panel reactive antibody
PRN	*pro re nata* (as needed)
PROMM	proximal myotonic myopathy
PSA	prostate specific antigen
PT	prothrombin time
PTHrP	parathyroid hormone-related peptide
PVD	posterior vitreous detachment
RA	rheumatoid arthritis
RCN	radio contrast media induced nephropathy
RET	REarranged during Transfection
RPS	Renal Pathology Society
RYR1	Ryanodine receptor
SCC	squamous cell carcinomas
SCLC	small cell lung carcinoma
SIADH	syndrome of inappropriate antidiuretic hormone secretion
SIH	spontaneous intracranial hypotension
SLE	systemic lupus erythematosus
SLICC	Systemic Lupus International Collaborating Clinics
SNRI	serotonin and noradrenaline reuptake inhibitor
SSc	systemic sclerosis
SSPE	subacute sclerosing pan-encephalitis
STEC	Shiga toxin-producing *Escherichia coli*
SUNA	short-lasting unilateral neuralgiform headache attacks with cranial autonomic symptoms
TAC	trigeminal autonomic cephalalgia
TB	tuberculosis
TCA	tricyclic antidepressant
THR	total hip replacement
TIA	transient ischaemic attack
TINU	tubulointerstitial nephritis and uveitis
TLCO	transfer factor of the lung for CO

TMA	thrombotic microangiopathies
TMD	thin membrane disease
TNM	tumour, nodes, metastases
TPA	tissue plasminogen activator
TPMT	thiopurine methyltransferase
TTP	thrombocytopaenic purpura
UFH	unfractionated heparin
V_A	alveolar volume
VEGF	vascular endothelial growth factor
VEP	visual evoked potential
VIP	vasoactive intestinal peptide
VTE	venous thromboembolism
vWF	von Willebrand factor
VZV	varicella zoster virus

CONTRIBUTORS

Dr Michelle E Allan
Specialist Registrar in Renal and General Internal Medicine
Royal London Hospital, Barts NHS Trust, London, UK

Dr Nicola Ambrose
Consultant Medical Oncologist and Consultant in Oncogenetics
The Royal Marsden Hospital, London, UK

Dr Abhishek Das
Senior Registrar in Microbiology
University College London Hospital, London, UK

Dr Angela George
Consultant Medical Oncologist and Consultant in Oncogenetics
The Royal Marsden Hospital, London, UK

Dr Theodore Gouliouris
Consultant in Microbiology and Infectious Diseases
Cambridge University Hospitals NHS Foundation Trust, Cambridge, UK

Dr Maria Ibrahim
Renal Registrar
Guy's and St Thomas' NHS Trust, London, UK

Dr Bilal Iqbal
Consultant Interventional Cardiologist
Royal Jubilee Hospital, Victoria, British Columbia, Canada
Professor of Medicine
University of Victoria Faculty of Medicine, University of British Columbia, Canada
Honorary Consultant Interventional Cardiologist
Royal Brompton and Harefield Hospitals, Middlesex, UK

Dr Emon Khan
Consultant Rheumatologist
University College London Hospital, London, UK

Dr Daniel Marks
Consultant Physician
University College London Hospital, London, UK

Dr Gautam Mehta
Associate Professor of Hepatology
University College London, London, UK

Professor Philip I Murray
Professor of Ophthalmology
University of Birmingham, Birmingham, UK

Dr Akshay Nair
Speciality Trainee in General and Older Adult Psychiatry
South London and Maudsley NHS Trust, London, UK

Dr Amin Oomatia
Specialist Registrar in Nephrology
Royal Free Hospital, London, UK

Dr Thomas Stoker
Specialty Registrar in Neurology
Addenbrooke's Hospital, Cambridge, UK

Dr John Waters
Consultant in Acute Medicine and Nephrology
Addenbrooke's Hospital, Cambridge, UK

Dr Mike Zandi
Consultant Neurologist, National Hospital for Neurology and Neurosurgery, and Honorary
Associate Professor, UCL Queen Square Institute of Neurology, London, UK

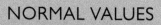

NORMAL VALUES

Category	Test	Unit	Range (All/Male)	Range Female
Haematology	Hb	g/L	130–180	115–160
	MCV	fL	80–98	
	WCC	× 10⁹/L	4.0–11.0	
	Plt	× 10⁹/L	150–400	
	Neut	× 10⁹/L	1.5–7.0	
	Lymph	× 10⁹/L	1.5–4.0	
	HCT	%	38.8–50	34.9–44.5
	MCV	fL/Red cell	79–98	
	MCH	pg/cell	27–33	
Urea and electrolytes	Sodium	mmol/L	135–145	
	Potassium	mmol/L	3.5–5.5	
	Creatinine	μmol/L	60–120	
	Urea	mmol/L	2.5–7.0	
	eGFR (MDRD)	mL/min/1.73m²	>60	
	Bicarbonate	mmol/L	20–28	
	Chloride	mmol/L	95–107	
	Magnesium	mmol/L	0.6–1.0	
Bone	Corrected Ca2+	mmol/L	2.2–2.6	
	Phosphate	mmol/L	0.8–1.4	
	PTH	pmmol/L	0.9–5.4	
Liver	ALT	iU/L	1–31	
	AST	iU/L	1–31	
	GGT	iU/L	<50	
	ALP	iU/L	45–105	
	Bilirubin	μmol/L	1–22	
	Albumin	g/L	37–49	
	Amylase	iU/L	60–180	

Category	Test	Unit	Range (All/Male)	Range Female
Clotting	PT	s	11.5–15.5	
	APTT	s	30–40	
	INR		0.9–1.1	
	Fibrinogen	g/L	1.8–5.4	
Special haem	Reticulocyte	%	<2	
	HbA2	%	<2.5	
	HbF	%	0.3–4.4	
Misc	CRP	mg/L	<10	
	ESR	mm/1st Hr	<15	<20
	CK	iU/L	24–195	
	LDH	iU/L	10–250	
	Troponin T	ng/L	<14	
	Urate	µmol/L	200–420	
Endo	TSH	mU/L	0.4–5.0	
	T4 Serum free	pmol/L	10.0–22.0	
	T3 Serum free	pmol/L	3.0–70	
	HbA1c	mmol/mol	20–42	
	ACTH (9 am)	pmol/L	<18.0	
	Cortisol	nmol/L	138–635	
Lipids	Fasting glucose	mmol/L	4.0–7.0	
	Normal glucose	mmol/L	4.0–11.0	
	LDL	mmol/L	<3.36	
	HDL	mmol/L	>1.55	
	Total cholesterol	mmol/L	<5.2	
	Triglycerides	mmol/L	0.45–1.69	
CSF	Opening pressure	mmH20	12–250	
	Total protein	g/L	0.15–0.45	
	Glucose	mmol/L	2.5–4.4 (60–70% of serum glucose)	
Haematinics	Serum iron	µmol/L	12–30	
	TIBC (serum total iron binding capacity)	µmol/L	45–75	
	Transferrin saturation	%	15–50	

Category	Test	Unit	Range (All/Male)	Range Female	
	Ferritin	µg/L	15–300		
	Transferrin	g/L	2.0–4.0		
	Serum B12	ng/L	16–760		
	Serum Folate	µg/L	2.0–11.0		
	Serum haptoglobin	g/L	0.13–1.63		
Autoimmune serology	Rheumatoid factor	iU/mL	<14		
ABG	pO2	kPa	11.3–12.6		
	pCO2	kPa	4.7–6.0		
	pH		7.35–7.45		
	HCO3-	mmol/L	21–29		
	H+	nmmol/L	35–45		
	BE	mmol/L	+/−2		
Antibodies	Total IgA	g/L	0.8–3		
	Total IgG	g/L	6.0–13.0		
	Total IgM	g/L	0.4–2.5		
Anti-cardio lipin	IgG	iU/L	<10		
	IgM	iU/L	<10		
	C3	g/L	0.8–1.6		
	C4	g/L	0.16–0.48		
Anti-TTG	<7 U/mL	Negative	>10 U/mL	Positive	In between Equivocal
Testosterone	Male	11–36	nmol/L		
	Female	0.8–3.1	nmol/L		
LH	Male	1.8–12	iU/L		
	Pregnant female	<1.5	iU/L		
	Post-menopausal	15–62	iU/L		
	Menstruating female, varies	Varies	iU/L		
FSH	Male	1.5–12.4	iU/L		
	Pregnant female		iU/L		
	Post-menopausal	25–135	iU/L		
	Menstruating female, varies	Varies	iU/L		

Category	Test	Unit	Range (All/Male)	Range Female
Oestradiol	Male	20–100	pmol/L	
Prolactin	Male	<450	miU/L	
	Non-pregnant women	100–550	miU/L	
	Pregnant women	1700–8500	miU/L	

132. **A 43-year-old gentleman developed an episode of recurrent right-sided face and head pain lasting three weeks, associated with ipsilateral nasal stuffiness, ptosis, and a red eye. The headache was particularly severe and made him agitated. Each headache lasted two hours and they occurred up to twice daily during the three-week period. There was no history of fevers and he had no family history. He had previously ten such bouts over six years. His GP had tried codeine without success. Neurological examination was normal. ESR was 34 mm/hr.**

What is the likely diagnosis?

A. Cluster headache

B. Migraine with aura

C. SUNA (short-lasting unilateral neuralgiform headache attacks with cranial autonomic symptoms)

D. Symptomatic headache due to posterior communicating (PCOM) artery aneurysm

E. Temporal arteritis

133. **A 20-year-old man had a history of mild developmental delay—walking and running slightly later than his peers. In his teens he developed stiffness in his legs, and noticed towards the end of the day that his right foot would start to twist inwards. His symptoms progressed, but a diurnal variation remained, with symptoms progressing throughout the day. There were no sensory or sphincter symptoms. His father had similar but milder problems. Examination revealed only mild cogwheeling at the wrists, a slightly inward posturing of the right hand and foot, brisk reflexes, and spasticity in the legs with down-going plantar responses. General medical examination was unremarkable and serum CK, ESR, ANA, B$_{12}$, TSH, and CXR were normal.**

What is the likely diagnosis?

A. Dopa-responsive dystonia

B. Early onset idiopathic Parkinson's disease

C. Juvenile Huntington's disease (HD)

D. Primary progressive multiple sclerosis (PPMS)

E. Wilson's disease

134. **A 23-year-old woman developed paranoid delusions and was noted by her family to have changed in character. She had recently had a short-lived self-limiting viral illness and headache a few days before her behavioural change. A week later she complained of visual and auditory formed hallucinations. Subsequently she developed a subtle difficulty walking and writing. Two weeks later she had two generalized convulsions and was admitted to A&E. She required intubation and ventilation and was unable to be weaned from sedation. Rhythmic dystonic movements of her mouth and limbs were noted. Pupils were reactive and fundi normal. There were no other focal signs, but plantars were mute. General physical examination was unremarkable. MRI brain was normal. Cerebrospinal fluid (CSF) demonstrated 5 × 10⁶ lymphocytes/L, normal protein and glucose. Herpes simplex virus, enterovirus, and varicella zoster PCRs were negative. There were no acid-fast bacilli seen on prolonged culture, cryptococcal antigen was negative and an HIV test was negative. Electroencephalogram revealed frontal and temporal slowing with some sharp elements. CXR was normal.**

    What is the most likely clinical diagnosis?

    A. CNS vasculitis secondary to cocaine
    B. Hyperammonaemic encephalopathy
    C. NMDA receptor encephalitis with an underlying ovarian teratoma
    D. Subacute sclerosing pan-encephalitis (SSPE)
    E. Whipple's disease

135. **A 60-year-old, right-handed, plumber's family noted him to have become withdrawn over the previous two years. He developed a sweet tooth and some obsessional behaviour. He would make inappropriate comments at social gatherings and his 'memory' seemed poor. Communication with his family became difficult and subsequently he lost his ability to work and became increasingly withdrawn. Examination revealed some fasciculations around the shoulder girdle. He was orientated in place and time, but had difficulty reading words aloud. He read out 'pint' phonetically. He could encode and recall three words after three minutes. Presented with a picture of objects, he could name a watch, but not a kangaroo. The rest of the neurological examination was normal. MRI revealed asymmetric atrophy of the temporal lobes.**

    What is the likely diagnosis?

    A. Alzheimer's disease
    B. Creutzfeldt-Jacob disease
    C. Dementia with Lewy bodies
    D. Depression
    E. Frontotemporal dementia

136. A 65-year-old smoker had noticed two months previously that his right foot would slap while walking. He developed aching around the calf. A few weeks later his left foot was similarly affected. He found walking progressively difficult, and a few weeks before noticed difficulty holding a cup of tea with his left hand. He felt constitutionally unwell and had lost weight. He would nearly fall over on closing his eyes. His symptoms progressed rapidly and he now required a wheelchair. Examination revealed weakness of left first dorsal interosseus (FDIO), abductor digiti minimi (ADM), flexor pollicis longus (FPL), flexor digitorum profundi I and II (FDP I and II), abductor pollicis brevis (APB), reduced pin to the dorsum of the right hand, and bilateral ankle dorsiflexion at 2/5 on the Medical Research Council (MRC) scale. Vibration sense was reduced to both knees. ESR was raised at 65 mm/hr. Antinuclear antibody (ANA), anti-neutrophil cytoplasm antibodies (ANCA), extractable nuclear antigens (ENA), rheumatoid factor, paraneoplastic antibodies, B1, B6, B12, homocysteine, methylmalonic acid, and copper were all normal or negative. Nerve conduction studies demonstrated patchy reduced amplitudes with normal conduction velocities in motor and sensory nerves in both the upper and lower limbs.

What is the most likely diagnosis?

A. Diabetic neuropathy
B. Lyme disease
C. Lymphomatous neuropathy
D. POEMS
E. Vasculitic neuropathy

137. A 45-year-old, right handed gardener experienced a sudden onset severe headache associated with vomiting. The headache persisted and was severe. Neurological examination was normal. The next day, he developed tingling and weakness in his left hand and noticed that rooms and corridors looked longer than he knew they were. He became drowsy. He had a mild flaccid weakness of his left face, arm, and leg. He smoked 20 cigarettes a day and had two paternal uncles who had had deep vein thromboses. CT scan of the head done at a peripheral hospital showed blood in the right parietal lobe with some mass effect. Routine blood tests, ECG, and CXR were all normal.

What is the most likely diagnosis?

A. Aneurysmal subarachnoid haemorrhage with vasospasm
B. Bleed into a primary or secondary brain tumour
C. Cerebral vein thrombosis with venous infarct and haemorrhage
D. Right middle cerebral artery thrombotic stroke with haemorrhagic transformation
E. Spontaneous intracranial hypotension

138. **An 18-year-old female student awoke in A&E. She had bitten her tongue. A witness gave an account of her earlier that day suddenly falling to the ground and developing rhythmic 'tonic clonic' movements of her arms and legs. Her lips turned blue. She was drowsy for several hours and had no recollection of the event, or of any preceding symptoms. She had noticed jerking of her upper limbs on occasion over the preceding two years, occasionally causing her to drop a cup of tea. There was no family history or history of perinatal birth injury, meningitis, or developmental delay. Neurological and cardiovascular examination was normal. There was no abnormality of facies. A twelve-lead ECG was normal, with a normal corrected QT and PR interval. A CT of her head was normal.**

What is the diagnosis and most appropriate therapy?

A. Hippocampal sclerosis with focal seizures and secondary generalization, lamotrigine

B. Hippocampal sclerosis with focal seizures and secondary generalization, sodium valproate

C. Juvenile myoclonic epilepsy, phenytoin

D. Juvenile myoclonic epilepsy, sodium valproate

E. Neuronal migration disorder, levetiracetam (Keppra)

139. **A 45-year-old right-handed smoker noticed severe left posterior neck pain for one week and then, while walking, suddenly developed right face, arm, and leg weakness. He fell to the ground, and was taken to A&E. Examination revealed a blood pressure of 200/95 mmHg, BM 4.5, saturations 96% on air, weakness of the right face, dense flaccid weakness of his right arm, and mild weakness of the leg. His speech was non-fluent with comprehension errors. He could not name common bedside items. Reflexes were absent and plantars down-going. He had a left Horner's syndrome. He was rushed for urgent brain imaging to exclude haemorrhage in consideration of intravenous thrombolysis of an ischaemic stroke.**

What is the most likely clinical diagnosis at this stage?

A. Left middle and anterior cerebral artery territory infarct secondary to left carotid dissection

B. Left middle cerebral artery territory infarct secondary to cardiac embolism

C. Left middle cerebral artery territory infarct secondary to left carotid dissection

D. Left vertebral artery dissection and left posterior circulation infarct

E. Primary intracranial haemorrhage (basal ganglia)

140. **A 32-year-old left-handed electrician found increasing difficulty rising from a chair, followed a few years later by fatigue and difficulty walking and lifting heavy objects, which sometimes varied throughout the day. Exercise often led to muscle aching and cramps. In the past, he had participated in sports at school, but was never 'one of the best'. There was no family history. He took no regular medication. Examination revealed normal cranial nerves, in particular no ptosis or bulbar weakness. Head flexion and extension was strong. There was mild wasting of the upper chest muscles and quadriceps. The calves were prominent. Shoulder abduction, adduction, and elbow flexion were weak at 4+/5 on the MRC scale. Hip flexion and extension, and knee extension were weak at 4/5. Ankle dorsiflexion was also weak at 4+/5. There were no sensory changes. Reflexes were present and normal. TSH was normal. Creatinine kinase was elevated at 2400 U/L (normal range 31–125 U/L).**

    What is the diagnosis?

    A. Becker muscular dystrophy
    B. Duchenne muscular dystrophy
    C. Myasthenia gravis
    D. Myotonia congenita (Becker's)
    E. Ryanodine receptor (RYR1) mutation and congenital myopathy

141. **A 28-year-old, right-handed woman presented with painless visual loss of the right eye, developing over three days. At first she noticed that the visual image seemed less vivid in colour. At three days she could only detect the outline of objects. She then noticed onset of visual loss in the left eye, developing over two days, to the same severity. At the onset of the first eye's visual loss she noticed tingling and a sense of 'water lapping' on the outside of her left leg. The sensation progressed in intensity over two days, at which point she had difficulty walking down stairs, and noticed that her left leg dragged while she walked. Over 24 hours she developed urinary urgency and found that she could not stand unaided. On examination, visual acuity was 6/60 in the right eye, no perception of light in the left eye. There was no relative afferent pupillary defect in either eye. Both optic discs were slightly swollen. Reflexes were normal, but plantars were up-going. Power was reduced in both legs to 3/5 (MRC grade). There was a sensory level to T4.**

    What is the most likely clinical diagnosis?

    A. Devic's disease (neuromyelitis optica)
    B. Guillain-Barré syndrome (GBS)
    C. Multiple sclerosis (MS)
    D. Neuro-Behçet's with bilateral uveitis
    E. Neurofibromatosis type 1

142. A 62-year-old lady with motor neuron disease attended clinic for follow-up. She had significant weakness, and was dependent on a wheelchair when going out. Her regular medications included baclofen for muscle spasms and citalopram for depression. She had also been suffering from morning headaches for the previous month, which were felt all over her scalp. She did not feel refreshed after sleeping, and was often tired during the day. Her swallowing was normal, and she reported no other new symptoms.

On examination fasciculations and muscle wasting were seen in all limbs. Her upper limb reflexes were absent, knee jerks were symmetrical and normal, and she had bilateral extensor plantar responses. Ocular movements were unremarkable. Palatal movement and voice were normal, and jaw jerk could not be elicited. There was no dysphagia on bedside swallow test.

Which intervention is most likely to confer the greatest survival benefit in this lady?

A. Diaphragmatic pacing
B. Feeding via percutaneous endoscopic gastrostomy
C. Home oxygen
D. Non-invasive ventilation
E. Riluzole

143. A 16-year-old boy was referred to the neurology clinic for assessment. His mother had taken him to see his GP as he had been reporting increasing problems with muscle stiffness. He enjoyed playing football, but found this increasingly difficult due to stiffness in his legs. He found that after about 20 minutes, the stiffness improved and he was able to carry on playing. He did not report any pain, or other neurological symptoms. He was otherwise well with no significant history. There was no family history of neurological illness, but his mother mentioned that his father had suffered from muscle cramps, which prompted him to give up sports.

On examination he appeared well, with normal observations. He had a well-defined musculature and his power was normal throughout. There was a delay when he tried to extend his fingers from a tight fist, though this improved after several trials. His pupillary reflexes and eye movements were normal, as was fundoscopy. There was no sensory deficit.

Which of the following is the most likely diagnosis?

A. Becker's muscular dystrophy
B. Hypokalaemic periodic paralysis
C. McArdle's disease
D. Myotonia congenita
E. Myotonic dystrophy

144. **A 65-year-old gentleman presented to the emergency department with a cough. He was commenced on intravenous antibiotics for pneumonia. At his initial assessment he was noted to have a tremor of his right arm. This had been present for the past year, but did not interfere with his activities. On examination there was a rest tremor in his right hand. There was increased tone in this arm, and he had difficulty performing rapid alternating movements with both hands, more so on the right side. There was no other focal neurology, and his gait was normal, other than being slowed. These symptoms did not concern him. He was referred to the neurology team for assessment of his tremor.**

Which of the following is the most appropriate management option?

A. Benzhexol
B. Beta blockers
C. Levodopa
D. Observation and follow-up
E. Ropinirole

145. **A 17-year-old boy was referred to the neurology department with a history of abnormal movements. He had noticed a tremor in his hands over the previous six months, but this had not caused any problems and he had put it down to stress due to his exams. Over the three months prior to assessment he had developed uncontrollable movements affecting his limbs and trunk, which had been progressively getting worse. He had previously achieved well at school but had been having difficulty over the past year, having been reported for angry behaviour on a few occasions. He had been commenced on fluoxetine for low mood. He had no other significant past medical history. His family history was unremarkable other than a history of dementia in his paternal grandfather.**

On examination, he was sweaty and there were generalized continuous random uncontrollable movements affecting his extremities, with occasional similar movements occurring in his neck and trunk. He was unable to keep his tongue fully protruded for five seconds. Power was normal and there were no sensory deficits. Spider naevi were noted on the upper chest, but examination was otherwise unremarkable.

Investigations:

Hb	122 g/l	
WCC	6.2 × 10⁹/l	
Platelets	82 × 10⁹/l	
MCV	85 fl	
Reticulocyte count	2.5%	(0.5–1.5%)
Albumin	30 g/l	
Alanine transaminase	52 iU/l	
Alkaline phosphatase	115 iU/l	
Bilirubin	20 μmol/l	
Na⁺	135 mmol/l	
K⁺	4.1 mmol/l	
Creatinine	72 μmol/l	
Urea	5.2 mmol/l	
TSH	1.2 mU/l	(0.5–3.0 mU/l)
Serum free T4	14 pmol/l	(10–22 pmol/l)

Which of the following investigations is most likely to reveal the underlying diagnosis?

A. A 24-hour urinary copper excretion
B. Anti-phospholipid antibodies
C. Huntingtin gene trinucleotide CAG repeat number
D. Magnetic resonance imaging brain
E. Peripheral blood film

146. **A 58-year-old male presented to the emergency department with difficulty walking. He had noticed pins and needles in his fingers when he went to bed two nights before. When he woke on the morning of presentation his legs felt weak and he had difficulty standing. He also reported some lower back pain radiating into his buttocks which he put down to having been moving heavy boxes a few days before. His weakness had progressed and he had fallen over whilst trying to get to the bathroom in the morning, prompting his presentation to the emergency department. His past medical history included type II diabetes mellitus for which he took metformin, and he had recently had two days off work with food poisoning.**

On examination he was hypertensive, with blood pressure 185/100 mmHg. He was apyrexial and his other observations were within normal limits. Knee and ankle jerks were absent, and plantar reflexes were equivocal. His upper limb reflexes could not be elicited. Power was reduced to 4/5 in ankle flexion and dorsiflexion, as well as finger extension. He had a proprioceptive deficit in his lower limb extremities.

Which of the following should be performed next?

A. Anti-ganglioside antibodies
B. Electromyography
C. Forced vital capacity
D. Lumbar puncture
E. Nerve conduction studies

147. **A 42-year-old lady was referred to the neurology clinic after seeing her GP with a two-month history of intermittent double vision. It tended to occur at the end of the day, and she had put it down to tiredness. Her husband commented that her eyelids had been drooping towards the end of the day. She denied any limb weakness or difficulty swallowing. Her past medical history included only hyperthyroidism, for which she took carbimazole.**

On examination she had bilateral partial ptosis, and she sat with her neck partially extended to compensate for this. Her ptosis was worse after sustaining upward gaze for 15 seconds. There was no overt ophthalmoplegia, but she reported diplopia in multiple directions. Palatal movement was equal on both sides, and there were no abnormalities in tongue movements. Tone, power, reflexes, and sensation were normal in the upper and lower limbs.

Which of the following is the most appropriate initial management?

A. Azathioprine
B. Intravenous immunoglobulin
C. Mycophenolate mofetil
D. Pyridostigmine plus prednisolone
E. Thymectomy

148. A 42-year-old man from South Africa was brought to the emergency department with a reduced conscious level. Collateral history revealed that he had been complaining of headaches for the preceding few days, but he had become drowsy that afternoon. He had been feeling unwell for two weeks, with fevers, lethargy, and intermittent headaches. His GP had prescribed a course of antibiotics but this did not help. He had moved to the UK two years previously, and his past medical history included pneumonia, requiring hospital admission shortly after arriving in the country, and shingles.

On examination he was of thin habitus and was drowsy, with a Glasgow Coma Score of 12/15, but there was no focal neurological deficit. Neck stiffness was noted and he was seen to have oral thrush and cervical lymphadenopathy. His observations were: temperature 38.1°C, heart rate 92, respiratory rate 24, blood pressure 122/84 mmHg, SpO2 on air 95%.

The admitting team organized a CT head, followed by lumbar puncture, with the results as follows:

```
CT head:
    Mild generalized atrophy, no space-occupying lesions or
    mass effect. No acute pathology.
Cerebrospinal fluid:
    Opening pressure              23 cmH₂O (10-20 cmH₂O)
    Polymorphs                    11 cells/mm³ (0 cells/mm³)
    Lymphocytes                   72 cells/mm³ (0-3 cells/mm³)
    Red cells                     7 cells/mm³ (0 cells/mm³)
    Gram-stain                    no organisms seen
    Protein                       62 mg/dl (15-45 mg/dl)
    Cerebrospinal fluid glucose   2.3 mmol/l (3.3-4.4 mmol/l)
```

Which of the following investigations is most likely to reveal the cause?

A. Cryptococcal antigen testing
B. Herpes simplex virus PCR
C. India ink positive
D. Meningococcal PCR
E. Venereal disease research laboratory test (VDRL)

149. A 45-year-old Afro-Caribbean female was referred to the emergency neurology clinic with right-sided facial weakness, causing slurring of her speech for the preceding four days. She had noticed that both of her eyes had been red and uncomfortable for about a week, and she was taking chloramphenicol eye drops for this. Her past medical history was unremarkable, other than a self-limiting painful rash on her shins two months previously, which lasted seven days.

On examination there was facial asymmetry, with right-sided facial droop and loss of the right naso-labial fold. She was unable to fully close her right eye. Both eyes were erythematous. She was noted to have bilateral parotid gland swelling, and the glands were firm but not tender. Neurological examination was otherwise unremarkable.

```
Investigations:
  Hb                        142 g/l
  WCC                       10.7 × 10⁹/l
  Platelets                 220 × 10⁹/l
  Albumin                   37 g/l
  Alanine transaminase      40 iU/l
  Alkaline phosphatase      72 iU/l
  Bilirubin                 5 µmol/l
  Creatinine                84 µmol/l
  Urea                      4.2 mmol/l
  Na⁺                       139 mmol/l
  K⁺                        3.9 mmol/l
  Corrected Ca²⁺            2.9 mmol/l
  PO₄⁻                      1.2 mmol/l
```

What is the most likely cause of her facial weakness?

A. Bell's palsy

B. Left anterior circulation ischaemic stroke

C. Ramsay Hunt syndrome

D. Sarcoidosis

E. Vasculitis

150. **A 32-year-old man presented to the emergency department with a sudden onset of severe generalized headache. He had occasional tension headaches brought on by working with computers, but reported that he had never had a headache of this severity. He had taken ibuprofen and paracetamol, but these had not helped. He had been well prior to this.**

On examination, there was no focal neurological deficit. Photophobia was demonstrated on attempting to assess his pupillary reflexes. There was no neck stiffness or rash. His observations were as follows: pulse rate 96, respiratory rate 18, blood pressure 100/72 mmHg, SpO$_2$ 96% on room air, temperature 37.4°C.

His initial blood tests were unremarkable, and CT head was performed, which is shown in Figure 7.1

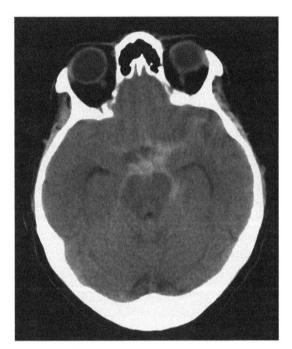

Figure 7.1 Non-contrast CT head.

Reproduced with permission from *Oxford Handbook of Medical Imaging*, edited by Darby M, Barron D, Hyland R, Fig. 10.2, p. 145, Oxford University Press, Oxford, UK, Copyright © 2011.

Which of the following options would be most appropriate in his initial management?

A. Intravenous 0.9% saline

B. Intravenous ceftriaxone

C. Oral nimodipine

D. Oxygen via non-rebreathe mask

E. Subcutaneous sumatriptan

151. A 52-year-old female presented with a two-month history of progressive hearing loss in her right ear. She also had noticed altered sensation on the right side of her face. She had not had any headaches and her vision was normal. Her past medical history included hyperthyroidism, for which she took carbimazole, but she was otherwise well.

On examination she was alert and oriented. Fundoscopy, pupillary reflexes, and visual acuity were all normal. There was a full range of eye movements, but nystagmus was noted on right horizontal gaze. Power was normal in all limbs, though there was a degree of dysmetria in the right upper limb. Her hearing was reduced in her right ear, with results of Rinne's and Weber's tests below. Sensation was reduced on the right side of her face, and her corneal reflex was absent.

```
Rinne's test:
Right ear: air conduction > bone conduction
Left ear: air conduction > bone conduction
Weber's test: lateralizes to left side
```

What is the most likely diagnosis?

A. Cerebellar haemorrhage

B. Cholesteatoma

C. Multiple sclerosis

D. Sarcoidosis

E. Vestibular schwannoma

152. **A 19-year-old female presented to the emergency department with a 36-hour history of headache. The headache was generalized, and she described it as a severe tightness. She reported having a fever during the day and thought she had developed flu. She had recently started studying at university. She was previously fit and well and had only been to hospital once when she had an anaphylactic reaction to penicillin, which she had been prescribed for tonsillitis when she was eight years old.**

On examination her temperature was 38.5°C, pulse rate was 100, respiratory rate was 20, blood pressure was 122/84 mmHg, and oxygen saturations were 95% on air. There was no focal neurological deficit, though pupil reflexes and fundoscopy were difficult to perform as the bright light caused discomfort. She also had nuchal rigidity. There were no skin changes observed.

Blood, including full blood count, C-reactive protein, urea and electrolytes, prothrombin time, and liver function tests were taken and sent to the laboratory, and lumbar puncture was performed.

What is the most appropriate initial treatment whilst awaiting initial investigation results?

A. Acyclovir
B. Benzylpenicillin
C. Ceftriaxone
D. Chloramphenicol
E. Meropenem

153. **A 41-year-old female, insulin-dependent diabetic presented to A&E complaining of loss of vision in her right eye. She reported upon waking that morning she could not see properly because of a mass of dark spots/blobs obscuring her vision. She did not complain of any pain. She had been otherwise well, without any prior problems with her vision, but was very short sighted for which she wore contact lenses. Her past medical history included hypertension and she had a 20-pack year smoking history. Her visual acuity was 6/36. Her pupils reacted normally, the eye was white but there was a reduced red reflex and on fundoscopy there was a limited view of the retina.**

What is the most likely cause of her vision loss?

A. Cataract
B. Central retinal vein occlusion
C. Posterior vitreous detachment
D. Retinal detachment
E. Vitreous haemorrhage

154. A 72-year-old woman complained of painless gradual loss of vision in both eyes for nine months. When looking at people she could not see the centre part of their faces, but had reasonably good peripheral vision. She was now unable to see the prices in the shops and could only read the headlines in a newspaper. Her vision at the optometrist was 6/24 in the right eye and 6/36 in the left eye. She was told that new glasses would not help. She had suffered with rheumatoid arthritis for many years. Her medications included methotrexate 15 mg/week and prednisolone 5 mg od.

What is the most likely cause for her poor vision?

A. Age-related macular degeneration
B. Cataract
C. Central retinal artery occlusion
D. Keratoconjunctivitis sicca
E. Primary open angle glaucoma

155. An 84-year-old woman complained of sudden loss of vision in her left eye. For the preceding six months she experienced pain when lifting objects, but this had eased since she had been taking prednisolone 7.5 mg od prescribed by her GP. Over the preceding few weeks she had had pain chewing her food, some discomfort when brushing her hair, and the left side of her head ached, especially when lying on her left side in bed. On examination her left visual acuity was only perception of light, there was a left relative afferent pupillary defect, and her optic disc was pale and swollen.

What is the most likely diagnosis?

A. Amaurosis fugax
B. Anterior ischaemic optic neuropathy
C. Glaucomatous optic neuropathy
D. Optic neuritis
E. Scleritis

156. A 35-year-old Afro-Caribbean man attended A&E with a week's history of a painful, red, light-sensitive left eye with blurred vision. He had been prescribed chloramphenicol eye drops but they had not helped. He usually had perfect vision. On examination, his vision was 6/12 in his left eye. Using fluorescein drops and a blue light the cornea looked normal but his left pupil was smaller than the right and did not look completely round. Fundoscopy revealed a healthy optic disc and macula.

What treatment would he likely to be prescribed for his eye problem?

A. Ganciclovir gel
B. Corticosteroid eye drops, for example prednisolone acetate 1%
C. Ofloxacin eye drops
D. Oral aciclovir
E. Oral prednisolone

132. A) Cluster headache

The autonomic symptoms and the strictly unilateral pain are classic of a type of trigeminal autonomic cephalalgia (TAC)—a category which includes cluster headache or short-lasting unilateral neuralgiform (SUNA) from the listed options. The two-hour duration of symptoms with bouts and strong autonomic symptoms make cluster headache (15–180 minutes duration) the likeliest diagnosis. By contrast, SUNA attacks last 5–200 seconds.

Epidemiologically, most headaches are likely to be migraine, but in this case, agitation makes TAC highly likely, whereas migraine makes people want to lie down in a dark room and is generally more of a progressive pounding headache, often with nausea, photophobia, phonophobia, and in some people an aura. A PCOM aneurysm may leak and cause subarachnoid haemorrhage with a pupil involving (though not always) third nerve palsy and ptosis (which may both be partial), but the history in this case is not of a thunderclap immediate onset to full intensity headache. Temporal arteritis is not likely given to the young age of the patient and episodic nature of symptoms. The slightly raised ESR is non-specific in this case.

Tutorial

Cluster headache, SUNA, and paroxysmal hemicrania constitute the TACs, and are generally strictly unilateral. Their key features are summarized in Table 7.1. There is an overlap with migraine, which remains the most common cause of headache. Secondary headaches, such as temporal arteritis, an erosive facial bone tumour, and trigeminal neuralgia are in the key differential diagnosis. Temporal arteritis is rare under the age of 60, and classical symptoms include tenderness of the scalp, jaw claudication, and raised ESR, CRP, and ALT. Corticosteroid therapy generally is initiated immediately, and temporal artery biopsy sought within ten days of steroid initiation, to reduce the risk of visual loss. A structural lesion should be excluded with MR imaging in TAC. Functional MRI suggests a role of the posterior hypothalamic grey matter in cluster headache. The headaches in these disorders are typically highly severe and cause significant morbidity.

Table 7.1. Key differentiating features of the trigeminal autonomic cephalalgias

	SUNA	**Paroxysmal hemicrania**	**Cluster headache**
Duration of attack	5–200 seconds	2–45 minutes	15–180 minutes
Attack frequency	Typically >10 a day up to 30/hour	1–20/day	1–8/day

A response to a trial of indomethacin suggests the rarer paroxysmal hemicrania, and is often a necessary step in making a diagnosis of cluster headache, in particular with symptoms of 15–45 minutes duration. Subcutaneous sumatriptan is a useful abortive treatment of cluster headache, or high flow oxygen, as oral abortive agents generally take too long to act. Verapamil (with ECG monitoring), lithium, topiramate, greater occipital nerve blocks, and occasionally neurosurgical procedures, are useful preventative therapy. Episodic cluster headache is that of bouts lasting from seven days to one year separated by pain-free periods lasting one month or more, and chronic cluster headache is of attacks lasting more than one year without remission, or with less than a month between attacks. Greater occipital nerve blocks may be useful. SUNA is classically responsive to lamotrigine. Medication overuse headache is a generally dull featureless headache associated with regular use of opiate medications and even regular paracetamol and ibuprofen. In general, opiates should be avoided for all headaches, primary or secondary.

Further Reading

Benoliel R (2012). Trigeminal autonomic cephalgias. *British Journal of Pain* 6(3): 106–123.

The International Headache Society classification—ICHD-II. Open access available at http://ihs-classification.org/en/

133. A) Dopa-responsive dystonia

The inward posturing of the foot and hand are due to sustained muscle contraction—dystonia, which may be primary or secondary. The progressive symptoms in this case, with diurnal variation, is classically seen (but not always present) in dopa-responsive dystonia. The condition is important to consider due to the striking resolution of symptoms and signs with small doses of levodopa, and is often missed.

The other listed conditions are reasonably in the differential diagnosis. Early onset Parkinson's disease is often genetic and recessive in inheritance, but usually resembles typical Parkinson's disease with bradykinesia, rigidity, tremor, and postural instability. PPMS often is associated with a progressive cord syndrome over five or so years, often with associated signs such as an internuclear ophthalmoplegia. There are no relapses in PPMS, and the disease takes a more aggressive course than 'regular' relapsing remitting multiple sclerosis. The Westphal variant of HD is young onset HD with prominent parkinsonism and dystonia. The neuropsychiatric features and chorea typical of HD can manifest later. Wilson's disease is hepatolenticular degeneration due to mutations in a copper transporter (ATP7B), and should be considered in any young (<50 years old) patient with any movement disorder, as it is treatable with copper chelation therapy.

Tutorial

Mutations in GTP cyclohydrolase 1 (GCH1) are associated with dopa-responsive dystonia (DYT5), and transmission is autosomal dominant.

Dystonia may be primary and genetic, or secondary and either genetic or acquired. The key to diagnosis of dystonia is to consider a broad differential: infective, autoimmune, metabolic, degenerative. Treatable conditions should be excluded: Wilson's disease (exclude in any movement disorder in a patient under 50), spinal cord lesions such as arteriovenous malformations, or extrinsic tumours. Huntington's disease, the spinocerebellar ataxias, multiple systems atrophy, progressive supranuclear palsy, and corticobasal degeneration may all be associated with dystonia. Neuronal brain iron accumulation disorders are also associated with dystonia and parkinsonism and have typical MR imaging with iron deposition seen in the basal ganglia. Unilateral dystonia requires urgent brain imaging to exclude a structural lesion. It is most useful clinically to generate a differential diagnosis by looking for associated signs. For example, dystonia and parkinsonism (neuronal brain iron accumulation, neuroacanthocytosis, rapid onset dystonia parkinsonism), eye movement disorder (Niemann Pick C), ataxia (Friedreich's ataxia), neuropathy (mitochondrial, metachromatic leukodystrophy). Dopamine transporter (DAT) scanning is expensive, and generally reserved for the differentiation between organic and non-organic (or non-extrapyramidal) pathology.

A comprehensive list of the causes of parkinsonism, and their distinguishing features can be found in Table 7.2.

Table 7.2 A comprehensive list of the causes of Parkinsonism, and their distinguishing features

Category	Cause	Distinguishing feature(s)
Heredodegenerative	Idiopathic Parkinson's disease	Generally unilateral onset Bradykinesia is defining feature
	Progressive supranuclear palsy	Early falls and rigidity, supranuclear gaze palsy
	Multiple systems atrophy	Autonomic failure and cerebellar involvement
	Lewy body dementia	Dementia may present before or with 18 months of neurological symptoms Visual hallucinations
	Huntington's disease	Presence of chorea Neuropsychiatric features
Metabolic disorders	Wilson's disease	Co-existing liver cirrhosis
	Manganese toxicity	Dystonia
	Leukodystrophies	Pyramidal signs
	Mitochondrial disease, e.g. Leigh's disease	Other symptoms of mitochondrial disorders: deafness, seizures.
	Carbon monoxide poisoning	Acute/subacute onset, basal ganglia hypointensities on CT
Drugs	Dopamine receptor blocking drugs, e.g. metoclopramide	
	Sodium valproate	Generally symmetrical symptoms
	Post traumatic	
Miscellaneous	Post-infectious	
	Functional	
Mimics	'Vascular parkinsonism'	Mainly that of a gait apraxia with shuffling steps, little evidence of parkinsonism in the upper limbs. Other co-existing deficits from vascular insults to the brain.

Further Reading

Edwards MJ, Stamelou M, Quinn N, Bhatia K (2016). *Parkinson's Disease and Other Movement Disorders* (Oxford Specialist Handbooks in Neurology), Second Edition. Oxford University Press, Oxford.

Geyer HL, Bressman SB (2006). The diagnosis of dystonia. *Lancet Neurology* 5(9): 780–790.

134. C) NMDA receptor encephalitis with an underlying ovarian teratoma

Psychosis, behavioural and cognitive change, seizures, and coma with rhythmic dystonic movements are highly suggestive of NMDA receptor encephalitis, an autoimmune encephalitis associated with antibodies to the N-methyl-D-aspartate receptor. Cases in young women are often paraneoplastic, associated with an underlying ovarian teratoma.

The main differential is CNS infection, and, in slightly older patients, a paraneoplastic encephalitis due to other occult tumour. Metabolic encephalopathies and mitochondrial disease are in the differential. A CNS vasculopathy and vasculitis can occur with cocaine, but commonly causes stroke-like episodes due to vasoconstriction. An encephalopathy can occur, but the history of this patient is not typical for this. Hyperammonaemic encephalopathy is commonly seen in hepatic encephalopathy, but can also be seen in urea cycle inborn errors of metabolism. The clinical course may be fluctuant and of a delirium and encephalopathy. SSPE shares many features with NMDAR encephalitis and is rare; if rarer, though, it is generally associated with myoclonus and white matter changes on MR imaging. CNS infection with *Tropheryma whipplei* is rare but associated with an oculomasticatory myorhythmia (OMM), and potentially treatable, so should be sought.

Tutorial

Non-infective encephalitis has been recognized since at least the 1960s, but many cases have been unexplained, and often grouped into disparate entities like Hashimoto's encephalopathy. Tumours of neuroectodermal origin are associated with an immune response against the tumour, which may trigger an immune reaction against neuronal elements. Small cell lung cancer (SCLC) is the most common tumour association. Historically such syndromes did not appear to be responsive to immunotherapy and tumour removal, but novel CNS syndromes, which in many cases have no underlying tumour, have been discovered in the last decade, associated with serum antibodies to neuronal channels or associated cell surface proteins and excellent response to immunotherapy. NMDA receptor antibodies are most commonly found, and strikingly associated with psychosis and other psychiatric symptoms at presentation. Exclusion of CNS infections is necessary, as is searching for an underlying tumour.

Tumours commonly associated with paraneoplastic encephalitis are listed in Box 7.1, and causes of CNS encephalitis are listed in Table 7.3.

Box 7.1 Tumours commonly associated with paraneoplastic encephalitis

Neuroectodermal tumours
Small cell lung cancer
Hodgkin's disease
Testicular tumours
Thymoma
Pancreatic cancer
Paraneoplastic antibodies are useful in predicting tumour, but generally are not predictive of clinical syndrome (e.g. encephalitis versus neuropathy, cerebellar degeneration or opsoclonus-myoclonus—the classical paraneoplastic syndromes.

Table 7.3 Common causes of encephalitis in the UK.

Infectious	Auto-immune
• Herpes simplex virus	• Acute disseminated encephalomyelitis (ADEM)
• TB	• NMDA receptor encephalitis
• Zoster	• Potassium channel-complex associated encephalitis
• Streptococci	• Paraneoplastic (a panel of paraneoplastic antibodies should include Hu,
• Dual infection	Yo, Ri, Tr, CV2/CRMP5, amphiphysin, glycine, voltage gated calcium
• Influenza A	channel, AMPAR, GABA(B)R)
• HIV	
• JC virus	
• Listeria	
• Measles	

Further Reading

Granerod J, Ambrose H, Davies N, et al. (2010). Causes of encephalitis and differences in their clinical presentations in England: a multicentre, population-based prospective study. *Lancet Infectious Diseases* 10(12): 835–844.

Vincent A, Bien C, Irani S, Waters P (2011). Autoantibodies associated with diseases of the CNS: new developments and future challenges. *Lancet Neurology* 10(8): 759–772.

135. E) Frontotemporal dementia

He has behavioural change, semantic difficulties, and his pronunciation error is termed 'surface dyslexia'. Memory is, in fact, well preserved, though most patients and their families will describe any cognitive complaint as a problem with 'memory'. The localization of such features is to the frontal and temporal lobes. The MRI features can be striking late in the disease. He was found to have a mutation in the *tau* gene.

Alzheimer's disease, though epidemiologically the most likely diagnosis, remains a possibility, but the classic pattern of atrophy and prominent frontal and temporal features with preserved anterograde memory make this less likely. The clinical course is too long for genetic, sporadic, or new variant prion disease, which are generally quite aggressive and rapidly progressive conditions, associated with myoclonus, ataxia, and triphasic sharp waves on EEG (though this on its own is a non-specific finding). Dementia with Lewy bodies is an alpha-synucleinopathy and is associated with REM sleep disturbance and fluctuating course, with visual hallucinations, and in many cases, early parkinsonism. Depression can mimic dementia (depressive 'pseudo-dementia') but is likely to lead to slowing of responses and no clear focal pattern.

Tutorial

Dementia is cognitive impairment sufficient to impact upon work and social function, and is generally progressive. Delirium may predict dementia, being more likely to occur in individuals with subclinical neurodegeneration. There are treatable reversible causes of dementia, for example limbic encephalitis, normal pressure hydrocephalus, and 'pseudodementias', for instance due to depression. Rare dementias such as prion disease and genetic young onset dementias (mentioned in the answer) should be considered. The key to the diagnosis of dementia is in looking for focal cognitive deficits, for dementia is not a 'global process' as was the textbook view for much of the 20th century. There has been a recent explosion in the understanding of the molecular basis of dementias, and the frontotemporal dementias share a pathological basis with motor neurone disease. Treatable conditions should be the focus of investigations (tumours, hydrocephalus, HIV, Wilson's, NMDAR and VGKC antibodies, hypothyroidism).

The most common dementias and their presenting features:

- Alzheimer's disease—anterograde amnesia with preserved distant autobiographical memory. Posterior cortical atrophy is a form with predominant visuospatial dysfunction. MR imaging may show hippocampal atrophy. Acetylcholinesterase inhibitors (donepezil, rivastigmine, galantamine) are useful symptomatic therapy.
- Frontotemporal dementia (FTD)—behaviour change, preference for sweet foods, decline in care of appearance, progressive non-fluent aphasia, or isolated loss of semantic knowledge (which may be subtle)—or any combination of the above. Coronal MR imaging classically shows asymmetric atrophy of the temporal lobes. FTD is associated with motor neuron disease, with often only fasciculations around the shoulders seen early on.
- Dementia with Lewy bodies—REM sleep disturbance, vivid dreams, visual hallucinations, and parkinsonism. Responds sometimes strikingly to rivastigmine and galantamine.

- Vascular dementia—with 'vascular parkinsonism' or frontal gait ignition failure and apraxia. May co-exist with other pathologies, especially neurological deficits from other previous cerebrovascular insults. A step-wise decline is often apparent from the history.

For a further comprehensive summary and discussion of the clinical features of the common types of dementia, see the tutorial for Question 187.

Further Reading

Rossor M, Fox N, Mummery C, Schott J, Warren J (2010). The diagnosis of young-onset dementia. *Lancet Neurology* 9(8): 793–806. Review.

136. E) Vasculitic neuropathy

The patchy involvement, axonal nerve conduction studies rather than demyelinating (prolonged velocities, normal amplitudes) with individual nerves being 'picked off', and the feeling of being constitutionally unwell, along with a raised ESR, makes vasculitis the most likely diagnosis here. Both common peroneal nerves, the right superficial radial and the left high median (because of the involvement of FPL, and FDP I and II, the long finger flexors supplied by the anterior interosseus nerve) are clinically involved in his case.

Diabetes is common and can cause various patterns of neuropathy, but generally causes a mild length dependent and symmetrical axonal neuropathy. Lymphomatous infiltration is a possibility in this case and clinically can mimic vasculitis, though commonly would affect more proximal nerves and the brachial or lumbar plexus. If no clear supportive evidence of vasculitis is found then a CT of the body for lymphoma and a nerve biopsy are often necessary to distinguish between the two. Lyme disease is underdiagnosed and the prevalence is related strongly to the geographical location. The diagnosis is possible here, but overall less likely. Lyme serology is routinely tested for in the investigation of most neuropathies. The rapidity, patchiness, and severity are unusual for diabetes. Polyneuropathy, organomegaly, endocrinopathy, M-band, and skin changes (POEMS syndrome) is underdiagnosed, and requires aggressive treatment, often directly with stem cell transplant. Serum VEGF levels are raised and the M band may only be found with immunofixation. POEMS is less likely to be associated with clear patchy axonal change and generally has clearly associated other clinical features.

Tutorial

There are a myriad of causes of neuropathy. Focal and initial upper limb symptoms suggest inflammation. Burning pain, paraesthesiae, and lancinating pains are common symptoms, but often the initial symptoms could point to a central cause, and the examination findings (hyporeflexia, atrophy) and nerve conduction studies are key to guiding investigations.

Nerve conduction studies (to look for axonal involvement—vasculitis, versus demyelination—CIDP, paraproteinaemic neuropathies, MAG-antibody associated neuropathy) are key, as is EMG for denervation, CSF examination, and in many cases nerve biopsy. Large volumes of CSF (10 ml on three occasions) are sometimes required to diagnose lymphoma.

Peripheral nervous system vasculitis may be secondary to drugs, infection (HIV, hepatitis C-associated cryoglobulinaemic vasculitis), paraneoplastic, associated with systemic vasculitis (Churg-Strauss, Wegener's, or other ANCA-associated vasculitides, such as systemic lupus erythematosus (SLE), polyarteritis nodosa (PAN). Isolated peripheral nerve vasculitis is relatively rare, and patients may be ANCA-negative and feel constitutionally well. Patients with a patchy axonal neuropathy with no clear cause may benefit from nerve biopsy to exclude vasculitis. Thorough investigation to exclude vasculitic mimics is necessary. Treatment consists of aggressive immunotherapy, often with high-dose corticosteroids, cyclophosphamide, and maintenance azathioprine.

Further Reading

Lunn M, Willison H (2009). Diagnosis and treatment in inflammatory neuropathies. *Journal of Neurology, Neurosurgery, and Psychiatry* 80(3): 249–58. Erratum in *Journal of Neurology, Neurosurgery, and Psychiatry* 2009 80(5): 584. Dosage error in article text.

Said G (2010). Vasculitic neuropathy, Advances in Clinical Neuroscience and Rehabilitation (ACNR). Available at: http://www.acnr.co.uk/SO10/ACNRSO10_10_review_said.pdf)

137. C) Cerebral vein thrombosis with venous infarct and haemorrhage

There are several causes of thunderclap headache, but in this case the sudden onset, with later focal neurology, and blood seen on scan is either: (1) subarachnoid haemorrhage complicated by arterial vasospasm and focal ischaemia, or (2) cerebral venous sinus thrombosis with venous congestion and venous haemorrhagic infarction. The visual phenomena in this patient are parietal. In this case, cerebral vein thrombosis is slightly more likely in a patient who is relatively well at onset, and in whom the scan shows haemorrhage with mass effect, and in whom there is a family history of thrombosis.

Answers B) and D) would be associated with weakness at the onset of symptoms. The headache of spontaneous intracranial hypotension (SIH) is similar to a post lumbar puncture headache— low pressure: a headache brought on and exacerbated by vertical posture, and nearly completely alleviated by lying down. This occurs spontaneously due to a spontaneous CSF tear (e.g. after prolonged coughing). The patient often remembers the exact date of onset, and has a severe headache precipitated by standing, relieved by lying down. If there is no response to one week's strict bed rest a blood patch is often required, performed by an anaesthetist. Other causes of thunderclap headache include migraine (a diagnosis of exclusion), carotid artery dissection, and CNS vasculopathies.

Tutorial

Thunderclap headache, with (though not exclusively) papilloedema (late), focal symptoms, and drowsiness is suggestive of venous sinus thrombosis. Venous congestion can lead to haemorrhage and infarcts, often mistaken for arterial intracranial haemorrhage. As the management is so different to that of arterial haemorrhage the diagnosis should be considered often and urgent venography obtained. Most if not all district general hospitals are able to perform CT venography out of hours. Contrast CT venography usually shows a filling defect in the straight, sagittal, or transverse sinuses, but more than one sinus can be affected, and deeper vein thromboses (e.g. vein of Galen) are associated with coma and worse neurological outcome.

The management is urgent anticoagulation after a confident diagnosis is made, which often requires a neuroradiologist's review of the scans. Superficial or cortical vein thromboses are associated with focal seizures, which may secondarily generalize. Blood for a full thrombophilia screen, including genetic causes and anti-phospholipid antibodies, should ideally be taken prior to the commencement of heparin (but should not delay therapy). Like any deep vein thrombosis, an occult tumour may be the predisposing factor. Thromboses clinically not responsive to low molecular weight heparin (LMWH), that is, progressing to coma, should be considered for local tissue plasminogen activator (TPA) therapy at an experienced centre. Decompressive craniectomy may also be required to allow brain swelling time to develop and recede.

Further Reading

Bousser M, Ferro J (2007). Cerebral venous thrombosis: an update. *Lancet Neurology* 6(2): 162–170.

Ferro J, Canhão P, Stam J, Bousser M, Barinagarrementeria F, and ISCVT Investigators (2004). Prognosis of cerebral vein and dural sinus thrombosis: results of the International Study on Cerebral Vein and Dural Sinus Thrombosis (ISCVT). *Stroke* 35(3): 664–670. Open access.

138. D) Juvenile myoclonic epilepsy, sodium valproate

The generalized discharges and myoclonus make juvenile myoclonic epilepsy (JME) the likely diagnosis.

By contrast, hippocampal sclerosis is common but patients will not have myoclonus and often will have focal temporal seizures with déjà vu, motor, and gustatory automatisms prior to generalized seizures. Neuronal migration disorder presents with focal and localization related generalized seizures, often without clear focal seizures, or with frontal lobe seizures.

The diagnosis is difficult, but interictal EEG is often normal and high resolution MRI is key to diagnosis. Sodium valproate was shown in the SANAD I study to be the most efficacious drug for this form of epilepsy. Phenytoin, a sodium channel blocker, makes the myoclonus of JME worse and is to be avoided.

Tutorial

Epilepsy is more than one seizure, due to any cause. There are a myriad of causes, genetic (channel mutations associated with febrile convulsions, paediatric metabolic syndromes, the progressive myoclonic epilepsies (Unverricht-Lundborg), neuronal ceroid lipofuscinosis, sialidosis, mitochondrial cytopathies, dentatorubral-pallidoluysian atrophy

(DRPLA)), congenital (neuronal migration defects), and acquired (e.g. CNS tumours, infection, autoimmune). The most useful clinical distinction is between idiopathic generalized epilepsy (IGE, including JME and childhood absence) and epilepsy due to a structural focal cause which can lead to both partial (simple or complex, the latter with altered awareness) and secondary generalized seizures. This distinction has the greatest impact on the choice of drug. The SANAD studies have been useful in providing evidence for the use of anticonvulsants. Valproate, though the drug of choice for JME is associated with significant cognitive impairment in the children born to mothers taking the drug, so alternatives are sometimes used—namely lamotrigine or levetiracetam. Valproate is one of the best drugs for IGE (not to be confused with secondarily generalized epilepsy), and lamotrigine or carbamazepine for focal seizures (with or without generalization). Levetiracetam is gaining favour among neurosurgical centres for use for tumours and epilepsy. Refractory focal epilepsies, having tried three or more drugs, should be referred for consideration of resective surgery early. EEG telemetry and functional MRI and PET are useful in localizing focal epilepsy in the assessment of refractory cases for resective surgery.

Sudden death, driving, and pregnancy in epilepsy are all important topics to discuss with patients. The data of safety of anticonvulsants is in rapid flux, so liaise closely with neurologists. The treatment of status epilepticus is not covered in this tutorial but is a common neurological emergency. Urgent anaesthetic review and detection of non-convulsive status are necessary.

The common pitfalls in A&E, general practice, and general medicine are in assuming loss of consciousness is due to a seizure, when in fact serious cardiac causes are equally important to exclude. A twelve-lead ECG to look for Wolff-Parkinson-White, and prolonged QT intervals among others are necessary, and referral to a cardiologist for sometimes prolonged cardiac loop monitoring is often necessary with unexplained loss of consciousness.

Further Reading

Marson A, Al-Kharusi A, Alwaidh M, et al., SANAD Study group (2007). The SANAD study of effectiveness of carbamazepine, gabapentin, lamotrigine, oxcarbazepine, or topiramate for treatment of partial epilepsy: an unblinded randomised controlled trial. *Lancet* 369(9566): 1000–1015.

Marson A, Al-Kharusi A, Alwaidh M, et al., SANAD Study group (2007). The SANAD study of effectiveness of valproate, lamotrigine, or topiramate for generalised and unclassifiable epilepsy: an unblinded randomised controlled trial. *Lancet* 369(9566): 1016–1026.

139. C) Left middle cerebral artery territory infarct secondary to left carotid dissection

Weakness of face and arm, greater than leg, is typical of a middle cerebral artery territory involvement. The neck pain and Horner's syndrome suggest a neck vessel dissection on the left.

A smoker with a Horner's may have an apical lung lesion and have a raised risk of stroke, or a Horner's may be incidental. Embolic stroke without dissection therefore is possible in this case but less likely. A vertebral dissection and posterior circulation infarct may give a Horner's as part of a lateral medullary syndrome. If the leg was involved as severely as the arm then the anterior cerebral artery territory may be involved too.

Tutorial

This case, if the scan had excluded a bleed, it would be suitable for urgent thrombolysis. Familiarize yourself with the rapidly evolving criteria for stroke thrombolysis (currently up to 4.5 hours after onset of stroke, with suspected cases increasingly being taken directly to neurological centres with hyperacute-stroke units), major stroke syndromes (see Table 7.4), and indications and timing for decompressive hemicraniectomy (the malignant MCA syndrome within 72 hours, the malignant posterior fossa syndrome requires posterior decompression within 24 hours to allow survival). There is data that supports the view that decompressive surgery is associated with good functional improvement and quality of life. Local thrombolysis— or even thrombectomy in specialist centres—performed by a neurovascular interventional neuroradiologist should be available and considered in cases not responding rapidly to systemic thrombolysis.

In the treatment of extracranial artery dissection, there is no hard evidence for anticoagulation over antiplatelet therapy, but clinical practice varies. Carotid and large vessel disease are associated with platelet aggregation and therefore antiplatelet therapy is intuitively likely to be more effective, whereas stroke associated with atrial fibrillation requires anticoagulation once the period of risk of intracranial haemorrhagic transformation is over and assuming there are no contraindications. National guidelines for stroke thrombolysis can be found here: <LINK>http://www.rcplondon. ac.uk/resources/stroke-guidelines.

Common stroke and TIA syndromes and their prominent clinical findings are listed in Table 7.4.

Table 7.4 Common stroke and TIA syndromes and their prominent clinical findings

Type of stroke	Artery affected	Distinguishing clinical feature
Anterior circulation	Carotid artery	Amaurosis fugax
	Anterior choroidal	Hemiparesis, hemisensory loss, and field defect
	Anterior cerebral artery syndrome	Deficit more pronounced in legs compared to arms
	Middle cerebral artery	M1, M2, M3 segments)—face and arm, dominant hemisphere aphasia
	Thalamic—anterior/polar/ tuberothalamic (from posterior communicating artery)	Amnesia and emotional involvement
Posterior circulation	Posterior cerebral artery	Visual field defect

Table 7.4 Continued

Type of stroke	Artery affected	Distinguishing clinical feature
	Vertebral artery and posterior inferior cerebellar artery (PICA)	Lateral medullary syndrome* Vestibular disturbance—vertigo/vomiting/nystagmus Ipsilateral cerebellar signs Ipsilateral laryngeal and pharyngeal weakness (X nerve)—dysphagia, hoarse voice, and absent gag reflex Ipsilateral pain and temperature deficit *in face* Contralateral pain and temperature deficit *in body* Ipsilateral Horner's syndrome.
	Anterior spinal artery	Medial medullary syndrome* Ipsilateral XII nerve palsy Contralateral limb weakness Contralateral loss of proprioception, vibration, and discriminative touch
	Tip of the basilar	Quadriparesis and ophthalmoplegia, dysarthria, dysphagia
	Midbrain	Vertical ophthalmoplegia
	Pontine	Horizontal ophthalmoplegia (or locked in syndrome if bilateral)
	Thalamic	Overlap with lacunar infarcts Can cause coma if bilateral
Lacunar	Perforating vessels occlusion	Can vary depending on location but can include: Pure hemiparesis Pure hemisensory loss Mixed motor and sensory loss 'Clumsy hand dysarthria' syndrome Ataxic-hemiparesis

*In cases of lateral and medial medullary syndrome, the exact clinical presentation may vary depending on which artery is affected, at which location the occlusion lies, and variation of blood supply between individuals.

Further Reading

Kim J, Caplan L (2016). Clinical stroke syndromes. *Frontiers in Neurology and Neuroscience* 40: 72–92.

Lyrer P, Engelter S (2010). Antithrombotic drugs for carotid artery dissection. *Cochrane Database Systematic Reviews* 6(10): CD000255.

140. A) Becker muscular dystrophy

The long-standing history, with poor performance at school sports, but progressive muscle weakness, calf hypertrophy, and quadriceps wasting is typical of Becker muscular dystrophy.

Duchenne muscular dystrophy (also due to mutations in the *dystrophin* gene) has similar clinical features to Becker muscular dystrophy but is of greater clinical severity. It affects boys, with most unable to walk at all in their teens, and most succumbing to the disease in their twenties and thirties. The disorder is also one of a mutation in the dystrophin gene. A neuromuscular junction problem such as myasthenia gravis is often difficult to distinguish from a myopathy, and fatigability is not specific to myasthenia, but the atrophy and markedly raised CK make myasthenia unlikely. Becker's myotonia congenita is a channelopathy which leads to severe cramps and episodic muscle weakness, due to mutations in the chloride channel gene CLCN1. The congenital myopathy central core disease is due to RYR1 mutations which also cause malignant hyperthermia. The disease is one of a slowly progressive or non-progressive proximal weakness, often presenting with hypotonia in childhood and with weakness that can involve facial muscles, and may be associated with spinal deformities.

Tutorial

Becker and Duchenne's muscular dystrophy are currently untreatable X-linked dystrophinopathies. Novel therapies (exon skipping and viral vectors) aimed at increasing muscle dystrophin are in development. Co-ordinated care and careful transition from paediatric to adult care in Duchenne's are associated with better survival and outcome. The associated cardiomyopathy is important to recognize and in counselling to female carriers.

Diagnosing muscle disease is difficult and often requires a biopsy and interpretation by experienced muscle histopathologists. The history remains the cornerstone of diagnosis, with elucidation of impairment in early life pointing to a congenital disorder. Inflammatory syndromes include polymyositis, dermatomyositis, SRP-antibody associated necrotizing myositis, and inclusion body myositis (IBM). IBM is the most commonly acquired myopathy of late adult life, and has an inflammatory and degenerative component in its pathophysiology. Nerve conduction studies are useful in identifying a co-existing neuropathy in the diagnostic workup. Electromyography is non-specific in many myopathies but useful in the diagnosis of the muscle channelopathies. The arrival at a correct diagnosis is important for many of the untreatable genetic myopathies to be able to assess the risk of cardiac involvement and in the counselling of possible carriers. HyperCKaemia in asymptomatic individuals, if over three times the normal range, requires muscle biopsy, in particular in females who may be dystrophin carriers.

Further Reading

Matthews E, Hanna M (2008). Recent advances in genetic muscle disease—possible new treatments in muscular dystrophy. ACNR. Open access online journal. http://www.acnr.co.uk/mar_apr_2008/ACNRMA08_recent.pdf

Washington University Neuromuscular website: http://neuromuscular.wustl.edu/ (an excellent site used by general neurologists and neuromuscular specialists).

141. A) Devic's disease (neuromyelitis optica)

The development of symptoms over days is suggestive of an inflammatory process. The constellation of bilateral optic nerve involvement and cord involvement with such severity is highly suggestive of neuromyelitis optica (NMO).

GBS is an acute demyelinating syndrome of the peripheral nervous system, and although a false sensory level is sometimes seen, the patient principally has ascending motor symptoms. Visual symptoms are not seen, though it is worth noting that ophthalmoplegias do occur in the Miller-Fisher variant of GBS. Though MS remains more common than NMO such severe and bilateral optic neuropathies are unusual as a presentation of MS. NF-1 is rarely associated with intramedullary spinal tumours or optic nerve involvement.

Neuro-Behçet's is rare and may be over-diagnosed. The presence of uveitis and oral and genital ulcers would support this diagnosis for which there is no diagnostic serological test. It also requires the exclusion of other inflammatory conditions such as MS and NMO which would require further neuro-imaging and CSF analysis.

Important criteria for NMO are listed in Boxes 7.2 and 7.3.

Box 7.2 Differentials for neuromyelitis optica presenting with acute bilateral visual loss

- Ocular pathology, for example glaucoma
- CNS tumour
- Multiple sclerosis
- Paraneoplastic optic nerve degeneration
- Leber's hereditary optic neuropathy (mitochondrial)
- Vasculitis
- SLE, Sjögren's
- Anti-phospholipid syndrome
- HIV
- Syphilis
- Sarcoidosis
- Lyme disease

Box 7.3 Differentials for neuromyelitis optica presenting with cord syndrome

- Epidural haematoma or abscess
- Dural arteriovenous fistula (DAVF)
- Arteriovenous malformation
- Multiple sclerosis
- Intramedullary cavernoma, tumour, or abscess
- Primary CNS or intravascular lymphoma
- Paraneoplastic
- SLE, Sjögren's
- Anti-phospholipid syndrome
- HIV
- HTLV-1
- HSV2
- Lyme
- Schistosomiasis

Tutorial

In NMO, brain imaging is usually normal or may show brainstem high signal on MRI and radiological evidence of swollen optic nerves. The cord signal on MRI is characteristically 'longitudinally extensive', leading to the term 'longitudinally extensive transverse myelitis' or LETM. CSF may be inflammatory, and oligoclonal bands may be present or not, with no discriminatory value. Visual evoked potentials (VEPs) are prolonged. VEPs are sometimes used to look for subclinical optic nerve involvement in LETM. A thorough ocular examination and ophthalmological review is mandatory to exclude foreign bodies, retained contact lenses, uveitis, and retinal pathology.

There remains debate over whether NMO should be considered a form of multiple sclerosis or a separate disease entity. Serum antibodies to the water channel, aquaporin 4 (AQ4) are specific to the disease, not found in multiple sclerosis, and have evidence of pathogenicity from passive transfer models. If one defines the disease by antibodies alone a broader phenotype is seen, including optic nerve involvement alone. There are no large randomized controlled trials of therapy in NMO, but there is case report evidence that conventional therapies for MS, such as beta-interferon, can make the disease worse, and that therapies such as steroids or plasma exchange in the acute phase, or rituximab can impact on the disease.

Many cases of SLE and Sjögren's associated LETM have been reported to have AQ4 antibodies, which suggests that SLE and Sjögren's simply raise susceptibility to this probable B-cell driven disease. Severe CNS inflammation in any pattern is often a presenting sign of remote cancer (paraneoplastic). CV2/CRMP5 antibodies are associated with a NMO phenotype and cancer. If the phenotype is unusual for NMO, severe and progressive, and AQ4 antibodies are absent, a thorough search for cancer, including full skin, breast, and testes examination, CXR, CT body, and positron emission tomography (PET) should be undertaken. The focus of the investigations should be first to exclude surgical emergencies and infectious diseases, and then to confirm the diagnosis and allow early treatment.

Further Reading

Compston A, Coles A (2008). Multiple sclerosis. *Lancet* 372(9648): 1502–1517.

Lennon V, Wingerchuk D, Kryzer T, et al. (2004). A serum autoantibody marker of neuromyelitis optica: distinction from multiple sclerosis. *Lancet* 364(9451): 2106–2112.

Sellner J, Boggild M, Clanet M, et al. (2010). EFNS guidelines on diagnosis and management of neuromyelitis optica. *European Journal of Neurology* 17(8): 1019–1032.

142. D) Non-invasive ventilation

This patient has a progressive generalized weakness, with a mixture of upper and lower motor neuron signs. The preservation of her knee jerks in the presence of generalized wasting may be considered an upper motor neuron sign. There does not seem to be significant bulbar involvement, so her condition is most consistent with the amyotrophic lateral sclerosis variant of motor neuron disease.

The morning headaches and daytime somnolence indicate respiratory muscle compromise. Diaphragmatic weakness results in hypoventilation and carbon dioxide retention, causing cerebral vasodilation and headache. Non-invasive ventilation improves quality of life and confers a survival benefit in patients with respiratory impairment in motor neuron disease, particularly when there is no bulbar involvement. Trials of diaphragmatic pacing have been disappointing; hence it has not been adopted widely.

Riluzole offers a modest survival benefit in motor neuron disease, increasing life expectancy by on average two to four months. She does not have any dysphagia, so percutaneous endoscopic gastrostomy is unlikely to provide any benefit. Since the respiratory impairment in motor neuron disease is due to ventilatory failure, home oxygen therapy is not indicated.

Tutorial

Motor neuron disease is a relentlessly progressive neurological disease in which there is degeneration of the anterior horn cells, resulting in lower motor neuron weakness, and/or neurons of the motor cortex and corticospinal tract, resulting in upper motor neuron weakness. Additionally, bulbar cranial nerve nuclei may be involved, resulting in dysphagia and vocal dysfunction. The extra-ocular muscles and sphincters are spared, and any sensory involvement should prompt consideration of an alternative diagnosis. The rate of progression varies, but average survival time is about three years. The incidence is approximately 2 per 100,000 per year, with peak age of onset about 60 years. Most cases occur sporadically but 5–10% of cases are familial (Box 7.4).

Box 7.4 Genetic causes of motor neuron disease

- *C9orf72* (>30% familial cases)
- *SOD1* (20% familial cases)
- *TARDBP* (5% familial cases)
- *FUS* (1–5% familial cases)

Rare: angiogenin, ataxin-2, optineurin, ubiquilin-2, P62, *VCP*, *FIG4*

There are four recognized patterns of motor neuron disease (Table 7.5), though there is considerable overlap between these syndromes. Three quarters present with asymmetric weakness affecting the extremities, whilst about a quarter present with bulbar dysfunction. The differential diagnosis is broad, and depends on the presence or absence of lower or upper motor neuron sign predominance (Box 7.5).

Table 7.5 Motor neuron disease subtypes

Motor neuron disease subtype	Pathology and features
Amyotrophic lateral sclerosis	Degeneration of the anterior horn cells, motor cortex, and corticospinal tract, resulting in a combination of upper and lower motor neuron signs
Progressive bulbar palsy	Degeneration of the lower cranial nerve nuclei, resulting in lower motor neuron bulbar dysfunction
Progressive muscular atrophy	Degeneration of the anterior horn cells resulting in lower motor neuron signs
Primary lateral sclerosis	Degeneration of the motor cortex and corticospinal tract resulting in upper motor neuron signs

---

Box 7.5 Main differential diagnoses of motor neuron disease

Lower motor neuron signs predominant:

- Myopathies (e.g. inclusion body myositis)
- Multifocal motor neuropathy with conduction block
- Spinal muscular atrophy
- Chronic inflammatory demyelinating polyneuropathy (motor-predominant)
- Benign fasciculations
- Neuralgic amyotrophy
- Post-polio syndrome

Upper motor neuron signs predominant:

- Primary progressive multiple sclerosis
- Hereditary spastic paraplegia

Mixed upper and lower motor neuron signs:

• Cervical radiculomyelopathy

Bulbar signs predominant:

• Myasthenia gravis
• Brainstem tumour
• Oculopharyngeal dystrophy

The combination of upper and lower motor neuron signs may occur in other conditions, which may be accompanied by sensory features. Examples include subacute combined degeneration of the cord, lesions at the conus medullaris, taboparesis, and Friedrich's ataxia. Combined pathology (e.g. peripheral neuropathy and stroke, both of which may be associated with diabetes mellitus) may also result in mixed motor signs.

There is no diagnostic test for motor neuron disease, and the diagnosis is made clinically. Investigations are concerned primarily with excluding treatable conditions, such as multifocal motor neuropathy with conduction block, and determining the need for supportive therapies such as non-invasive ventilation. These should be performed as early as possible to prevent unnecessary delays in management.

Brain and cervical spine MRI should be performed to exclude treatable mimics such as cervical disc disease. Creatine kinase may be modestly elevated in motor neuron disease. Nerve conduction studies demonstrate normal motor conduction velocity with reduced compound muscle action potentials, while electromyography shows denervation and fibrillation potentials. Additional tests such as lumbar puncture, muscle or nerve biopsy, and anti-acetylcholine receptors may be performed to exclude alternative diagnoses. Pulmonary function tests are important in determining the need for ventilatory support, and these should be repeated frequently to detect the onset of respiratory weakness.

Treatment of motor neuron disease is predominantly supportive. This should occur in a multidisciplinary setting, involving neurology, physiotherapy, occupational therapy, dietetic, and speech and language therapy input. Riluzole is the only medication licensed for motor neuron disease, which has a modest effect on disease course, increasing survival by 2–4 months. Bulbar impairment results in risk of aspiration pneumonia, which is reduced by insertion of a percutaneous endoscopic gastrostomy. When the patient cannot lie flat or cannot be sedated safely, radiologically inserted gastrostomy may be necessary. As the disease progresses to involve ventilatory muscles, non-invasive ventilation may be required. This should be considered when there are features of respiratory compromise, which are summarized in Table 7.6.

Table 7.6 Features of ventilatory impairment in motor neuron disease

Symptoms	Signs
Breathlessness/orthopnoea	Tachypnoea
Recurrent pneumonias	Shallow breathing/reduced chest expansion
Non-refreshing/disturbed sleep	Weak cough
Daytime somnolence	Weak sniff
Poor concentration/memory	Use of accessory muscles
Morning headaches	Abdominal paradox
Confusion	
Hallucinations	
Fatigue	
Poor appetite	

Further Reading

Bäumer D, Talbot K, Turner M (2014). Advances in motor neuron disease. *Journal Royal Society of Medicine* 107(1): 14–21.

Kiernan M, Vucic S, Cheah B, et al. (2011). Amyotrophic lateral sclerosis. *Lancet* 377(9769): 942–955.

National Institute for Clinical Excellence (2019). Motor neurone disease: assessment and management [NG42]. February 2016, updated July 2019. Available at: https://www.nice.org.uk/guidance/ng42

Turner M, Talbot K (2013). Mimics and chameleons in motor neuron disease. *Practical Neurology* 13(3): 153–164.

143. D) Myotonia congenita

This boy presents with muscle stiffness which improves with exercise, with a possible family history of similar problems. The examination reveals evidence of myotonia, which improves on repeated attempts (warm-up myotonia). This phenomenon is a characteristic feature of myotonia congenita, which is further supported by the 'well-defined musculature', with patients with this condition often described to have a Herculean appearance. In the absence of other features of myotonic dystrophy, and with the characteristic warm-up myotonia, myotonia congenita is the more probable diagnosis.

Becker's muscular dystrophy would be more likely to result in weakness rather than stiffness, and McArdle's disease is characterized by painful muscle cramps on exercise. The periodic paralyses are characterized by episodes of profound weakness, rather than muscle stiffness.

Tutorial

Myotonia refers to the phenomenon of delayed muscle relaxation following contraction. On electromyography, myotonia is typically described as a 'dive-bomber' pattern, due to the sound produced.

Myotonia most commonly occurs in the autosomal dominant genetic condition, myotonic dystrophy. This occurs due to a trinucleotide CTG repeat expansion in the myotonin kinase gene. It is an example of a genetic condition that demonstrates anticipation, with subsequent generations presenting earlier and being affected more severely. The severe congenital form usually occurs in neonates with affected mothers, so genetic counselling is particularly important in female patients. Clinical severity is highly variable, ranging from a severe congenital myopathy to isolated late-onset cataracts. Clinical manifestations are summarized in Box 7.6, but include predominantly distal myopathy, cataracts, cardiomyopathy, and cognitive deficits, for example. Treatment is generally supportive, ensuring appropriate multidisciplinary professionals are involved. Cardiac screening with regular electrocardiograms is very important. Myotonia may be treated with mexiletine or phenytoin if it is problematic, and daytime somnolence may warrant treatment with stimulants such as modafinil.

Box 7.6 Clinical features of myotonic dystrophy

- Motor—myotonia and myopathy (predominantly distal)
- Cardiomyopathy
- Respiratory muscle weakness
- Endocrine disturbance—diabetes mellitus and thyroid disease
- Hair loss
- Cognitive slowing
- Daytime somnolence
- Bowel dysmotility

The diagnosis of myotonic dystrophy can usually be made on clinical grounds, but genetic testing is available. If the genetic test is negative, the similar condition proximal myotonic myopathy (PROMM) should be considered. Features are similar to myotonic dystrophy, though the weakness tends to be proximal rather than distal. Myalgia is more suggestive of PROMM than myotonic dystrophy.

Myotonia congenita is another genetic condition which is characterized by warm-up myotonia. There is often stiffness at the onset of exercise, which improves with continued activity. It may be inherited in dominant (Thomsen's disease) or recessive (Becker's disease) fashion. Due to excess muscle contraction, these patients develop a well-defined musculature. Power at rest is usually normal. Myotonia congenita occurs due to a mutation in the voltage-gated chloride channel *CLCN1*.

In contrast, the genetic condition paramyotonia congenita is characterized by episodes of muscle stiffness that get worse on continued exercise, due to mutations in the voltage-gated skeletal muscle sodium channel subunit *SCN4A*. Episodes may also be precipitated by cold temperatures. Mexiletine can be used to treat symptoms.

Further Reading

Gardiner A, Jaffer F, Dale R, et al. (2015). The clinical and genetic heterogeneity of paroxysmal dyskinesias. *Brain* 138(12): 3567–3580.

Ryan A, Matthews E, Hanna M (2007). Skeletal-muscle channelopathies: periodic paralysis and nondystrophic myotonias. *Current Opinions in Neurology* 20(5): 558–563.

Udd B, Krahe R (2012). The myotonic dystrophies: molecular, clinical, and therapeutic challenges. *Lancet Neurology* 11(10): 891–905.

Walters R (2014). Muscle diseases: mimics and chameleons. *Practical Neurology* 14(5):288–298.

144. D) Observation and follow-up

This patient has been incidentally found to have asymmetric parkinsonism. In this age group, asymmetric parkinsonism is nearly always due to idiopathic Parkinson's disease. Dopamine agonists (e.g. ropinirole or pramipexole), monoamine oxidase B inhibitors (e.g. rasagiline) and levodopa (a dopamine precursor) can all be used to treat motor symptoms early during the disease. However, they have several potential side effects, and generally treatment is commenced when the patient's symptoms become problematic. This gentleman is not troubled by his symptoms, so watching and waiting would be appropriate at this stage

Tutorial

Parkinson's disease is a neurodegenerative condition characterized clinically by a typical motor disorder consisting of bradykinesia, rigidity, and rest tremor, as a consequence of loss of dopaminergic neurons in the substantia nigra pars compacta. Other causes of parkinsonism are discussed in the tutorial for question 133. In addition to the motor disorder, other manifestations of Parkinson's disease include anosmia, cognitive deficits and dementia, neuropsychiatric manifestations including depression and anxiety, and sleep disturbance (e.g. rapid eye movement sleep behaviour disorder). Diagnosis can be made on clinical grounds, with investigations only warranted in atypical cases.

The motor disorder responds well to dopaminergic medications. These can have significant side effects, including dyskinesias, off-target effects such as impulse control behaviours and cognitive dysfunction, and on-off cycling. These adverse effects constitute a significant aspect of advancing Parkinson's disease, and as such treatment is usually delayed until the motor symptoms become problematic.

Classically, treatment is initiated with a dopamine agonist or a monoamine oxidase B inhibitor. The rationale for this is that it delays the need for levodopa-based therapies, which ultimately herald problematic dyskinesias and on-off cycling. However, increasingly levodopa is commenced as the first agent. This is usually in combination with a dopa-decarboxylase inhibitor which does not cross the blood-brain barrier, limiting peripheral side effects, whilst allowing for activity within the central nervous system. Catechol-O-methyl transferase inhibitors (e.g. entacapone) may also be used in combination with levodopa, boosting the available dopaminergic dose. Apomorphine is a potent dopamine agonist that can be used parenterally to alleviate Parkinsonian crisis, or as a maintenance therapy via a subcutaneous pump.

Other medications used include anticholinergics (e.g. benzhexol) or beta blockers for tremor, and indeed in tremor predominant cases this may be all that is necessary. However, they may precipitate hallucination in patients with cortical pathology, so their use is generally limited to young patients without cognitive impairment. Rivastigmine is licensed for treatment of dementia in the setting of Parkinson's disease. Deep brain stimulation is also an effective in controlling the movement disorder in patients that had previously demonstrated a good response to levodopa. Amantadine may also be used for the treatment of dyskinesias. A list of treatments and their main side effects is listed in Table 7.7.

Table 7.7 Dopaminergic therapies for Parkinson's disease and their main side effects

Class	Examples	Main side effects
Levodopa-based preparations	Co-careldopa (levodopa + carbidopa) Co-beneldopa (levodopa + benserazide) Stalevo (co-careldopa + entacapone) Duodopa (intestinal gel)	Nausea Dyskinesia On-off fluctuations Psychosis Cognitive dysfunction
Dopamine agonists	Ropinirole Pramipexole Rotigotine Apomorphine	Nausea Psychosis Impulse control behaviours Peripheral oedema
Monoamine oxidase B inhibitors	Rasagiline Selegiline	Worsening of dyskinesia Risk of serotonin syndrome when co-prescribed with selective serotonin reuptake inhibitors or tramadol for example
Catechol-O-methyl transferase inhibitors	Entacapone Tolcapone	Increased severity of levodopa-induced side effects Gastrointestinal upset Hepatotoxicity (tolcapone)

Impulse control disorder, characterized by compulsive behaviours such as gambling, shopping, hypersexuality, and excessive eating, is a significant adverse effect. It is most commonly seen with dopamine agonists, but can occur with levodopa. Treatment generally involves withdrawal of dopamine agonist therapy, prior to commencement of alternative agents. This must be done cautiously, due to the risk of dopamine agonist withdrawal syndrome (DAWS), which manifests with anxiety, depression sweating, orthostatic hypotension, generalized pain, and drug cravings, for example.

Further Reading

Ali K, Morris H (2015). Parkinson's disease: chameleons and mimics. *Practical Neurology* 5(1): 14–25.

Kalia L, Lang A (2015). Parkinson's disease. *Lancet* 386(9996): 896–912.

Kalia S, Sankar T, Lozano A (2013). Deep brain stimulation for Parkinson's disease and other movement disorders. *Current Opinions in Neurology* 26(4):374–380.

National Institute for Clinical Excellence (2017). Parkinson's disease in adults [NG71]. July 2017. Available at: https://www.nice.org.uk/guidance/ng71

145. A) A 24-hour urinary copper excretion

This young male has presented with a progressive movement disorder in the setting of antecedent behavioural abnormalities. His blood tests reveal mildly deranged liver function. The normocytic anaemia in association with raised reticulocyte count suggests haemolytic anaemia. The combination of neurological and hepatic findings point to a diagnosis of Wilson's disease, in which haemolytic anaemia may occur. The diagnosis of Wilson's disease may be suggested by low caeruloplasmin levels or elevated urinary copper excretion.

It is important to consider Huntington's disease in cases of chorea, and his family history of dementia may point one towards this. However, this would not account for the abnormal blood results, and usually does not manifest until the fourth decade. Anti-phospholipid syndrome is another cause of chorea, but there is nothing in the history to suggest this is the diagnosis.

Tutorial

Chorea refers to excessive spontaneous movements which are random and smooth. The most common cause of chorea is Huntington's disease; other causes are listed in Table 7.8. An abrupt onset of chorea is more suggestive of acquired causes, whereas inherited chorea may develop insidiously.

Table 7.8 Causes of chorea

Inherited	Acquired
Huntington's disease	Sydenham's chorea (post-streptococcal)
Benign hereditary chorea	Pregnancy (chorea gravidarum)
Spinocerebellar ataxia (types 1, 2, 3, and 17)	Drug-induced (antipsychotics, levodopa, dopamine
Wilson's disease	agonists, anticholinergics)
Neuro-acanthocytosis	Systemic lupus erythematosus
Friedrich's ataxia	Antiphospholipid syndrome
Ataxia telangiectasia	Striatal lesions (e.g. stroke, tumour)
Lysosomal storage diseases	Thyrotoxicosis
Neuroferritinopathy	Polycythaemia rubra vera
	Human immunodeficiency virus
	Herpes simplex encephalitis
	Variant Creutzfeldt-Jakob disease

Huntington's disease is an autosomal dominant disorder with high penetrance. It occurs due to a trinucleotide CAG repeat expansion in the huntingtin gene. Onset of the movement disorder tends to occur around age 40, though there may be prodromal psychiatric and cognitive manifestations, such as depression. As progression ensues, the choreiform movement disorder often degenerates into a Parkinsonian picture, accompanied by cognitive decline and dementia. The juvenile Westphal variant is characterized by an akinetic-rigid syndrome with dystonia and little chorea. Diagnosis can be made with a genetic test for the trinucleotide repeat number. There is no disease-modifying treatment for Huntington's disease, so genetic counselling is paramount prior to undertaking genetic testing.

Wilson's disease is an important cause of chorea, as it is treatable, but can be fatal if not managed appropriately. It is an autosomal recessive disorder caused by mutations in the *ATP7B* gene which encodes a transmembrane copper transporter. Presentation is usually within the first two decades. Although many systems can be affected, the most important manifestations are hepatic disease and neurological dysfunction. Presentation may be with acute hepatic failure, hepatitis, or cirrhosis. Neurological manifestations may include neuropsychiatric disturbance, dysarthria, or a movement disorder, which may take the form of tremor, chorea, or an akinetic-rigid syndrome, often with autonomic features. Rarely, haemolytic anaemia may be the presenting manifestation. Copper deposition in the cornea results in Kayser-Fleischer rings, which can be detected on slit-lamp examination and are useful diagnostically. Laboratory tests indicating Wilson's disease include a low serum caeruloplasmin level, high 24-hour urinary copper excretion, or increased hepatic copper content, though these must be taken into account alongside clinical features. The disease can be successfully treated using copper-chelators. Penicillamine is generally considered the first-line treatment, though the alternative trientine is often used as the treatment of choice in neurological presentations.

Further Reading

Ala A, Walker A, Ahskan K, et al. (2007). Wilson's disease. *Lancet* 369(9559): 397–408.

Cardoso F (2004). Chorea: non-genetic causes. *Current Opinions in Neurology* 17: 433–436.

Phillips W, Shannon K, Barker R (2008). The current clinical management of Huntington's disease. *Movement Disorders* 23(11): 1491–1504.

Walker F (2007). Huntington's disease. *Lancet* 369(9557): 218–228.

146. C) Forced vital capacity

This gentleman presents with an acute progressive peripheral neuropathy, as evidenced by distal motor and sensory impairment, with global areflexia. The likely diagnosis here is GBS, in which a degree of back pain is often seen in addition to the weakness. The antecedent gastrointestinal illness (which he had considered to be 'food poisoning') also supports the diagnosis. Though the other tests may be important in his subsequent work up, the priority is establishing his ventilatory status so that higher level care can be arranged if necessary—hence forced vital capacity should be performed as soon as possible.

Tutorial

GBS refers to an acute onset predominantly motor neuropathy. Typically, the pathological basis of GBS is an acute demyelinating polyneuropathy/polyradiculopathy, though it is now recognized that axonal variants exist (Table 7.9). Classically, onset occurs 2–4 weeks following a gastrointestinal or respiratory infection (see Box 7.7 for a list of common causative organisms), with peripheral neurological symptoms (sensory disturbance or weakness) which progress in an ascending symmetrical pattern over hours or days. Weakness can progress to involve the ventilatory muscles, so monitoring forced vital capacity is necessary, and elective intubation is often necessary to avoid impending respiratory failure. Weakness may progress over a few weeks, with the mean time to clinical nadir being 12 days. Cranial nerve involvement may result in lower motor neuron facial weakness, diplopia, and bulbar dysfunction. Pain in the back, shoulder-girdle, or buttocks is common. Autonomic disturbance is a frequent and significant problem, and most commonly manifests as a labile hypertension. Tachy- and bradyarrhythmias may occur, warranting cardiac monitoring. Other autonomic features may include urinary retention, ileus and facial flushing, for example. Mortality in GBS remains about 5%, and about 20–30% of patients are left with a permanent deficit.

Table 7.9 Patterns of Guillain-Barré syndrome

Clinical patterns of Guillain-Barré syndrome

Classic	Ascending tetraparesis with or without cranial nerve involvement
Pharyngeal-cervical-brachial variant	Bulbar, cervical, and shoulder/upper limb weakness
Paraparetic variant	Lower limb weakness
Bilateral facial weakness with paraesthesias	Bilateral lower motor neuron facial weakness and peripheral sensory disturbance
Miller-Fisher syndrome	Ophthalmoplegia, ataxia and areflexia, without limb weakness
Bickerstaff's brainstem encephalitis	As for Miller-Fisher syndrome, with additional hypersomnolence due to involvement of the reticular formation

Electrophysiological patterns of Guillain-Barré syndrome

- Acute inflammatory demyelinating polyneuropathy
- Acute motor and sensory axonal neuropathy (associated with anti-GM1, anti-GM1b, and anti-GD1a antibodies)
- Acute motor axonal neuropathy (associated with anti-GM1, anti-GM1b, anti-GD1a, and anti-GalNac-GD1a antibodies)
- Acute sensory neuropathy (associated with anti-GD1b antibodies)
- Acute pandysautonomia

Box 7.7 Infectious agents associated with Guillain-Barré syndrome

- *Campylobacter jejuni*
- *Mycoplasma pneumonia*
- *Haemophilus influenzae*
- *Cytomegalovirus*
- Epstein-Barr virus
- Human immunodeficiency virus

GBS is usually diagnosed on clinical grounds, with supportive investigative evidence coming later. The typical CSF picture is that of albuminocytological dissociation—protein is elevated, with less than 10 cells/mm³. The rise in protein may take a week to occur, so a repeat, delayed lumbar puncture is often performed (it should be noted that if the patient has received intravenous immunoglobulin therapy, then a rise in lymphocytes may be seen secondary to an aseptic meningitis). Nerve conduction studies can be helpful, and typically demonstrate features of proximal and distal demyelination, including delayed distal latencies, with slow conduction velocities and prolonged F-waves. However, electrophysiology may be normal early in the course of disease, so a normal result does not exclude GBS. Serological tests for antecedent infection may be performed, for example for *Campylobacter jejuni*, *Mycoplasma pneumoniae*, *Cytomegalovirus* (CMV), and Epstein-Barr virus (EBV) amongst others. Additionally, HIV testing should be performed, as GBS may occur as a seroconversion illness. Anti-ganglioside antibodies (anti-GD3, anti-GM1, and anti-GQ1b) are identified in over half of cases. Anti-GM1 in particular is associated with *C. jejuni* infection, and anti-GQ1b occurs in association with the Miller-Fisher variant of GBS, characterized by ophthalmoplegia, areflexia, and ataxia.

Management consists of monitoring, supportive measures, and targeting pathological antibodies. Cardiac and blood pressure monitoring is important, along with regular forced vital capacity assessment. A fall in forced vital capacity to less than 15–20 ml/kg or 1.2 l should prompt elective intensive care admission and intubation. Intravenous immunoglobulin (0.4 g/kg/day for five days) is the first-line treatment for GBS, with plasma exchange being an alternative approach. There is no evidence for the use of steroids.

Further Reading

Garg N, Park S, Vucic S, et al. (2016). Differentiating lower motor neuron syndromes. *Journal of Neurology, Neurosurgery and Psychiatry* 88(6): 474–483.

Goodfellow J, Willison H (2016). Guillain-Barré syndrome: a century of progress. *Nature Reviews Neurology* 12(12): 723–731.

Pritchard J (2006). What's new in Guillain-Barré Syndrome? *Practical Neurology* 6: 208–217.

Wakerley B, Yuki N (2015). Mimics and chameleons in Guillain-Barré and Miller Fisher syndromes. *Practical Neurology* 15(2): 90–99.

147. D) Pyridostigmine plus prednisolone

This patient presented with diplopia and bilateral ptosis. There is evidence of fatiguability on examination, which explains why her symptoms are worse at the end of the day. In the absence of limb weakness, her diagnosis is therefore most likely to be ocular myasthenia gravis. The treatment options for myasthenia gravis are discussed below, but given that she does not have any bulbar or generalized features, an acetylcholinesterase inhibitor such as pyridostigmine would be the most appropriate treatment of those listed. Though ocular myasthenia is sometimes treated with pyridostigmine alone, most patients convert to generalized myasthenia, so prednisolone is often commenced from the outset.

Steroid-sparing agents such as azathioprine and mycophenolate mofetil are used as maintenance, to allow for steroid-related side effects to be minimized. Intravenous immunoglobulin or plasma exchange are indicated in myasthenic crises. The role of thymectomy is still not clearly defined. It may be performed in younger patients, in which it may result in disease remission. Older patients may undergo thymectomy if a thymoma is identified, though the rationale for treatment in this group is to remove the tumour, rather than with a view to improving neurological symptoms.

Tutorial

Myasthenia gravis is an autoimmune disorder caused by (in the majority of cases) antibodies against the post-synaptic nicotinic acetylcholine receptor, resulting in dysfunction of the neuromuscular junction. The clinical hallmark is muscle weakness with fatiguability, which may be demonstrated on examination. The differential diagnoses of neuromuscular dysfunction and ocular myasthenia are listed in Boxes 7.8 and 7.9 respectively.

Box 7.8 Causes of neuromuscular junction dysfunction

- Myasthenia gravis
- Lambert-Eaton myasthenic syndrome
- Congenital myasthenia
- Cholinergic crisis/organophosphate poisoning
- Botulism
- Snake venom

Box 7.9 Differentials of ocular myasthenia

- Thyroid eye disease
- Mitochondrial disease
- Cranial nerve palsies
- Multiple sclerosis
- Oculopharyngeal muscular dystrophy
- Guillain-Barré syndrome

There is an association with other autoimmune disorders, and also with thymoma. The spectrum of clinical severity is broad, with symptoms in some cases being limited to the extra-ocular muscles, and in others causing bulbar dysfunction and generalized weakness. Presentation may be acute, in the form of myasthenic crisis in which the ventilatory muscles may be involved. Crises are most commonly precipitated by infections, but several medications can exacerbate symptoms (aminoglycosides, ciprofloxacin, erythromycin, chloroquine, lithium, procainamide, verapamil, beta blockers, and penicillamine). There is also a significant risk of deterioration in the post-partum period.

Diagnosis can be supported by identification of the anti-acetylcholine receptor antibody which is present in up to 90% of patients with generalized myasthenia. In antibody negative cases, the anti-muscle specific kinase (anti-MuSK) antibodies should be sought, which are identified in about half of 'seronegative' cases. Neurophysiology is also useful in confirming a diagnosis. The electrophysiological correlate of fatiguability is a decremental response in the compound muscle action potential on nerve conduction studies with repetitive stimulation, and single-fibre electromyography demonstrates increased jitter (variability in time intervals of depolarization between fibres within a motor unit). It is also important to perform thyroid function tests, as autoimmune thyroid disease occurs concomitantly in about 10% of cases. Mediastinal imaging should also be performed to exclude thymoma, which is present in 10–15% of patients (10% of which have malignant features).

The management of myasthenia depends on the severity. Disease limited to the extra-ocular muscles may be treated with the acetylcholinesterase inhibitor, pyridostigmine, which increases the amount of acetylcholine available in the neuromuscular junction. In generalized disease, or in refractory cases, suppression of the immunological pathology is necessary. This is performed with steroids, titrated up to the minimum dose that alleviates symptoms. Once remission has been achieved for at least 2–3 months, the dose may be tapered to the minimum effective dose. Steroid-sparing agents such as azathioprine, mycophenolate mofetil, and methotrexate may be necessary to allow weaning of steroids to an acceptable level. There is some evidence that thymectomy is useful in achieving remission in younger patients though there are still no clear guidelines on when this should be performed. Myasthenic crises warrant treatment with intravenous immunoglobulin or plasma exchange, along with high-dose steroids. Respiratory function should be closely monitored, and ventilatory support is often necessary. Cholinesterase inhibitors should be discontinued in suspected myasthenic crisis, as abrupt generalized weakness may also occur in cholinergic crisis, which is an important differential to consider. This diagnosis may be supported clinically by the presence of cholinergic 'SLUDGE' symptoms (salivation, lacrimation, urinary incontinence, diaphoresis, gastrointestinal upset, and emesis).

Further Reading

Sanders D, Wolf G, Benatar M, et al. (2016). International consensus guidance for management of myasthenia gravis: Executive summary. *Neurology* 87(4): 419–425.

Sussman J, Farrugia M, Maddison P, et al. (2015). Myasthenia gravis: Association of British Neurologists' management guidelines. *Practical Neurology* 15(3): 199–206.

148. A) Cryptococcal antigen testing

This patient has presented with meningism, fever, and reduced conscious level, on a background of non-specific symptoms occurring in the previous weeks. The identification of oral thrush in association with his history of shingles raises suspicion of HIV, which is also supported by the cervical lymphadenopathy. The CSF lymphocytosis, low glucose, and raised protein is most consistent with cryptococcal meningitis, though tuberculous meningitis could cause a similar picture. The most sensitive test for cryptococcal meningitis is CSF cryptococcal antigen testing, which is positive in over 95% of cases. India ink staining may help with diagnosis of cryptococcal meningitis, but is only positive in 25–50% of cases.

The long prodrome and CSF findings would not be consistent with herpes simplex meningoencephalitis or meningococcal meningitis. The VDRL is a serological test for syphilis, which may cause an aseptic meningitis.

Tutorial

HIV is associated with a many neurological conditions, due to opportunistic infections or the HIV virus itself (Table 7.10).

Toxoplasmosis, caused by the protozoan *Toxoplasma gondii*, is the commonest opportunistic infection affecting the central nervous system in HIV. Most cases occur due to reactivation of a latent infection, so it is important to test for *Toxoplasma* serology routinely, with seropositive patients receiving prophylaxis in the form of co-trimoxazole. Presentation is usually with focal neurological symptoms secondary to multifocal mass lesions, though encephalitis is also possible, and may involve the brainstem. Negative serology does not exclude the diagnosis, and brain biopsy is required for confirmation, though diagnosis is often made on the basis of a response to treatment with pyrimethamine and sulphadiazine (with folinic acid supplementation). Thallium SPECT is negative, which helps to distinguish toxoplasmosis from primary central nervous system lymphoma (PCNSL).

Progressive multifocal leukoencephalopathy (PML) is caused by reactivation of the JC virus, which replicates in oligodendrocytes, resulting in demyelination. PML has subacute onset and involves a combination of focal signs in addition to progressive cognitive decline. Diagnosis can usually be made with CSF PCR, though brain biopsy may be necessary. Neuroimaging demonstrates a single or multiple lesions, without mass effect.

Cryptococcal meningitis usually occurs when CD4 cell count falls below 100 cells/mm^3. Clinical features include headache, fever, and drowsiness. Only about one third develop overt meningism. Onset may be acute or subacute with headaches, fevers, and constitutional symptoms. Cryptococcal antigen testing is the most sensitive method of diagnosis, and fungal hyphae can sometimes be detected with India ink staining. Raised opening pressure on lumbar puncture is a poor prognostic sign. CSF shows a lymphocytosis, raised protein, and low glucose, similar to findings seen with tuberculosis. Treatment is with amphotericin B, sometimes with adjuvant flucytosine.

Tuberculosis is common in HIV patients. Often there are pulmonary manifestations, but neurological involvement may occur in the form of a basal meningitis, which may result in cranial nerve palsies, or the formation of space-occupying lesions (tuberculomas) which can cause focal neurological deficits.

Herpes viruses can also result in neurological disease in HIV patients. Varicella zoster virus (VZV) reactivation results in shingles, causing pain and vesicles in a dermatomal distribution. CMV may cause disease when CD4 counts fall to below 50 cells/mm^3, with CMV retinitis being a significant cause of blindness in HIV patients. It may also result in an acute encephalitis.

PCNSL is associated with EBV infection and is the second most common cause of mass lesions, after toxoplasmosis. Presentation is with focal neurological deficit and headache, and seizures may occur. There is no effective treatment for PCNSL, though radiotherapy and steroids may be employed. Unlike toxoplasmosis, the thallium SPECT scan demonstrates high uptake.

HIV itself can cause neuropathology. At seroconversion 10% of patients have neurological involvement, which may take the form of aseptic meningitis, acute disseminated encephalomyelitis, transverse myelitis, or brachial neuritis. Later on in the course of disease, HIV can result in a subcortical dementia, though the incidence of this has decreased significantly since the introduction of highly active anti-retroviral therapy (HAART). This cognitive impairment progresses from subtle changes such as altered concentration, to significant memory impairment, personality change, and sometimes motor deficits.

HIV may also result in spinal cord involvement (vacuolar myelopathy), resulting in a progressive spastic paraparesis, with sensory ataxia and sphincter dysfunction, resembling subacute combined degeneration of the cord. This occurs in up to 10% of patients. Other direct effects of HIV include peripheral neuropathy and polymyositis. It should be remembered that peripheral neuropathy may also result from treatment with HAART.

Table 7.10 Important neurological manifestations of HIV

Direct effects	Opportunistic infections
HIV seroconversion	*Toxoplasmosis*
Aseptic meningitis	Focal deficits
Acute disseminated encephalomyelitis (ADEM)	Thallium SPECT scan negative
Brachial neuritis	*Tuberculosis*
Transverse myelitis	Meningitis
Vacuolar myelopathy	Tuberculomas
Progressive spastic paraparesis	*Cryptococcal meningitis*
Dorsal column involvement—sensory ataxia	Headache
Sphincter dysfunction	Fever
Peripheral neuropathy	Drowsiness
Distal sensory neuropathy	Raised opening pressure on lumbar puncture
Guillain-Barré syndrome	Meningism in 1/3
Mononeuritis multiplex	*Primary central nervous system lymphoma*
HIV-associated dementia (AIDS dementia complex)	Focal deficits
Altered concentration	Headache
Memory loss	Seizures
Personality change	Thallium SPECT scan positive
Motor impairment	*Progressive multifocal leukoencephalopathy*
	Subacute progressive focal deficits
	Cognitive impairment
	No mass effect on neuroimaging
	Cytomegalovirus
	Retinitis
	Encephalitis
	Varicella zoster virus
	Shingles

Further Reading

McArthur J, Brew B, Nath A (2005). Neurological complications of HIV infection. *Lancet Neurology* 4(9): 543–555.

Tan I, Smith B, von Geldern G, et al. (2012). HIV-associated opportunistic infections of the CNS. *Lancet Neurology* 11(7): 605–617.

Williamson P, Jarvis J, Panackal A, et al. (2017). Cryptococcal meningitis: epidemiology, immunology, diagnosis and therapy. *Nature Reviews Neurology* 13(1): 13–24.

149. D) Sarcoidosis

This patient has presented with a subacute lower motor neuron facial weakness, as evidenced by the involvement of orbicularis oculi in addition to the lower facial muscles. Additional features of parotid swelling and ocular inflammation are pointers towards uveoparotid fever (Heerfordt's syndrome) as a cause of her facial palsy, which usually responds to steroids. This is a rare presentation of sarcoidosis, which is supported by the previous lower limb rash which was probably erythema nodosum.

Bell's palsy, Ramsay Hunt syndrome, and vasculitis can all cause lower motor neuron facial weakness, and the factors that would lead one to these alternative diagnoses are discussed below. Anterior circulation strokes cause facial weakness of an upper motor neuron distribution, sparing the muscles of the upper part of the face. Rarely, posterior circulation strokes involving the facial nerve nucleus in the pons could cause a lower motor neuron facial weakness.

Tutorial

The facial nerve motor nucleus is in the pons, which gives supply to muscles of the face and to stapedius in the ear. The facial nerve also carries parasympathetic fibres to the lacrimal and salivary glands, sensory afferents from the external ear, and special sensory fibres for taste from the anterior two thirds of the tongue (in the chorda tympani). The nerve exits the skull though the internal auditory meatus, and passes through the parotid gland, where it divides into five regional branches to supply the facial muscles. These anatomical features are reflected in the clinical manifestations of facial nerve palsy.

Bell's palsy is often considered to be the cause of lower motor neuron facial weakness when no other cause is identified. However, a positive diagnosis can be made, based on the presence of characteristic findings. Clinical features include unilateral lower motor neuron facial weakness, mild-moderate pain around the ipsilateral ear, hyperacusis (involvement of stapedius), and abrupt (but not sudden) onset, with peak weakness occurring within 72 hours. Ipsilateral loss of taste on the anterior two thirds of the tongue confirms a peripheral facial nerve palsy, most likely in the facial canal. Recovery begins by three weeks, and prolonged or progressive weakness should prompt consideration of an alternative diagnosis. About 20% of patients are left with some deficit. Treatment involves protection of the unblinking eye with patching and lubricating eye drops, and prognosis is improved with a short course of steroids. There is no clear evidence for use of antivirals, though this is often used.

Ramsay Hunt syndrome occurs due to reactivation of the varicella zoster virus, and results in unilateral facial nerve weakness. Pain is more severe than that seen in Bell's palsy, and there are usually herpetic vesicles in or around the ear, or on the tongue or hard palate. These may follow the facial weakness, and in some cases are not detected (Ramsay Hunt sine herpeticum). Ramsay Hunt syndrome is treated with a combination of steroids and anti-viral agent. Prognosis is worse than Bell's palsy, with about 50% of patients making a full recovery.

Brainstem lesions (pontine tumour or stroke, or demyelination) can cause dysfunction of the facial nerve nucleus, resulting in lower motor neuron facial weakness. Due to proximity of other structures, there are usually associated findings, such as abducens nerve palsy or impaired conscious level. Likewise, the nerve may be compressed by cerebellopontine angle tumours (most commonly vestibular schwannomas) as it exits the brainstem. Again, one would expect other findings, including palsies of the vestibulocochlear and trigeminal nerves. In these central causes of facial nerve palsy, taste is not affected.

Parotid gland pathology (tumours, sarcoidosis) can result in lower motor neuron weakness, damaging the nerve as it passes through the glands. Bilateral facial weakness may raise suspicion of GBS, myasthenia gravis, or myopathies. Taste is not affected in these conditions.

Further Reading

Fuller G, Morgan C (2016). Bell's palsy syndrome: mimics and chameleons. *Practical Neurology* 16(6): 439–444.

Krumholz A, Stern B (2014). Neurologic manifestations of sarcoidosis. *Handbook of Clinical Neurology* 119: 305–333.

Sweeney C, Gilden (2001). Ramsay Hunt syndrome. *Journal of Neurology, Neurosurgery, and Psychiatry* 71: 149–154.

150. C) Oral nimodipine

The CT scan and clinical story are consistent with a subarachnoid haemorrhage. The majority of subarachnoid haemorrhages occur due to rupture of a berry aneurysm, and after initial resuscitation, urgent neurosurgical referral is required to arrange endovascular coiling, or surgical clipping of the aneurysm (or arterio-venous malformation). A significant early complication of subarachnoid haemorrhage is vasospasm, with the resulting cerebral ischaemia contributing to further morbidity and mortality. The treatment of choice for preventing vasospasm is regular nimodipine (a calcium channel blocker).

Intravenous saline may be used in subarachnoid haemorrhage in order to maintain cerebral perfusion, after the aneurysm has been secured, but is not the correct answer in this case. The history is not consistent with meningitis, so ceftriaxone is not indicated. Subcutaneous sumatriptan may be useful in migraine or cluster headache, but plays no role in the management of subarachnoid haemorrhage. Oxygen therapy is useful in acute management of cluster headache, but is not indicated in this case.

Tutorial

Subarachnoid haemorrhage occurs in most cases due to rupture of a berry aneurysm, causing arterial bleeding into the subarachnoid space. Other causes include arteriovenous malformations, vasculitis, tumours, and trauma. Berry aneurysms may be associated with diseases that affect connective tissues, including autosomal dominant polycystic kidney disease, pseudoxanthoma elasticum, Marfan syndrome and Ehlers-Danlos syndrome, for example. Aneurysmal subarachnoid haemorrhage carries a high morbidity and mortality, with overall survival about 50%.

Clinical presentation is typically with a sudden onset severe headache, often described as thunderclap. Maximal severity is usually at onset, but may take up to five minutes to develop. Consciousness is often reduced, and meningism may be present. CT imaging of the head demonstrates subarachnoid blood in about 95% of cases within 48 hours. The diagnosis can be secured in CT-negative cases by performing a lumbar puncture (delayed by at least 12 hours after onset) which demonstrates xanthochromia (a measure of the breakdown products of blood) for up to two weeks.

Where the patient is well and presents more than two weeks after the onset of the headache, they should be investigated with a CT angiogram. This does not show if subarachnoid haemorrhage has occurred but demonstrates if there is a lesion that might predispose to further haemorrhage.

Complications of subarachnoid haemorrhage are summarized in Box 7.10. Cerebral vasospasm is a significant problem, resulting in ischaemic damage, and further neurological deficit.

Box 7.10 Complications of subarachnoid haemorrhage

Vascular
Re-bleeding
Vasospasm

Metabolic
Hyponatraemia (syndrome of inappropriate ADH release or cerebral salt-wasting)
Hyperglycaemia

Neurological
Seizures
Hydrocephalus

Immobility
Pressure ulceration
Venous thromboembolism
Infections

Medical
Pulmonary oedema
Cardiac arrhythmias

Initial management involves urgent referral to neurosurgery for consideration of options for securing an aneurysm. Historically this was achieved with surgically placed clips, though increasingly endovascular aneurysm coiling is employed. Prior to neurosurgical intervention, management is supportive and aimed at preventing complications. The risk of vasospasm is reduced by the use of regular nimodipine 60 mg every four hours (the dose may need to be reduced in hypotensive patients).

Further Reading

Raya A, Diringer M (2014). Treatment of subarachnoid hemorrhage. *Critical Care Clinics* 30(4): 719–733.

Schwedt T, Matharu M, Dodick D (2006). Thunderclap headache. *Lancet Neurology* 5(7): 621–631.

van Gijn J, Kerr R, Rinkel G (2007). Subarachnoid haemorrhage. *Lancet* 369(9558): 306–318.

151. E) Vestibular schwannoma

This patient presents with progressive hearing loss. Examination is suggestive of sensorineural hearing loss, associated with a right-sided trigeminal nerve palsy (facial sensory deficit and absent corneal reflex) and right-sided cerebellar signs. This constellation would be in keeping with a cerebello-pontine angle lesion, of which the most common would be vestibular schwannoma.

Tutorial

There are several structures in close anatomical proximity at the cerebellopontine angle, which may be damaged by compressive lesions. Cerebellopontine angle lesions may result in lesions of the trigeminal, facial, and vestibulocochlear cranial nerves, and cerebellar dysfunction. Equally, these structures may be damaged during surgical treatment of the offending cause. Patients may develop sensorineural hearing loss or tinnitus, disequilibrium, speech disturbance, and facial weakness, for example.

Most commonly, cerebellopontine angle lesions are vestibular schwannomas (also referred to as acoustic neuromas), which may occur bilaterally in the inherited neurocutaneous condition neurofibromatosis type II. Other causes include basal meningioma, metastases, cholesteatoma, or intracranial aneurysms.

Rinne's and Weber's tests provide a bedside measure of whether hearing loss is conductive or sensorineural. This should be performed with a 512 Hz tuning fork and the expected findings are summarized in the table below. In Weber's test the tuning fork is held centrally in the forehead, and the patient asked which side the sound lateralizes to. In Rinne's test, air conduction is compared to bone conduction, with the former being louder in normal circumstances (Table 7.11). These tests are not 100% reliable and any patient with progressive unilateral hearing loss or hearing loss with other neurological symptoms, should have an MRI of the internal auditory meatus.

Table 7.11 Interpretation of Rinne and Weber's tests

	Normal	Sensorineural hearing loss	Conductive hearing loss
Rinne's test	Air conduction louder than bone conduction	Air conduction louder than bone conduction	Bone conduction louder than air conduction
Weber's test	No lateralization	Lateralizes to contralateral side	Lateralizes to ipsilateral side

Further Reading

Davies R (2004). The essentials of bedside neuro-otological examination and interpretation of commonly used investigations. Neurology in practice review. *Journal of Neurology, Neurosurgery and Psychiatry* 75(4): 32–44.

Keane J (2005). Multiple cranial nerve palsies: analysis of 979 cases. *Archives of Neurology* 62(11): 1714–1717.

Starr A, Picton T, Sininger Y, et al. (1994). Auditory neuropathy. *Brain* 119: 741–753.

152. D) Chloramphenicol

This patient presented with a short history of headache and fever, associated with objective evidence of meningism. This presentation is typical of acute bacterial meningitis, with the most likely causative organism being *Neisseria meningococcus*. Prompt antibiotic treatment is important, and the agent used must have good central nervous system penetration. Ceftriaxone is a broad-spectrum antibiotic that is generally used as a first-line agent for bacterial meningitis. There is a cross-reactivity between penicillins and cephalosporins, and it is reported that 10% of patients with a penicillin allergy are allergic to cephalosporins. Though this figure is lower for third-generation cephalosporins such as ceftriaxone, her previous documented anaphylactic reaction to penicillin would be a relative contraindication to using cephalosporins. The second-line agent for meningococcal meningitis is intravenous chloramphenicol, and would be the most appropriate option in this case. Meropenem has good central nervous system penetration, but carbapenems are also associated with cross-reactivity in true penicillin allergy. Benzylpenicillin is clearly contraindicated. Acyclovir may be given empirically to cover for herpes simplex encephalitis, but her presentation is much more suggestive of bacterial meningitis.

Tutorial

Meningitis may be caused by bacterial, viral, or fungal infection, malignancy, inflammatory conditions such as Behçet's disease or SLE, or medical intervention (e.g. intravenous immunoglobulin). The most common infectious causes of meningitis are listed in Box 7.11. Other organisms including *Staphylococcus aureus*, *Staphylococcus epidermidis*, and Gram-negative bacteria may cause meningitis in association with CSF shunts, skull fracture, or penetrating trauma.

Box 7.11 Infectious causes of meningitis

Bacterial

Neonates:

- *Escherichia coli*
- Group B streptococcus
- *Listeria monocytogenes*

Children:

- *Neisseria meningitidis*
- *Haemophilus influenzae*
- *Streptococcus pneumoniae*

Adults:

- *Neisseria meningitidis*
- *Streptococcus pneumoniae*
- *Listeria monocytogenes* (>50 years old or immunocompromised)

Viral

Enteroviruses

Herpes simplex virus (more commonly type II)

Mumps

Varicella zoster virus

Human immunodeficiency virus

Lymphocytic choriomeningitis virus

Mycobacterial

Mycobacterium tuberculosis

Fungal

Cryptococcus neoformans

The most useful investigation for determining the cause of meningitis is CSF analysis. The typical CSF findings in meningitis are indicated in Table 7.12.

Table 7.12 Cerebrospinal fluid findings in meningitis

	Acute bacterial	Viral	Cryptococcal	Tuberculous
Appearance	Cloudy/turbid	Clear	Clear	Clear
Cells	Polymorphs	Lymphocytes	Lymphocytes	Lymphocytes
Protein	↑	↑ or normal	↑	↑↑
Glucose	↓	Normal (↓ in mumps)	↓↓	↓↓
Opening pressure	↑	Normal	↑ (poor prognosis) or normal	↑
Stains	Gram stain	Nil	Silver stain	Ziehl-Nielsen stain Auramine stain
Other	CSF and blood culture	PCR*	Cryptococcal antigen testing	Prolonged culture

PCR = polymerase chain reaction

The clinical features of meningitis include fever, headache, neck stiffness, photophobia, nausea, and vomiting. Seizures may occur, and there may be evidence of systemic sepsis and disseminated intravascular coagulation, particularly in meningococcal meningitis. Long-term sequalae such as sensorineural deafness or hydrocephalus are more common in pneumococcal meningitis. Acute bacterial meningitis usually develops over hours to days, whereas cryptococcal and tuberculous meningitis may develop more insidiously over weeks.

Bacterial meningitis must be treated initially with a broad-spectrum antibiotic with good central nervous system penetrance. A third-generation cephalosporin such as ceftriaxone is generally used empirically as a first-line agent, with ampicillin added in if *Listeria monocytogenes* is a possibility. In cases of true penicillin allergy, when the risk of cross-reactivity with cephalosporins is considered too high, intravenous chloramphenicol may be used. Once the causative organism has been identified, antibiotic treatment may be refined. Dexamethasone is also recommended in cases of suspected bacterial meningitis and should be commenced before or with the first dose of antibiotics. In meningococcal meningitis, household contacts should be treated with rifampicin or ciprofloxacin to eradicate nasopharyngeal carriage.

Further Reading

McGill F, Heyderman R, Michael B, et al. (2016). The UK joint specialist societies guideline on the diagnosis and management of acute meningitis and meningococcal sepsis in immunocompetent adults. *Journal of Infection* 72: 405–438.

Van de Beek D, de Gans J, Tunkel A, Wijdicks E (2006). Community-acquired bacterial meningitis in adults. *New England Journal of Medicine* 354(1): 44–53.

Weisfelt M, de Gans J, van der Poll T, van de Beek D (2006). Pneumococcal meningitis in adults: new approaches to management and prevention. *Lancet Neurology* 5(4): 332–342.

153. E) Vitreous haemorrhage

The patient's symptoms of a mass of dark spots and blobs are due to vitreous opacities/floaters. In a young insulin dependent diabetic patient who smokes, and with a sudden onset of these symptoms, the most likely cause of the spots/blobs is a vitreous haemorrhage secondary to proliferative diabetic retinopathy.

A posterior vitreous detachment (PVD) causes photopsia (flashing lights) and some floaters and usually occurs in patients >60 years where the vitreous humour starts to shrink and pulls away from its retinal attachment. It can also occur in high myopes at a younger age. A PVD usually has no sequelae but if the vitreous pulls away from a thin/weak area of retina then this could result in a retinal tear and subsequently a retinal detachment. Occasionally as the vitreous detaches it pulls on a small retinal vein to cause a vitreous haemorrhage. With a retinal detachment the patient sees what appears to be a curtain coming across the vision and is usually preceded by symptoms of photopsia and floaters. If the retina is detached in the macular region then the vision will be very poor. A central retinal vein occlusion (CRVO) will also result in painless, sudden loss of vision but normally worse than 6/36. It can be associated with diabetes, hypertension, glaucoma, and smoking. Although there are retinal haemorrhages a CRVO does not cause a vitreous haemorrhage or floaters. A cataract causes gradual, painless loss of vision and a reduced red reflex but not floaters. It would commonly occur in people >65 years but can occur at a younger age if diabetic.

This patient requires urgent referral to an ophthalmologist for further assessment. If the vitreous haemorrhage fails to resolve spontaneously then a vitrectomy with endolaser photocoagulation is required. If spontaneous resolution occurs then panretinal laser photocoagulation is undertaken. It is vital that the patient understands the importance of strict glycaemic control.

Tutorial

Diabetic retinopathy is an increasingly common condition due to the rising prevalence of diabetes in the UK, as well as global, population. The NHS has a screening programme for all patients affected and whilst exact pathways may differ by region, it is worth familiarizing oneself with the stages and grading of diabetic eye disease and the management at the various stages. These are summarized in Tables 7.13 and 7.14.

Table 7.13 Definitions in diabetic eye disease

Retinopathy	
Background (low risk)	Microaneurysms, small haemorrhages, hard exudates, occasional CWS
Pre-proliferative (high risk)	IRMAs, venous beading/loops, clusters of large blot haemorrhages, multiple CWS
Proliferative	
NVD	New vessels at the disc or within 1DD of the disc ('high risk': NVD >1/3 disc area or any NVD with vitreous or preretinal haemorrhage)
NVE	New vessels elsewhere in the retina ('high risk': NVE >1/2 disc area with vitreous or preretinal haemorrhage)
Maculopathy	
Focal	Well-circumscribed areas of leakage, with oedema and full/part rings of exudates often surrounding a microaneurysm
Diffuse	Generalized leakage with oedema
Ischaemic	↓VA with relatively normal clinical appearance, but macular ischaemia on FFA
Mixed	Combination, e.g. of diffuse and ischaemic
Clinically significant macular oedema (CSMO)	• Retinal thickening at or within 500 microns of the centre of the macula • Hard exudates at or within 500 microns of the centre of the macula if associated with adjacent retinal thickening • Retinal thickening of >1 disc area, any part of which is within 1DD of the centre of the macula
Centre-involving DMO	Thickening involving the foveal centre. If >400 microns, anti-VEGF should be considered

Reproduced with permission from *Oxford Handbook of Ophthalmology*, Fourth Edition, Denniston A and Murray P, Table 13.5, Oxford University Press, Oxford, UK, Copyright © 2018.

Table 7.14 An approach to diabetic eye disease

Retinopathy	
None/background	Discharge to community screening service for annual review; if significant systemic disease, consider review at 9–12 months by hospital eye service.
Pre-proliferative	Observe 4–6-monthly (consider early PRP in select cases, e.g. in only eye where first eye lost to proliferative diabetic retinopathy or prior to cataract surgery).
Proliferative (active)	PRP (1–2 sessions × ≥1,000 × 200–500 microns × 0.1s; shorter durations, e.g. 20–30 ms with newer pattern lasers)—wherever possible, this should occur on the same day or within two weeks; evolving role for anti-VEGF therapies. In young patients with type I diabetes, PRP should be delivered over 3–4 sessions, as ↑ risk of macular oedema post-PRP if excess burns applied in single session.

Table 7.14 Continued

Proliferative (regressed)	Observe 4–6-monthly (signs of ↓ neovascularization activity include: regression of vessels ± fibrosis, resolution of retinal haemorrhages, decreases in retinal vessel dilatation and tortuosity).
Proliferative with coexisting diabetic macular oedema (DMO)	For 'high-risk' cases, consider combined macular laser and PRP (with completion of PRP over three sessions, rather than 1–2). For 'low-risk' cases, it may be possible to perform macular laser initially, with PRP at subsequent follow-up. Anti-VEGF therapies may be of particular use in this context, although practice guidelines are still evolving.
Maculopathy	
Focal leakage	Focal laser photocoagulation ($n \times$ 50–100 microns $\times$ 0.08–0.1 s; shorter durations, e.g. 10–20 ms with newer lasers); review at 3–4 months.
Diffuse leakage	Grid laser photocoagulation; review at 3–4 months; anti-VEGF now more commonly used for diffuse centre-involving leakage.
Centre-involving oedema	Anti-VEGF (ranibizumab and aflibercept) are approved if thickness >400 microns. Ranibizumab is given monthly until VA stable (on three consecutive visits). Aflibercept is given monthly for 5 months and then every 2 months, with intervals extended if appropriate after the first year. Dexamethasone implant (Ozurdex®) may be appropriate in pseudophakic eyes if unsuitable for, or failed, anti-VEGF. Can be repeated at 4 months (risk of intraocular pressure rise).
Ischaemic	Fundus fluorescence angiography (FFA) or optical coherence tomography angiography (OCTA) to confirm diagnosis; observation may be appropriate if significant ischaemia and/or no response to previous laser or anti-VEGF.
Persistent maculopathy	Consider intravitreal fluocinolone (Iluvien®) in pseudophakic eyes; consider vitrectomy if vitreomacular traction.
Rubeosis (neovascularisation of the iris)	
Rubeosis + clear media	Urgent PRP ± anti-VEGF therapies.
Rubeosis + vitreous haemorrhage	Vitrectomy + endolaser.
Rubeotic glaucoma	Urgent PRP/anti-VEGF therapies ↓IOP with topical medication/cyclodiode/augmented trabeculectomy/tubes.
Vitreous haemorrhage	
No view of fundus	US to ensure retina flat + review 2–4-weekly until adequate view.
Adequate view	Ensure retina flat + PRP.
Persistent	Vitrectomy + endolaser + anti-VEGF therapies.

PRP = Panretinal photocoagulation

Reproduced with permission from *Oxford Handbook of Ophthalmology*, Fourth Edition, Denniston A and Murray P, Table. 13.6, Oxford University Press, Oxford, UK, Copyright © 2018.

Further Reading

Denniston A, Murray P (2018). Ch. 13 Medical Retina. In: *Oxford Handbook of Ophthalmology*. Edited by Denniston A, Murray P. Fourth Edition. Oxford University Press, Oxford.

154. A) Age-related macular degeneration

This patient has a gradual onset of painless loss of vision affecting her central vision with peripheral sparing. Given her age, symptoms (difficulty seeing faces is a classic complaint as it requires high visuo-spatial resolution which is found only in the macula), and examination findings, age-related macular oedema is the most likely diagnosis here.

Although cataract causes gradual, painless loss of vision most people complain of cloudy/misty vision, colours being faded but not a loss of central vision. Keratoconjunctivitis sicca is associated with rheumatoid arthritis but it causes painful, red eyes and requires frequent artificial tear substitutes. Central retinal artery occlusion is an ophthalmic emergency resulting in devastating sudden loss of vision (total blindness—no perception of light) usually only in one eye. It can be a manifestation of giant cell arteritis, but more common causes include atherosclerosis and emboli from the carotid bifurcation. As the central retinal artery is an end artery, then if it is occluded there is no vascular supply to the retina so it infarcts. Primary open angle glaucoma also causes gradual vision loss, occurs in the older age group but would not affect central vision until very advanced in both eyes and by then would have resulted in a large degree of peripheral visual field loss.

Tutorial

Age-related macular degeneration (AMD) is the leading cause of blindness in people aged 60+ years in the western world. It is a multifactorial disease and risk factors include smoking and several loci in the complement factor H (CFH) gene. The commonest type is the dry form where there is a gradual loss of central vision in one or both eyes. It begins as white/cream coloured deposits called drusen in the base of the retina in the macular region that coalesce to form larger, 'soft' drusen, eventually resulting in atrophy of the surrounding retina. It does not cause a problem with the peripheral field of vision. There is no medical treatment and magnifiers are usually given and with this level of vision she would be eligible to be registered as sight impaired (previously known as partially sighted). The more devastating type is the wet type of AMD. Drusen are still the first signs but in this type a choroidal (the choroid is the layer between the retina and sclera) neovascular membrane forms with new blood vessels pushing up into the retina. These vessels bleed causing sudden, central vision loss, then with time form a 'disciform' scar. The first symptoms may be distortion of vision, with straight lines appearing bent.

Patients undergo fundus fluorescein angiography and optical coherence tomography (OCT) to visualize the choroidal neovascular membrane. The treatment to stabilize and/or improve vision is with a course of intravitreal anti-VEGF injections (ranibizumab, bevacizumab, and more recently aflibercept). OCT is used to monitor the effect of treatment. The AREDS and AREDS2 studies showed that certain vitamins and antioxidants delayed progression from intermediate to advanced AMD.

Further Reading

Denniston A, Murray P (2018). Ch. 13 Medical Retina. In: *Oxford Handbook of Ophthalmology*. Edited by Denniston A, Murray P. Fourth Edition. Oxford University Press, Oxford.

155. B) Anterior ischaemic optic neuropathy

This patient has many of the classic symptoms of giant cell (temporal) arteritis (GCA) with jaw claudication, scalp tenderness, and temporal headache. Her pain when lifting objects is likely to be due to polymyalgia rheumatica that is known to be associated with GCA. The commonest ocular complication of GCA is an anterior ischaemic optic neuropathy (AION).

Amaurosis fugax ('fleeting blindness') is a transient ischaemic attack (TIA) affecting only one eye. There is transient obstruction of the central retinal artery so the vision after a few seconds becomes black then it rapidly returns to normal. Usually this is due to an embolus passing through the artery (or rarely due to GCA). The embolus is likely to come from the carotid bifurcation, but possibly from the heart if the patient is in atrial fibrillation.

Glaucomatous optic neuropathy is characterized by an increase in the vertical cup:disc ratio of the optic disc, that is, the size of the pale central cup that contains no nerve fibres that allows the central retinal artery and central retinal vein to pass in and out of the eye, respectively, compared to the orange, pink neuroretinal rim. A normal optic disc has a vertical cup:disc ratio of about 0.4 or less but in a glaucomatously damaged optic disc the ratio is 0.5 or more. As the nerve fibres continue to be destroyed by the high pressure the cup appears to enlarge further and unless the intraocular pressure can be controlled, eventually all nerve fibres will be lost (i.e. a cup: disc ratio of 1.0) resulting in total blindness.

Optic neuritis usually occurs in a younger patient with vision loss, but not as profound as in AION. There is pain on moving the eye, an afferent pupillary defect, reduced red-green colour vision, and red desaturation. The optic disc may look normal as the part of the nerve that is inflamed is behind the eyeball, that is, retrobulbar neuritis. There is a strong association with multiple sclerosis. Scleritis is probably the most painful of all ocular conditions and is associated with an intensely red eye. It can give an associated headache around the eye. It is not associated with sudden loss of vision. About 40% of patients have an underlying systemic disease, such as rheumatoid arthritis, and granulomatosis with polyangiitis. Systemic therapy is the mainstay, initially corticosteroid, but systemic immunosuppression may be necessary.

Tutorial

Anterior ischaemic optic neuropathy can result in a devastating loss of vision to 'perception of light' or 'no perception of light'. As the optic nerve is involved there is a relative afferent pupillary defect and characteristically the optic disc is pale and swollen, then later there is optic atrophy.
The diagnosis of GCA is clinical and one should have a high suspicion of the condition. The condition affects over 50-year-olds, women more than men, and classically presents as a unilateral headache with tenderness over the scalp and temples. Other symptoms of GCA can include jaw claudication, sore throat and dysphagia, and problems with dizziness. However, it is important to note, that some patients may present with symptoms relating to their AION (e.g. diplopia or visual disturbance) and not have any of the classical symptoms of GCA.

There is normally a raised ESR and C-reactive protein. AION may be arteritic or non-arteritic. Missing a diagnosis of GCA and not starting urgent treatment means there is a 95% risk of AION happening in the second eye, thus leading to complete blindness in each eye. Patients are admitted and given three pulses of intravenous methylprednisolone 1 g and ideally a temporal artery biopsy should be undertaken within the next 48 hours. Oral prednisolone is then prescribed and titrated according to symptoms and inflammatory markers. Other complications of GCA include a TIA, stroke, myocardial infarction, cranial nerve palsies, mesenteric artery occlusion, thoracic artery aneurysms, and death.

Further Reading

Denniston A, Murray P (2018). Ch. 16 Neuro-ophthalmology. In: *Oxford Handbook of Ophthalmology*. Edited by Denniston A, Murray P. Fourth Edition. Oxford University Press, Oxford.

156. B) Corticosteroid eye drops, for example prednisolone acetate 1%

The symptoms are consistent with an anterior uveitis (iritis) and the small, irregular pupil—the latter due to adhesions between the iris and anterior lens capsule known as posterior synechiae—would also fit. The symptoms could be similar to a corneal ulcer, for example a herpes simplex dendritic ulcer, but examination did not reveal any fluorescein staining of the cornea.

Treatment for anterior uveitis is with corticosteroid eye drops as there would be good penetration into the anterior chamber. The frequency of drops would be determined by the amount of inflammation (the number of white blood cells) in the anterior chamber and anterior uveitis can only be correctly diagnosed using a slit-lamp microscope. One of the major complications of corticosteroid eye drops is causing a rise in intraocular pressure that could lead to glaucoma and irreversible optic nerve damage. Mydriatic (pupil dilating) drops are also prescribed to try and break any posterior synechiae to make the pupil round again and prevent discomfort from spasm of the ciliary muscle.

Oral corticosteroids would normally be reserved for when there is posterior uveitis as eye drops do not readily penetrate into the back of the eye. There is nothing to indicate that this is due to a herpes viral or bacterial infection (there is no purulent discharge), and so use of antibiotics or antivirals is not indicated.

Tutorial

Anterior uveitis accounts for around 75–90% of all cases of uveitis. It represents a wide spectrum of disease—it may be isolated, part of a panuveitis/intermediate uveitis, or part of a systemic disease. It is essential that all patients with anterior uveitis have pupils dilated and fundi examined to exclude any posterior segment inflammation. The classic symptoms are of pain, photophobia, redness, and/or blurred vision. On slit-lamp examination there is circumlimbal injection—the corneal limbus is the border of the cornea and sclera, along with the presence of cells, flare (protein release through inflamed vasculature of the eye) with keratic precipitates in the anterior chamber. In around 50% of cases, patients with anterior uveitis are HLA B27 positive (cf 8% of general population is HLA B27 positive in the UK), many of whom will have a pre-existing diagnosis of a seronegative arthropathy.

Anterior uveitis is also associated with various systemic conditions, which the patient's history, symptoms, and examination findings may provide clues, or there may be an infective cause. These are listed in Box 7.12.

Box 7.12 Conditions associated with anterior uveitis

- Seronegative spondyloarthropathies (HLA-B27 associated):
  - Ankylosing spondylitis
  - Psoriatic arthritis
  - Inflammatory bowel disease
  - Reactive arthritis
- Sarcoidosis
- Juvenile idiopathic arthritis (JIA)
- Behçet's syndrome
- Tubulointerstitial nephritis and uveitis (TINU)
- Diabetes (poorly controlled)
- Herpes viruses e.g. herpes simplex, varicella zoster
- Vasculitis

Further Reading

Denniston A, Murray P (2018). Ch. 11 Uveitis. In: Oxford *Handbook of Ophthalmology*. Edited by Denniston A, Murray P. Fourth Edition. Oxford University Press, Oxford.

157. A 34-year-old woman was referred with a four-week history of swelling, discomfort, and erythema of her left breast. She denied pruritis. She had been treated with oral flucloxacillin, followed by clarithromycin, with no improvement.

She had two children, aged four years and nine months, whom she had breastfed for six months. She had had several episodes of mastitis, but no other medical or family history of note. She took no regular medications. On examination, the left breast had diffuse erythema covering the lower two thirds with associated increased warmth. The skin appeared oedematous. There were no masses within the breast but she had several enlarged nodes in the left axilla; the rest of the examination was normal.

Which of the following investigations will be most helpful in determining her management?

A. Biopsy of affected area of the breast

B. CT scan of the thorax/abdomen/pelvis

C. Mammogram

D. MRI scan of breast

E. Skin swab and blood cultures with antibiotic sensitivity testing

158. **A 69-year-old woman presented with a two-week history of increasing shortness of breath on exertion. She denied chest pain but had noted a dry cough, especially in the evening. She first noticed the dyspnoea a week after returning from holiday in the USA. She was a non-smoker. She had a history of breast cancer treated four years previously, with a wide local excision, adjuvant radiation, and six cycles of anthracycline-based chemotherapy. She did not receive Herceptin but was currently taking tamoxifen. A CT scan performed two months previously of the thorax/abdomen/pelvis showed no evidence of recurrence.**

     On examination, she had a well-healed left wide local excision scar with no masses in the breasts. Lymph node examination was normal and she had dual heart sounds, with a heart rate of 105/minute and no murmurs. Auscultation of the lungs revealed only fine crepitations bibasally.

     Which of the following is the most likely diagnosis for her shortness of breath?

     A. Intraparenchymal lung metastases
     B. Left ventricular failure
     C. Lymphangitis carcinomatosis
     D. Malignant pleural effusion
     E. Pulmonary embolism

159. **A 63-year-old man was found to have an adenocarcinoma on colonoscopy following investigation for microcytic anaemia. He was seen in the oncology clinic to discuss the diagnosis and treatment options. He reported multiple members of his family had had colorectal cancer (CRC).**

     Which of the following features would be most consistent with underlying hereditary non-polyposis colorectal cancer (HNPCC)?

     A. A father diagnosed with colon cancer age 72
     B. An aunt with a germline MLH1 mutation
     C. K-ras mutation in tumour tissue
     D. The presence of microsatellite instability in his tumour tissue
     E. The presence of three synchronous polyps noted during his colonoscopy

160. **A 39-year-old woman presented with a six-week history of nausea, fatigue, loss of appetite, and abdominal pain. She had had a renal transplant 12 years previously for which she took ciclosporin and prednisone. Her only other medication was Depo-Provera (depot injection progesterone) for contraception and she reported irregular vaginal bleeding, a known side effect, since starting this 18 months previously. She was a non-smoker, and drank wine occasionally. There was no family history of note.**

On examination, she had hepatomegaly. An ultrasound scan confirmed multiple liver lesions consistent with metastatic disease.

The most likely primary tumour for this woman is:

A. Breast
B. Cervix
C. Lung
D. Ovary
E. Pancreas

161. **A 59-year-old woman presented acutely with shortness of breath nine days after her first cycle of primary chemotherapy for stage IIIC ovarian cancer. She had been treated with carboplatin and paclitaxel, and received ondansetron, dexamethasone, and metoclopramide anti-emetic cover.**

On examination, she was tachypnoeic, with oxygen saturations of 92% on room air and a sinus tachycardia of 105/min. There was moderate abdominal distension with positive succession splash, and a palpable omental cake. Auscultation of the lungs revealed decreased lung volumes, with no other abnormalities.

```
Investigations:
  Hb                      101 g/L
  WCC                     2.9 × 10⁹/L
  Neutrophils             1.5 × 10⁹/L
  Platelets               103 × 10⁹/L
```

What is the most likely cause of her shortness of breath?

A. Chemotherapy-induced left ventricular failure
B. Chemotherapy-induced pneumonitis
C. Neutropaenic sepsis
D. Occlusion of a bronchus from a pulmonary metastasis
E. Pulmonary embolus

162. **A 58-year-old woman was reviewed six months after completing six cycles of carboplatin/paclitaxel chemotherapy for stage IV non-small cell lung cancer, to which she had shown good treatment response. However, she complained of increasing cough, lassitude, and loss of appetite. A re-staging CT scan of the thorax/abdomen/pelvis demonstrated progression in the lung primary, and new liver metastases. She was keen to consider targeted treatments or second-line chemotherapy, and erlotinib (Tarceva) or doxetaxel (Taxotere) were being considered.**

    With regards to having second-line chemotherapy, which of the following statements is true for this woman?

    A. As her cancer has progressed within six months of first-line chemotherapy, her cancer is likely to be resistant to docetaxel
    B. Development of a maculopapular rash one week after initiating treatment with docetaxel is indicative of response
    C. Non-smokers with adenocarcinoma may do better with EGFR inhibitors such as erlotinib
    D. Second-line chemotherapy will extend her overall survival by 6–12 months
    E. The site of metastases will decrease her chance of responding to any treatment

163. **A 73-year-old retired builder with no past medical history presented with fatigue and weight loss. He had lost approximately 7 kg in the preceding three months. He smoked 20 cigarettes per day. On examination, his blood pressure was 171/92 mmHg.**

    ```
    Investigations:
        Hb                          164 g/L
        WCC                         11.9 × 10⁹/L
        Neutrophils                 7.3 × 10⁹/L
        Platelets                   433 × 10⁹/L
        Sodium                      135 mmol/L
        Creatinine                  111 μmol/L
        Urea                        7.9 mmol/L
        Potassium                   4.6
        ALT                         24 iU/L
        ALP                         196 iU/L
        GGT                         41 iU/L
        Albumin                     32 g/L
        Corrected calcium           2.7 mmol/L
    ```

    Which of the following investigations is most likely to be helpful?

    A. Bone scan
    B. CT thorax/abdomen/pelvis
    C. Myeloma screen
    D. Parathyroid hormone
    E. PSA (prostate specific antigen)

164. A 27-year-old man was admitted with significant nausea and vomiting, which had started five days after his first cycle of chemotherapy for stage IVB diffuse large B cell lymphoma (DLBCL). He had received CHOP chemotherapy (cyclophosphamide, doxorubicin, vincristine, prednisone) with prophylactic ondansetron, metoclopramide, and allopurinol.

Examination showed multiple enlarged lymph node masses involving the cervical, axillary, and inguinal chains, although his partner thought these were smaller than they were prior to the chemotherapy.

```
Investigations:
   Creatinine              364 µmol/L
   Urea                    12.0 mmol/L
   Sodium                  133 mmol/L
   Potassium               6.4 mmol/L
   Uric acid               1421 µmol/L
   Corrected calcium       1.4 mmol/L
   Phosphate               2.6 mmol/L
   Albumin                 38 g/L
```

Which is the first step in managing this?

A. Aggressive intravenous rehydration

B. Haemodialysis

C. Increase allopurinol

D. Insulin/dextrose infusion

E. Rasburicase

165. A 20-year-old male engineering student was referred to the respiratory physicians with shortness of breath and an abnormal chest X-ray. A CT scan of the thorax showed a large anterior mediastinal mass 12 × 10 cm in diameter which encased the major blood vessels. Tumour markers showed an LDH of 1857 iU/ml, β-hCG of 18,393 iU/ml and an α-fetoprotein of 14,694 iU/ml. Fine needle aspiration showed poorly differentiated carcinoma. An ultrasound of the testicles was unremarkable, and CT staging demonstrated no other disease.

He commenced chemotherapy but was concerned about the future, and wished to know his chances of being alive to complete his degree.

Which of the following best represents his chance of being alive in five years?

A. 30%

B. 50%

C. 75%

D. 85%

E. 95%

166. **A 62-year-old lifelong smoker presented with worsening cough and an episode of haemoptysis. Imaging showed a right upper lobe lesion and biopsy confirmed adenocarcinoma. A staging PET scan showed no evidence of metastatic disease or nodal involvement, and he was referred for surgical assessment. He had a normal performance status, and an FEV1 of 89% predicted. He underwent a right upper and middle lobectomy. Histology confirmed a completely excised poorly differentiated adenocarcinoma, positive for TTF-1. Two lymph nodes out of fifteen were involved.**

    He struggled to recover post-operatively with significant post-operative neuropathic pain, but his only co-morbidity was hypertension.

    Which of the following will increase his five-year survival?

    A. Adjuvant chemotherapy
    B. Adjuvant concurrent chemotherapy and radiation
    C. Adjuvant EGFR targeted agent
    D. Adjuvant radiotherapy
    E. There is no indication for adjuvant treatment

167. **A 76-year-old retired man presented with confusion and erratic behaviour. He complained of a one-week history of nausea and vomiting. He was a normally independent widower. He had type II diabetes mellitus, and took metformin and gliclazide. He was an ex-smoker with a 70-pack year history and drank several nips of whisky every night.**

On examination, he was appropriately dressed, with a mini-mental examination score of 8/10. Examination of the cardiorespiratory and abdomen was unremarkable, but he had a craggy 2 cm node in the left supraclavicular fossa.

```
Investigations:
  Hb                         101 g/L
  WCC                        14.0 × 10⁹/L
  Neutrophils                9.8 × 10⁹/L
  Platelets                  523 × 10⁹/L
  Sodium                     121 mmol/L
  Potassium                  3.6 mmol/L
  Urea                       5.8 mmol/L
  Creatinine                 91 µmol/L
  Corrected calcium          2.3 mmol/L
  Glucose                    7.1 mmol/L
  Chest X-ray:               enlarged hilum
  CT chest:                  right-sided hilar mass, left
                             supraclavicular mass, and a
                             5 cm liver metastasis
```

His hyponatraemia is most likely to respond to:

A. Chemotherapy

B. Radiation to lung primary

C. Surgery to resect liver and lung disease

D. Surgery to resect liver metastasis

E. Surgery to resect lung lesion only

168. **A 36-year-old woman presented with a self-detected lump in her left breast. A mammogram showed a sinister-appearing lump and biopsy confirmed a high-grade ductal carcinoma. A staging CT scan showed no evidence of distant metastases. Her past medical history included stage IIB nodular sclerosing Hodgkin's lymphoma 20 years previously, for which she received six cycles of ChlVIPP chemotherapy (chlorambucil, vincristine, prednisone) and mantle irradiation. She had been discharged from follow-up ten years previously and was on no regular medications.**

Regarding how her previous treatments could affect her treatment options for her new breast cancer, which of the following statements is true?

A. Her previous cancer has no impact on the choice of surgery and potential adjuvant treatment (chemotherapy or radiation)

B. Her previous chemotherapy will affect her ability to have adjuvant radiation treatment to the chest wall

C. Her previous chemotherapy will affect her response to hormone treatment if she is found to be oestrogen receptor (ER) positive

D. Her previous radiation will affect her ability to have adjuvant radiation treatment to the chest wall

E. She should not undergo surgery, but should undergo combination chemotherapy and radiation instead

169. A 44-year-old woman presented to with weight loss, abdominal pain, excessive thirst and polyuria. She had been previously fit and well, with no past medical history. On examination, she looked unwell and had an acetone scent to her breath. A finger-prick blood sugar level was 32 and she had ketones in her urine. She was treated for diabetic ketoacidosis as per local guidelines. Despite haemodynamic and biochemical stabilization over the next few days, she reported ongoing abdominal pains. A CT scan of the abdomen demonstrated a mass in the head of the pancreas. Further imaging revealed no evidence of metastatic disease, and she underwent a Whipple's resection (pancreaticoduodenectomy). Pathology confirmed a poorly differentiated ductal carcinoma of the pancreas, with three lymph nodes involved. The resection margins were clear. On further questioning, she reported that her mother had ovarian cancer at age 53, and her maternal grandfather had pancreatic cancer in his 70s.

Which of the following statements is false?

A. Diabetes or impaired glucose tolerance is present in at least 50% of patients
B. Testing for the BRCA2 mutation should be considered
C. The median survival for those with completely resected pancreatic tumours is 36–48 months
D. The use of adjuvant chemotherapy adds 3–5 months to overall survival in pancreatic cancer
E. Up to 10% of pancreatic cancer has an underlying inherited gene mutation

170. A 72-year-old man presented for his routine follow-up. Two years previously he had had a radical prostatectomy for a Gleason 3 + 4 adenocarcinoma of the prostate. His post-operative PSA was <0.1 ng/mL, and his last level three months previously was 0.3 ng/mL.

He reported feeling well but his PSA had risen to 32 ng/ml. A bone scan demonstrated several small bony metastases around 3 mm in size in the ribs and T10 vertebrae. He refused further surgery, but was willing to consider other treatment options.

He had a history of hypertension, mild asthma, and osteoarthritis. He had a right total hip replacement (THR) seven years previously, which was complicated by a post-operative DVT requiring six months of anticoagulation.

Which of the following would you recommend?

A. Commence hormone manipulation with a GnRH (gonadotrophin releasing hormone) agonist such as goserelin
B. Commence hormone manipulation with an oestrogen analogue (diethylstilbestrol)
C. Commence hormone manipulation with medroxyprogesterone (Megace)
D. Observation
E. Radiation to metastatic deposits

171. **A 12-year-old girl and her mother attended their GP to discuss concerns about her forthcoming human papillomavirus (HPV) vaccination with the bivalent vaccine (Cervarix). They were concerned after reading online reports questioning the safety and efficacy of the vaccine. She was in good health and denied being sexually active. The mother preferred to wait until her daughter was 18, when there would be more long-term data available and her daughter could choose for herself whether or not to be vaccinated.**

What would you advise them?

A. If she is vaccinated, she will also be protected against the common versions of the virus that cause anogenital warts

B. If she is vaccinated, she will require less frequent cervical smear screening

C. It makes no difference to the efficacy of the vaccine if she waits until age 18

D. The vaccine has not been tested in those over 18, and therefore she should be vaccinated now

E. The vaccine is most effective in those who have not been exposed to HPV and therefore she should be vaccinated now

172. **A 54-year-old woman with breast cancer presented with pain in the right clavicle. She was known to have a bony metastasis in this area, but had previously declined radiotherapy. She was taking regular paracetamol for the pain, with normal release oral morphine 5 mg on an as required (PRN) basis. However, she did not feel that the morphine had been particularly helpful, despite taking 4–5 doses per day, and moreover felt that it made her unacceptably nauseous. She was taking no other medications except tamoxifen, and was awaiting a restaging CT scan to assess her disease.**

```
Investigations:
   Sodium                136 mmol/L
   Potassium             3.9 mmol/L
   Urea                  3.4 mmol/L
   Creatinine            79 μmol/L
   Corrected calcium     2.3 mmol/L
   CXR:                  expansile mass in right mid-clavicle;
                         no evidence of pathological fracture
```

What would be the most reasonable first step to control her pain if she is to stop the morphine?

A. Continue paracetamol and add in diclofenac EC 50 mg TDS

B. Continue paracetamol and add in fentanyl transdermal patch 25 mcg/hr

C. Continue paracetamol and morphine but increase morphine to 7.5 mg PRN

D. Stop paracetamol and add in amitriptyline 25 mg ON

E. Stop paracetamol and add in morphine sulphate MR (Zomorph®) 30 mg bd

173. **A 75-year-old woman was admitted with nausea, abdominal pain, and vomiting. She had a long history of ovarian cancer, and had no further options for treatment. A CT scan showed multiple levels of obstruction secondary to disseminated peritoneal disease, including the first part of the duodenum, ileum, and transverse colon. The surgeons did not feel she would benefit from surgery given the multi-level obstruction.**

She was commenced on once daily subcutaneous dexamethasone and a syringe driver containing morphine and cyclizine. She was given intravenous fluids and a nasogastric tube was inserted. Her pain and nausea were under reasonable control, but she was troubled by distension and large volume aspirates from the nasogastric tube.

Which of the following may be helpful to improve her symptoms?

A. Chlorpromazine subcutaneous injection as required
B. Ketamine by continuous subcutaneous infusion
C. Levomepromazine (Nozinan) by continuous subcutaneous infusion
D. Metoclopramide by continuous subcutaneous infusion
E. Octreotide by continuous subcutaneous infusion

174. **A 79-year-old man with metastatic gastric cancer was admitted with large volume haematemesis. A gastroscopy confirmed ongoing oozing from his primary, not amenable to injection. His haemoglobin was 79 g/L for which he was transfused two units of red blood cells and kept nil by mouth whilst awaiting palliative irradiation.**

He had been on morphine sulphate MR capsules 70 mg twice daily, plus an average of two doses of 20 mg of normal release oral morphine per day. He reported his pain was well controlled. He also took regular metoclopramide 10 mg tds, lansoprazole 30 mg od and paracetamol 1g qds.

As he had ongoing vomiting, it was decided that a continuous subcutaneous infusion via syringe driver should be used to deliver his medication.

Which is the most appropriate combination for the syringe driver to run over 24 hours?

A. Morphine sulphate 70 mg plus metoclopramide 30 mg
B. Morphine sulphate 90 mg plus metoclopramide 30 mg
C. Morphine sulphate 90 mg plus metoclopramide 30 mg plus lansoprazole 30 mg
D. Morphine sulphate 140 mg plus metoclopramide 30 mg
E. Morphine sulphate 140 mg plus metoclopramide 30 mg plus lansoprazole 30 mg

175. A 41-year-old woman with metastatic cervical cancer was admitted with urosepsis. She had bilateral ureteric stents inserted six weeks previously for bilateral hydronephrosis secondary to peritoneal disease. She had extensive palliative care input to help manage her pain, and took Oxycontin (oxycodone MR) 50 mg bd, Oxynorm (oxycodone IR) as required, gabapentin and diclofenac.

On examination, she was drowsy and twitchy, with a GCS (Glasgow Coma Score) of 12. She was unable to follow instructions. Observations were: T36.6°C; HR 103/min; BP 110/90 mmHg; RR 10/min; and SpO$_2$ 93% in room air.

```
Investigations:
   Haemoglobin                91 g/L
   WCC                        14.3 × 10⁹/L
   Neutrophils                11.6 × 10⁹/L
   Creatinine                 302 µmol/L
   Urea                       8.3 mmol/L
   Sodium                     130 mmol/L
   Potassium                  5.4 mmol/L
   CRP                        303 mg/L
   Corrected calcium          2.2 mmol/L
   Glucose                    6.3 mmol/L
```

She was given small doses of naloxone which improved her GCS and respiratory rate, but she began to complain of severe pain. A CT scan confirmed unilateral hydronephrosis with perinephric fat stranding and she was started on intravenous antibiotics and made nil by mouth whilst awaiting surgical review.

What would be the most appropriate analgesic option to manage her pain?

A. Alfentanil subcutaneous infusion

B. Fentanyl transdermal patch

C. Intravenous pethidine as required

D. Ketamine intravenous infusion

E. Oxycodone subcutaneous infusion

176. **A 58-year-old man had locally recurrent rectal cancer with a large pelvic mass that caused significant pain. This was managed with a combination of paracetamol 1g qds, gabapentin 300 mg tds and morphine sulphate MR 60 mg bd. However, he complained of intolerable side effects on this regime, including drowsiness, resistant constipation, and nausea. Attempts to decrease his dose caused worsening pain, and he was keen to trial an alternative opioid. He was asked to consider a switch to Oxycontin (oxycodone MR). His blood tests showed normal renal and liver function.**

    Which of the following would be the appropriate dose?

    A. Oxycontin 20 mg bd and OxyNorm 5 mg PRN
    B. Oxycontin 30 mg bd and OxyNorm 10 mg PRN
    C. Oxycontin 60 mg bd and OxyNorm 20 mg PRN
    D. Oxycontin 90 mg bd and OxyNorm 30 mg PRN
    E. Oxycontin 120 mg bd and OxyNorm 40 mg PRN

157. A) Biopsy of affected area of the breast

This patient has a number of features suggestive of inflammatory breast cancer. The best way to confirm the diagnosis, and rule out drug resistant infection as a cause, is a biopsy of the breast.

A skin swab and blood cultures are unlikely to be helpful given there is no purulent discharge. A mammogram is unlikely to be particularly sensitive given her age and recent breastfeeding; in inflammatory breast cancer, both this and an MRI may show abnormalities, but will not confirm diagnosis or direct treatment as a biopsy would do in terms of drug choice. Equally, while a CT scan will reveal the presence or absence of metastatic disease, the biopsy is more important in giving information such as PR, ER, and HER2 receptor status which will be important in directing chemotherapy and treatment options.

Tutorial

Inflammatory breast cancer is the most aggressive form of breast cancer, and is often misdiagnosed as infection when patients first present. It should be considered in any patient who fails to respond to a week-long course of appropriate antibiotics, particularly if they have no other symptoms of systemic infection. It is more common in young women (age <40 years) than older women, and overall accounts for 3–5% of breast cancer.

The presentation of inflammatory breast cancer is generally that of a rapid onset of breast erythema, oedema or *peau d'orange* and increased warmth, with or without a palpable mass within the breast. Involvement of the nipple with retraction, crusting, or flattening is often also present, and many women describe an increase of up to two cup sizes over a short number of weeks in the affected breast. There is often regional lymph node involvement.

The characteristic appearance of inflammatory breast cancer is produced by the invasion of the dermal lymphatic system by cancer cells: they often grow in sheets rather than the discrete mass present in non-inflammatory breast cancer. Around 25% of patients will have a palpable mass within the breast. A biopsy of the affected area should be performed (usually under USS-guidance), which may be an FNA, core biopsy, or punch biopsy. Histological examination generally shows dilated dermal lympho-vascular spaces with tumour emboli, and should have receptor status performed for oestrogen and HER2. Guidelines advise against routine assessment of progesterone receptor status; however, most centres still perform this.

Imaging in inflammatory breast cancer may not be particularly helpful given the diffuse nature in many patients. Mammograms and ultrasounds often demonstrate the skin thickening/oedema and dilated lympho-vascular spaces, but may be reported as normal. MRI scans will generally show widespread abnormality, so are useful for demonstrating the extent of disease. Staging should be performed with CT thorax/abdomen/pelvis, as 30–50% of patients will have metastatic disease at presentation. All patients with inflammatory breast cancer are classified as T4 tumours in the American Joint Committee Cancer Staging system, due to the involvement of the skin.

The primary treatment for inflammatory breast cancer is neoadjuvant chemotherapy, with Herceptin (trastuzumab) added in the HER-2 positive patients. This is generally a course of 6–8 cycles of treatment, using both anthracyclines and taxanes. Those who have complete resolution of skin involvement should then undergo mastectomy followed by radiation; those who do not should undergo radiation first before considering the role of surgery.

The long-term survival in inflammatory breast cancer is poor, even in those with localized disease at presentation. The best survival is seen in those who get a pathological complete response in the breast and nodes from neoadjuvant treatment, with five-year survival rates of up to 40% in this group. Traditional rates of pathological complete response in the breast and local lymph nodes were 15–20% with standard chemotherapy, but have increased to 30–40% in the HER2 positive patients with the use of trastuzumab (Herceptin).

Further Reading

Dawood S, Merajver D, Viens P, et al. (2011). International expert panel on inflammatory breast cancer: consensus statement for standardised diagnosis and treatment. *Annals of Oncology* 22: 515–523.

Woodward W, Cristofanilli M (2009). Inflammatory breast cancer. *Seminars in Radiation Oncology* 19(4): 256–265.

158. B) Left ventricular failure

This woman has developed left ventricular failure, most likely contributed to by her previous treatment (left chest radiation and anthracycline chemotherapy). She has history and examination findings compatible with left ventricular failure.

The recent flight and tamoxifen are both risk factors for pulmonary embolism (PE), but the history of gradual onset is not classical for embolism and this does not explain the auscultatory findings. A malignant pleural effusion may cause shortness of breath, but you would expect to see some evidence of this on the CT scan, plus there should be dullness to percussion of the chest. Intraparenchymal lung metastases would have to be extensive to cause shortness of breath, or else causing obstruction, which again should have been visible on the CT scan, and would not generally cause crepitations. Lymphangitis carcinomatosis is a rare form of metastatic adenocarcinoma that can cause fine crepitations, but is much less likely to be the cause than left ventricular failure.

Tutorial

Anthracycline-induced cardiomyopathy is a well-recognized phenomenon in patients and is one of the most important long-term, life-limiting toxicities of treatment for curative malignancies, such as lymphoma and breast cancer (adjuvant treatment). The risk is related to total dose: it tends to manifest in those patients receiving a cumulative dose of ≥ 300 mg/m^2 of doxorubicin, or ≥ 600 mg/m^2 of epirubicin. Other contributing treatment factors include use of other concurrent cardiotoxic drugs (such as trastuzumab) and left-sided radiation treatment, which causes long-term vascular abnormalities.

A number of patient factors are also important in the risk of developing anthracycline-induced cardiomyopathy. The best validated are as follows:

- Age at treatment initiation (<18 or >65 years)
- Other cardiac risk factors (hypertension, pre-existing coronary artery disease, known left ventricular dysfunction)
- Pregnancy
- Ethnicity (higher rates in non-Caucasians)

There are three distinct types of anthracycline-induced cardiotoxicity:

1 Acute: occurs on the day of chemotherapy, and most commonly presents as arrhythmia
2 Subacute: presents with cardiac failure within six months, and is generally irreversible
3 Late: occurs beyond six months after completion of treatment

The late cardiotoxicity will often have some reversible component, as it is thought to be due to subclinical cardiotoxicity from the chemotherapy, compounded by further insults to the heart from factors such as hypertension, hyperlipidaemia, and diabetes. Therefore, good control of known cardiac risk factors can reduce the risk of developing significant late cardiotoxicity and aggressive treatment can improve the ejection fraction. There is, however, no current evidence that prophylactic treatment with medication such as beta blockers or angiotensin-converting enzyme (ACE) inhibitors is cardioprotective. All patients should have a baseline echocardiogram or assessment of cardiac function by a multi-gate acquisition (MUGA) scan, to ensure they have adequate reserve prior to treatment. In general, patients should have an ejection fraction of at least 50% to receive anthracyclines, although treatment, especially curative, at lower ejection fractions may be appropriate.

The presentation of cardiac failure in anthracycline-induced cardiomyopathy is no different from other causes of heart failure: pulmonary oedema in left ventricular failure and signs of right-sided heart failure in those with biventricular disease. Many of the patients developing these signs will be younger than the population presenting with ischaemic left ventricular failure, and therefore require a high index of suspicion to diagnose. The standard diagnostic test is an echocardiogram, while the mainstays of treatment remain ACE-inhibitors, beta blockers, and diuretics. There has been increasing use of left-ventricular assist devices to support cardiac function in recent years, with a modest improvement in life expectancy.

A number of strategies have been developed to try to decrease the risk of treatment-related cardiotoxicity. These include: the use of less cardiotoxic anthracyclines, such as epirubicin or liposomal formulations; the use of multi-agent chemotherapy regimens to reduce the exposure to anthracyclines; the use of alternative non-anthracycline based treatment in those at highest risk; and the use of free radical scavenger agents such as dexrazoxane. Though the latter reduces the effectiveness of the chemotherapy and therefore has not been widely used in many countries.

Further Reading

ASCO (2007). ASCO clinical evidence review on the ongoing care of adult cancer survivors: cardiac and pulmonary late effects—review summary. *Journal of Clinical Oncology* 4: 233–235.

Pinder M, Duan Z, Goodwin J, et al. (2007). Congestive heart failure in older women treated with adjuvant anthracycline chemotherapy for breast cancer. *Journal of Clinical Oncology* 25: 3808–3815.

159. B) An aunt with a germline MLH1 mutation

In order to have an inherited, or genetic, component there must be a germline mutation. Tumours can have mutations, such as the presence of microsatellite instability in his tumour tissue, but this does not imply an inherited mutation: it may be a somatic mutation. Germline mutations will also be present in normal tissue, rather than restricted to tumour. A first-degree relative who has an associated cancer is one of the Amsterdam criteria for diagnosing HNPCC, but there are two other criteria that must also be fulfilled. K-ras mutation in tumour tissue has no relationship to underlying germline mutations, and the presence of three synchronous polyps is not consistent with *non-polyposis* related cancer.

Tutorial

At least 20% of patients with CRC will have inherited an underlying genetic susceptibility to CRC. The most common of these is Lynch syndrome (HNPCC), where inactivation of the genes required for repair of the base-base mismatches in DNA is inherited. This mutation can also be acquired (or somatic), occurring just in the tumour. This occurs in approximately 15% of patients with non-familial colorectal cancer, where bi-allelic silencing of the promoter region of the MLH1 gene by promoter methylation inactivates mismatch repair.

Those with HNPCC germline defects (usually MLH1 and MSH2) have a lifetime CRC risk of 80%, but most will develop CRC by the age of 45 years. The genomic instability also causes much more rapid progression to cancer, and therefore annual colonoscopy is recommended for known carriers as the tumours may develop and metastasize within the three years recommended for standard colonoscopy surveillance.

The major features of HNPCC are:

- Autosomal dominant inheritance pattern
- Right-sided colon cancers—70–85% are proximal to splenic flexure
- Accelerated carcinogenesis (2–3 years versus 8–10 years in general population)
- High risk of additional colorectal malignancy (25–30% have second colorectal cancer)
- Increased risk of malignancy in other sites: endometrium (40–60%), ovary (12–15%), small bowel, hepatobiliary and pancreas, bladder (transitional cell carcinoma), and renal pelvis
- Poorly differentiated colorectal carcinoma
- Improved survival, compared stage for stage with non-HNPCC CRC

Diagnosis is made on identification of germline mutation in mismatch repair gene (generally MLH1, MSH2, or MSH6).

The guidelines commonly used to identify those at risk of developing Lynch syndrome are the modified Amsterdam II criteria (all of the following required):

- Three or more affected relatives with histologically verified Lynch syndrome associated cancers: one of whom must be a first-degree relative of the other two. Familial adenomatous polyposis must be excluded.
- Two successive generations affected.
- One or more cancers diagnosed before the age of 50.

Reprinted from *Gastroenterology*, 116, 6, Vasen et al., New clinical criteria for hereditary nonpolyposis colorectal cancer (HNPCC, Lynch syndrome) proposed by the International Collaborative group on HNPCC, pp. 1453-1456. Copyright 1999, with permission from Elsevier and the American Gastroenterological Association.

The criteria can be remembered by the '3-2-1 rule': 3 affected members, 2 generations, 1 under age 50.

Current screening recommendations for those known to carry a germline mutation are for annual colonoscopy to begin at age 20–25 years. Females should begin annual screening with a transvaginal ultrasound scan at age 30–35 years for endometrial and ovarian cancer, and may consider risk-reduction surgery with a hysterectomy and bilateral salpingo-oophorectomy after they have completed their families.

The presence of a mismatch repair gene mutation does not influence the choice for chemotherapy, or the chemotherapeutic agents used. However, the knowledge that a patient carries a germline mutation may influence the type of surgery performed, as there is a much higher risk of multiple tumours in such patients. Therefore more extensive surgery, such as a subtotal or total colectomy may be performed to reduce the risk of subsequent bowel malignancies. Stage for stage, patients with a mis-match repair gene germline mutation have improved rates of survival when compared with patients without mutations, and are likely to gain more benefit from standard adjuvant chemotherapy.

Further Reading

Vasen H, Watson P, Mecklin J, Lynch H (1999). New clinical criteria for hereditary nonpolyposis colorectal cancer (HNPCC, Lynch syndrome) proposed by the International Collaborative group on HNPCC. *Gastroenterology* 116(6): 1453–1456.

Cunningham D, Atkin W, Lenz H-J, et al. (2010). Colorectal cancer. *Lancet* 375: 1030–1047.

160. B) Cervix

This woman presents with symptomatic liver metastases, on a background of previous renal transplantation and long-term immunosuppression. Her risk is therefore greatest for cancers associated with immunosuppression. There is no strong association between immunosuppression and ovarian, breast, or pancreatic cancer; however, there is an association with lung and cervical cancer. Of these, the strongest association is with squamous cell carcinoma of the cervix, which is therefore the most likely primary. The risk of lung cancer is significantly higher in smokers compared with non-smokers.

The question mentions irregular vaginal bleeding, which is a frequent symptom of cervical carcinoma but is often discounted by patients with an irregular menstrual cycle. The cervical smear history is not mentioned, but cervical cancers often display rapid progression in those who are immunosuppressed, and therefore tumours may develop in between regular cervical smears if they are performed three yearly. The current recommendations for those on long-term immunosuppression suggest annual cervical smears, although compliance can be a problem.

Tutorial

Patients who have undergone a renal transplant and are on long-term immunosuppression have long been noted to have excess rates of some malignancies, particularly squamous cell carcinomas. These most commonly affect the skin, but in females the genital tract is also affected. More recently, patients treated with newer immunosuppressive agents such as mycophenolate mofetil and sirolimus appear to have much lower rates of malignancy than those treated with traditional agents, such as ciclosporin, prednisone, and azathioprine.

A number of cancers have been shown to be more common in these immunosuppressed patients; some (e.g. lymphomas) are likely to be partially driven by viruses such as EBV. This is also true of patients with cervical cancer, where the correlation between HPV and precancerous lesions and cancers is very well documented.

Squamous cell cancer of the skin is the most common malignancy in post-renal transplant patients. Men and women are affected equally and the risk has been shown to increase with age. Patients are much more likely to have multiple, rapidly progressive skin cancers, with early rates of metastatic disease. Some patients may have an improvement in their disease with reduction in their immunosuppression. Excess rates of melanoma and basal cell carcinoma are also well documented, and also show much more rapidly progressive courses than in immunocompetent patients.

Cervical cancer rates have been reported at up to 25 times the general population risk in post-transplant patients. All female patients should undergo annual screening smears to reduce the risk of late-stage disease. It is thought the excess risk is due to either latent reactivation of HPV, or the inability of the body to deal with a primary infection. Again, the rate of disease progression may decrease if the immunosuppression regime is reduced. It is possible that widespread HPV vaccination may reduce this risk in future by reducing the carrier rate of HPV, therefore removing the stimulus for the transplant-associated malignancy.

Native kidneys are at high risk of renal cell cancers. One study from Japan showed the rate of renal cell cancer was 80 times that of the general population, with similar results from Danish and

American studies. The most likely cause is acquired cystic kidney disease due to prolonged uraemia, which transforms into malignant disease. The renal cell carcinomas occurring in transplant patients also appear to behave much more aggressively.

Post-transplant lymphoproliferative disease has been recognized for more than 30 years as a complication of renal transplants. The most common malignancies are lymphomas (both Hodgkin's and non-Hodgkin's types), with higher rates in those who received anti-lymphocyte antibodies as prophylaxis against acute rejection. These lymphomas may go into remission with lessening of the immunosuppression, and may not require other treatments.

Further Reading

Hoshida Y, Tsukuma H, Yasunaga Y, et al. (1997). Cancer risk after renal transplantation in Japan. *International Journal of Cancer* 16: 517–520.

Kessler M, Jay N, Molle R, et al. (2006). Excess risk of cancer in renal transplant patients; *Transplant International* 19: 908–914.

161. E) Pulmonary embolus

The most likely cause for this woman is PE. Ovarian cancer is one of the most thrombogenic cancers, and many chemotherapy regimens have also been suggested to increase thrombotic risk.

With regards to occlusion of a bronchus from a pulmonary metastasis, stage IIIC ovarian cancer is localized to the peritoneum and therefore the patient would not have lung metastases. The above drugs would not cause left ventricular failure, and her examination findings are inconsistent with this. The patient's neutrophil count is too high to qualify for neutropenia; and while most chemotherapy drugs rarely cause pneumonitis, one would expect to hear crepitations on auscultation, and overall this would be a much less common cause than venous thromboembolism (VTE).

Tutorial

VTE is one of the most common complications of malignancy, and a frequent cause of morbidity and mortality. Patients may be at a higher risk for a number of reasons, including increased immobility and abnormal blood flow due to pressure from tumours. However, many tumours also release cytokines that potentiate clotting and procoagulant enzymes which may inappropriately initiate coagulation or cause a thrombocytosis.

There are a number of well-recognized risk factors for developing malignancy-associated thrombosis. These include increasing age, a prior personal history of VTE (especially with thrombophilias), concurrent infection (particularly neutropaenic sepsis) and increased BMI. Times when patients are most at risk include: at the time of initial cancer diagnosis; in the presence of metastatic disease; following major surgery; during prolonged admissions to hospital; and with certain malignancies.

Malignancies carrying the highest risk of VTE include:

1. Gynaecological malignancy (especially ovary)
2. Haematological malignancy (including lymphoma)
3. Renal cell carcinoma
4. Primary brain tumours
5. Lung carcinoma (both small cell and non-small cell)
6. Gastrointestinal malignancy (higher risk with upper GI, such as gastric and pancreatic carcinoma)

Treatment with chemotherapy, hormone treatment, targeted treatments, and erythropoietin can all increase the risk of thrombosis. There are particularly high rates associated with the hormone treatments tamoxifen and medroxyprogesterone (Megace), and anti-angiogenic treatments such as thalidomide and bevacizumab. Those with central venous access devices (CVADs), such as portacaths, Hickmann lines, and peripherally inserted central catheter (PICC) lines, also have a higher risk of thrombosis associated with the device (up to 5%). Trials in which low dose warfarin was prophylactically used to reduce this risk showed no reduction in the rate of CVAD-associated thrombosis.

While most patients with large, clinically significant thromboses will have symptoms, an increasing number of asymptomatic patients will have thromboses diagnosed on routine CT scans performed to assess response to treatment, or baseline scans performed at first presentation with malignancy. In general, all patients with a demonstrated genuine thrombus should be considered for anticoagulation unless there are contraindications such as active bleeding present. Inferior vena cava (IVC) filters may be used in some patients to prevent recurrent episodes of PE, and should be considered for those with thromboses undergoing surgery.

The preferred anticoagulant for patients with a confirmed thrombosis is LMWH. Those who are undergoing chemotherapy will often remain on once daily LMWH though this, as many chemotherapy regimens, will alter absorption of warfarin as well as platelet levels through the cycle. This can result in large fluctuations in the INR and put patients at a higher risk of further thrombotic episodes or bleeding. The use of LMWH also makes it easier to plan common interventions such as pleural and ascitic drains.

Patients with brain metastases who are diagnosed with DVT or PE are a common dilemma, as there is an increased risk of haemorrhage into brain metastases on anticoagulation. Therefore, the risk must be carefully weighed up on an individual basis when choosing whether or not to anticoagulate. Those with treated stable brain metastases have a lower risk on average than those who have untreated or progressive metastases.

Further Reading

Akl E, Labedi N, Barba M, et al. (2011). Anticoagulation for the long-term treatment of venous thromboembolism in patients with cancer. *Cochrane Database Systemic Review* 7: CD006650.

162. C) Non-smokers with adenocarcinoma may do better with EGFR inhibitors such as erlotinib

In non-small cell lung cancer (NSCLC), chemotherapy is helpful for symptomatic relief but only extends survival by an average of two months, not 6–12 months. The site of metastases has not been shown to influence chance of response except in brain metastases, where traditional chemotherapy does not reliably cross the blood-brain barrier. In some types of malignancy, such as ovarian cancer, progression within six months denotes resistance to drugs such as platinum agents, but this has not been shown to be true of lung cancer. The development of a maculopapular rash on epidermal growth factor receptor (EGFR) inhibitors is thought to be suggestive of response, but this is not true with chemotherapy including docetaxel. EGFR inhibitors such as erlotinib and gefitinib have a number of surrogate markers to suggest those who are more likely to respond. These include adenocarcinoma subtype, never-smokers, female gender, and Southeast Asian ethnicity.

Tutorial

The recognition of activating mutations in EGFR (also known as HER1) of some patients with lung cancer led to the trials of drugs targeting these receptors. There have now been a number of trials performed in the first, second, and subsequent lines of treatment with erlotinib and gefitinib. These are small molecule tyrosine kinase inhibitors which reversibly target the epidermal growth factor receptor. The EGFR signalling pathway is present in all tissues, but is activated in a number of different types of tumour cells. This may occur due to overexpression of EGFR, mutation of the EGFR receptors, or increased downstream signalling.

Amongst all patients with NSCLC, EGFR inhibitors have similar efficacy to second- and third-line chemotherapy, but are inferior to standard chemotherapy in the first line. However, some subgroups have been found to have much higher response rates and improved overall survival if treated with EGFR inhibitors, of which assessment of EGFR mutational status is the most reliable. To date, EGFR mutations have been found in 80% of those who respond to EGFR inhibitors, while those found to have *k-ras* mutations generally do not respond to either gefitinib or erlotinib. Assessment of gene mutation status, whilst becoming increasingly common, is still not widely available. For patients who have not had their mutation status assessed, there are a number of clinical indicators which have been shown in multiple trials to predict response. The most frequent responders have one or more of the following features:

- Female gender
- Southeast Asian ethnicity
- Adenocarcinoma histology
- Non-smoker

EGFR tyrosine kinase inhibitors are generally well tolerated, with the most common side effects being lethargy, diarrhoea (approximately 55%), and skin rash (~75%). Skin toxicity has been associated with improved overall survival and progression free survival in unselected patients, with theories including the skin as a surrogate indicator of EGFR inhibition; or a surrogate indicator of an immune-based inflammatory response which has an anti-tumour effect. The tablets are taken once daily, continuously, until progression or unacceptable toxicity.

Further Reading

Cataldo V, Gibbons D, Pérez-Soler R, et al. (2011). Treatment of non-small cell lung cancer with erlotinib or gefitinib. *New England Journal of Medicine* 364: 947–955.

National Institute for Clinical Excellence (2019). Lung cancer: diagnosis and management [NG122]. Available at: https://www.nice.org.uk/guidance/ng122

163. B) CT thorax/abdomen/pelvis

This patient presents with hypertension, weight loss, and lethargy, along with hypercalcaemia on blood tests. The differentials include malignancy such as renal cancer or myeloma, or hyperparathyroidism. However, hyperparathyroidism does not generally cause hypertension or weight loss; instead it presents either without any associated symptoms, or else with symptoms such as nephrolithiasis. Myeloma, whilst causing lytic bone lesions, does not cause a raised ALP and patients are usually anaemic. Prostate cancer, for which PSA may be a helpful marker, causes sclerotic bone lesion and does not typically cause hypercalcaemia. The patient most likely has a solid organ malignancy with bony metastases. The history of hypertension with borderline polycythaemia makes the diagnosis of renal cell carcinoma likely. A CT thorax/abdomen/pelvis would be most sensitive to detect this or other solid organ tumours such as lung that may metastasize to bone. A bone scan may show bony lesions, and is may be useful for staging but not diagnosis.

Tutorial

Renal cell carcinoma most commonly presents between the ages of 50 and 70, and has a male:female ratio of 2:1. It most commonly presents with hypertension, hypercalcaemia, erythrocytosis (secondary to increased erythropoietin), fever, or weight loss, although early tumours are often incidental findings on ultrasound or CT scans. There are three main histological subtypes: clear cell (70–80%), papillary (10–15%), and chromophobe (3–5%). Risk factors include smoking, genetic predisposition, cadmium or asbestos exposure, and acquired cystic kidney disease (resulting from end-stage renal disease and chronic dialysis). At presentation, 30% of patients will have metastatic disease, 25% of patients have locally advanced cancer, and 45% have localized disease. The rate of disease progression varies considerably amongst the patient population, but the anatomic extent of the disease is the most consistent factor that influences prognosis. The staging of renal cell carcinoma is generally made via CT scan, and uses the TNM (tumour, nodes, metastases) system as shown in Table 8.1.

Table 8.1 TNM classification of renal cell carcinoma

Tumour	
Tx	Primary tumour cannot be assessed
T0	No evidence of primary tumour
T1	Tumour <7 cm and confined to kidney
T2	Tumour >7 cm and confined to kidney
T3	Tumour invades major veins or perinephric tissues but not ipsilateral adrenal bland or beyond Gerota's fascia
T4	Tumour invades beyond Gerota's fascia (including adrenal)
Lymph nodes	
Nx	Regional lymph nodes cannot be assessed
N0	No regional lymph node metastasis
N1	Metastasis in one regional lymph node
N2	Metastases in more than one regional lymph node
Metastasis	
M0	No distant metastasis
M1	Distant metastasis present

Used with the permission of the American College of Surgeons. Amin MB, Edge, S.B., Greene FL, et al. (Eds.) *AJCC Cancer Staging Manual*, 8th Edition. Springer, New York, 2017.

Surgery is the mainstay of treatment for localized disease. Risk factors for disease recurrence include the stage and grade of tumour (the most important factors), performance status, and presence of paraneoplastic conditions. For those with metastatic disease, palliative nephrectomy has been shown to improve response to palliative treatments such as interferon, although the exact mechanism is unknown. There is also a documented rate of spontaneous regression of metastatic disease following palliative nephrectomy, in the region of 1–2%.

Renal cell cancer does not respond to standard chemotherapy, and response rates to radiation vary greatly from patient to patient; therefore for many years there has been little useful treatment for metastatic disease. Significant progress has been made in systemic treatment of metastatic renal cell carcinoma over the last few years, and there are now multiple novel biologic agents that have been shown to improve symptoms and progression free survival. These include sunitinib, and sorafenib (multi-targeted tyrosine kinase inhibitors); temsirolimus or everolimus (mTOR inhibitors); and bevacizumab (vascular endothelial growth factor inhibitor). Current trials are investigating the role of adjuvant targeted treatment following surgery to try to improve the outcome following resection of localized disease.

Hereditary renal cell carcinoma accounts for 2–3% of cases, the most common of which is von Hippel Lindau syndrome. This is associated with clear cell renal carcinoma, with sufferers also at risk of tumours in other organs including the brain, spine, adrenals (phaeochromocytoma), and pancreas (islet cell tumour). It is common for sufferers to develop hundreds of cysts at a young age, which can progress to tumours, with 40% of patients developing bilateral tumours.

Further Reading

Motzer R, Hutson T, Tomczak P, et al. (2007). Sunitinib versus interferon alfa in metastatic renal-cell carcinoma. *New England Journal of Medicine* 356: 115–124.

Rini B, Campbell S, Escudier B, et al. (2009). Renal cell carcinoma. *Lancet* 373: 1119–1132.

164. A) Aggressive intravenous rehydration

This patient has significant tumour lysis syndrome, an oncological emergency, as evidenced by hyperkalaemia, hyperuricaemia, hyperphosphataemia, and hypocalcaemia. He has significant renal dysfunction and the first step should be aggressive IV rehydration. Increasing the allopurinol, using an insulin/dextrose infusion to manage the potassium, rasburicase to bind the uric acid, and haemodialysis may be required depending on the response to fluids, but these are all secondary steps which should follow the fluids.

Tutorial

Tumour lysis syndrome is a set of metabolic abnormalities that arise from treatment of rapidly-proliferating, chemo-sensitive malignancies which can result in lactic acidosis, acute renal failure, and death. It generally occurs several hours to several days after commencing cytotoxic chemotherapy in those at risk. The highest risk malignancies are shown below:

- Acute leukaemias
- Burkitt's lymphoma
- Diffuse large B-cell lymphoma
- Germ cell tumours
- Small cell lung cancer

The rates can be up to 50% in haematological malignancies, although only 10% of these will be clinically significant. Tumour lysis has also been reported with these malignancies following radiation, targeted treatments such as rituximab, high-dose steroids, and stem cell transplant. The risk is generally highest with the first treatment, when there is the highest number of malignant cells to lyse. The other main risk factor is bulk of disease—particularly if there are multiple large lymph node groups, very high leucocyte count, or hepatosplenomegaly. An elevated uric acid level and pre-existing renal impairment also increase the risk, as does fluid depletion.

Tumour lysis syndrome is caused by the rapid breakdown of a large volume of tumour cells, releasing potassium, uric acid, phosphate, and other purine products in volumes greater than the kidneys can deal with. This leads to high serum levels of potassium, urate, and phosphate, which can cause a variety of symptoms including nausea, vomiting, diarrhoea, and ECG abnormalities.

The high phosphate causes hypocalcaemia, which in turn increases the parathyroid levels, causing increased phosphate reabsorption in the proximal tubule. This can cause renal dysfunction by increasing the risk of calcium phosphate crystals precipitating in the renal tubules. Uric acid excess (hyperuricaemia) is the most common finding, and may be the only finding in more mild cases.

The presentation of patients with tumour lysis syndrome varies with the degree of severity. Patients may be asymptomatic, with only mild-moderate electrolyte abnormalities; or in more severe conditions, can present with cardiac arrhythmias or oliguric renal failure. More commonly, moderate cases present with symptoms from the electrolyte abnormalities, such as nausea, vomiting, diarrhoea, tetany, weakness, paraesthesia, confusion, delirium, and seizures.

The best way to manage tumour lysis is to prevent it from occurring. All patients receiving treatment with bulky, rapidly growing tumours should begin treatment with allopurinol at least 24 hours before starting chemotherapy. Those at particularly high risk should always be treated as an inpatient for their first cycle of chemotherapy, so they can receive aggressive IV fluid hydration, starting prior to treatment and continuing throughout the cycle, with close monitoring of urine output and serum electrolytes. Adequate control of chemotherapy-induced nausea and vomiting is also important to reduce further fluid depletion.

In patients who do present with established tumour lysis syndrome, the single most important treatment is aggressive IV rehydration, with a minimum of 3 L per day. All patients should have the following tests performed:

- Renal function
- Sodium and potassium
- Calcium and phosphate
- Uric acid and LDH
- Serum glucose
- Liver function tests
- ECG

The next step is to treat the metabolite abnormalities, particularly significant hyperkalaemia with ECG changes. Calcium gluconate is useful in the short term both to improve the hyperkalaemia and hypocalcaemia, in addition to other standard treatments such as insulin/dextrose infusion. Hyperphosphataemia may require oral phosphate binders in severe cases.

If high dose allopurinol to reduce uric acid levels is not effective, intravenous rasburicase may be required. This is expensive and may not be readily available, but is useful for those with significant renal dysfunction due to hyperuricaemia. Finally, haemodialysis may be required for those with acute renal failure.

Overall, the mortality rate is around 15% for patients with clinically significant tumour lysis syndrome. Close monitoring of those at risk, and early recognition of the syndrome is the best way to prevent this.

Further Reading

Howard S, Jones D, Pui C-H, et al. (2011). The tumour lysis syndrome. *New England Journal of Medicine* 364: 1844–1854.

165. B) 50%

This patient has a primary mediastinal germ cell tumour, as evidenced by the tumour markers, CT results, and normal testicular ultrasound. This immediately puts him into the poor prognostic group of germ cell tumours, and drops his long-term survival to 50%. The confounding factor with this question is to realize that it is possible to get a primary mediastinal germ cell tumour without testicular involvement, and not to discount this as a diagnosis. There can be no other diagnosis with those tumour markers in a male patient.

Tutorial

Germ cell tumours most commonly present in men aged between 15 and 35 years, predominantly in Caucasians. There is an increased risk in those with a history of cryptorchidism or Klinefelter's syndrome. It generally presents as a testicular mass, either with or without pain, but patients may also present with metastatic disease.

Germ cell tumours can be divided into two main groups—seminomas and non-seminomatous tumours. Non-seminomas are generally a combination of histologies such as teratoma, yolk sac tumour, choriocarcinoma, and embryonal cell carcinoma. Of the two, seminomas are much more sensitive to radiation and overall have a better prognosis than non-seminomas. Tumour markers are more commonly present in non-seminomas, with α-fetoprotein elevated in 80–85% and β-hCG elevated in 80%. LDH may be elevated in both, but is more common in non-seminomas. Seminomas never have an elevated α-fetoprotein unless there is liver involvement, while a raised β-hCG is only present in 30%.

Germ cell primaries are most commonly in the testicles, but may also occur in the retroperitoneal or mediastinal areas, and these non-testicular primaries are associated with a worse outcome. They can be subdivided into prognostic groups by features which are summarized in Table 8.2.

Table 8.2 Germ cell primaries arranged by prognostic groups

Prognosis	Non-seminomas	Seminoma
Good	All of following: • Primary site not mediastinum • Absence of non-pulmonary visceral metastases • β-hCG <5000 iU/ml • AFP <1000 iU/ml • LDH <1.5 × ULN*	Absence of non-pulmonary visceral metastases

Intermediate	• Primary site not mediastinum, AND
	• Absence of non-pulmonary visceral metastases, AND
	• One of the following:
	  • β-hCG 5000–50,000 iU/ml
	  • AFP 1000–10000 iU/ml
	  • LDH 1.5–10 × ULN
		Presence of non-pulmonary visceral metastases

Poor prognosis	Any of the following: • Primary mediastinal site • Presence of non-pulmonary visceral metastases • B-hCG >50,000 iU/ml • AFP >10,000 iU/ml • LDH >10 × ULN	There are no poor prognosis seminomas

* ULN: upper limit of normal.

Prognosis for non-seminomas ranges from a five-year survival of 40–50% for high risk, to 90–95% for low risk. Seminoma survival rates ranged 75–90+%. The staging of germ cell tumours are summarized in Table 8.3.

Table 8.3 Staging of germ cell tumours

Stage	Features
I	Tumour is limited to the testis, spermatic cord, or scrotum, includes lympho-vascular invasion
II	Involves regional lymph nodes
III	Presence of distant metastatic disease

The primary treatment for localized disease is surgery to remove the testis. Those with stage I seminoma were traditionally treated with local radiation to the local lymph nodes (including the para-aortic nodes), although trials have now shown that one cycle of adjuvant chemotherapy with carboplatin is equivalent, and may have fewer long-term risks. An alternative, and now the generally preferred approach, is to use close surveillance rather than adjuvant treatment and treat at progression, with a relapse rate of 15–20%, generally within the first 15–18 months. Stage II disease is treated with adjuvant chemotherapy or radiotherapy, with reassessment of response post-treatment; options include surgery or further radiotherapy.

Treatment for advanced non-seminomatous tumours is generally with chemotherapy. The most common first-line regimen is BEP (bleomycin, etoposide, cisplatin) for 3–4 cycles followed by resection of any residual disease. Even those presenting with relapsed disease may be salvageable with second-line chemotherapy, radiation, or surgery. There is currently no role for targeted agents in germ cell tumours.

Further Reading

Feldman D, Bosl G, Sheinfeld J, et al. (2008). Medical treatment of advanced testicular cancer. *Journal of American Medical Association* 299: 672–684.

166. A) Adjuvant chemotherapy

Adjuvant chemotherapy has been shown to significantly improve outcome in patients with completely resected disease but with risk factors such as nodal involvement. There is currently no role for adjuvant radiation or EGFR treatment in resected lung cancer. There is a well-established role for chemo-radiation for unresectable locally advanced disease, but currently no improvement in survival with the combination in resected disease.

Tutorial

Lung cancer makes up 10–15% of cancer diagnoses in the UK and Europe, and accounts for 20% of cancer deaths. The underlying cause of 80% of lung cancer worldwide is smoking, with the remainder linked to other environmental factors such as radon, radiation, arsenic contamination of groundwater, and carcinogenic inhaled irritants such as asbestos. As smoking rates decline in some parts of the world (such as the USA, UK, and Australasia), it is anticipated that these countries will have a subsequent decline in smoking-related lung cancers over the next 20 years; however, rates of smoking remain high, or are indeed increasing, in most other parts of the world.

There are several main subtypes of non-small cell lung cancer—adenocarcinoma, squamous cell carcinoma, large cell carcinoma, and bronchoalveolar carcinoma. Overall, most patients present with symptoms such as chest pain, non-resolving cough, weight loss, or symptoms of metastatic disease such as bony pain, spinal cord compression, symptomatic brain metastases or paraneoplastic syndromes (Horner's syndrome, hypertrophic osteoarthropathy, hypercalcaemia). Some features are more strongly associated with specific subtypes.

Adenocarcinomas are more likely than other subtypes to occur in non-smokers, and their incidence has been increasing over the last 20 years. They are most often located in the periphery, and may therefore be easier than most lung cancers to see on chest X-ray. Sputum cytology tends to be negative as the cancers are generally well away from the large airways. Squamous cell carcinomas (SCC) have been decreasing in frequency as adenocarcinomas have become more common, and generally occur in smokers. They tend to occur centrally in the chest, and are most likely to give positive sputum cytology. SCCs are most likely to present with haemoptysis or hypercalcaemia.

Bronchoalveolar carcinoma is generally considered to be a subtype of slow-growing adenocarcinoma, and is often misdiagnosed on chest X-ray or CT scan as it manifests as a diffuse process, which may be mistaken for infection or inflammatory changes in the lungs. It is often difficult to biopsy because of the diffuse nature, with little in the way of large solid components to target for biopsy purposes. It commonly presents with bronchorrhoea (the profuse production of watery sputum).

Pre-operative staging with PET CT scan has improved the reliability of staging and decreased the need for pre-resection lymph node sampling, thus allowing better selection of surgical patients. Patients with stage IA–IIIA NSCLC have the best chance of survival if they can undergo surgical resection; however, many patients with lung cancer will be long-term smokers with poor lung function, poor performance status, and vascular disease. Patients who are unable to undergo surgical resection may be able to be treated with curative intent with radical radiation if they are able to tolerate the radiation.

The five-year survival of resected NSCLC remains poor, with rates between 25–73%. The LACE meta-analysis of platinum-based adjuvant chemotherapy published in 2008 showed a 5.3% overall survival benefit at five years, with no variation on the effect of chemotherapy with age, gender, type of surgery, histology subtype, and performance status. However, the benefit did vary by stage of cancer, with a negative effect with stage IA patients, 8% risk reduction for stage of IB, and 17% risk reduction for stage II and III. Current options for adjuvant chemotherapy include cisplatin/vinorelbine and cisplatin or carboplatin plus etoposide.

Those who have stage IIIB disease are generally considered un-resectable, and may be offered concurrent chemoradiation if they are well enough. This often includes Pancoast tumours. Concurrent regimens used include cisplatin/vinblastine and come with significant toxicity, so patients being considered must have adequate renal function and a good performance status.

Palliative chemotherapy is useful for improving symptoms in patients with metastatic NSCLC, but does not generally improve length of life. Traditionally, all patients with NSCLC have been treated in the same way, independent of histological subtype, although more recent trials have shown that histological subtype is important in choice of chemotherapy regimen. It is likely that further research will concentrate on selecting the best chemotherapy regimen for each subtype, as well as further research into maintenance treatments. There is also a role for targeted treatment with EGFR tyrosine kinase inhibitors, in those with EGFR mutations, for whom erlotinib and gefitinib are useful treatment options (discussed in more detail elsewhere in this chapter).

Further Reading

Albain K, Swann S, Rusch V, et al. (2009). Radiotherapy plus chemotherapy with or without resection for stage III non-small cell lung cancer: a phase III randomised controlled trial. *Lancet* 374: 379–386.

Goldstraw P, Ball D, Jett J, et al. (2011). Non-small-cell lung cancer. *Lancet* 378: 1727–1740.

167. A) Chemotherapy

The combination of a hilar mass and severe hyponatraemia in an ex-smoker should raise the possibility of SCLC, as this is one of the most common modes of presentation of this cancer. SCLC is exquisitely chemo-sensitive, and therefore the most appropriate option is chemotherapy. Radiation would only be used in SCLC if there were complete obstruction or significant haemoptysis requiring immediate treatment, or in those who cannot undergo chemotherapy due to other co-morbidities such as end-stage renal failure. There is no role for surgery in SCLC, as localized disease is treated with concurrent chemotherapy and radiation with curative intent.

Tutorial

SCLC currently makes up 10–15% of lung cancer, with the vast majority (>90%) occurring in current or prior heavy smokers. Risk increases with the increasing number of pack-years smoked. It is one of the most rapidly progressive malignancies, characterized by early spread to distant organs, with most patients having only an 8–12 week history of symptoms at diagnosis. Common presenting symptoms include increasing cough, wheeze, or shortness of breath, superior vena cava obstruction, haemoptysis, symptoms of metastatic disease (brain metastases, liver metastases), and paraneoplastic syndromes.

Small cell lung cancer is associated with the most paraneoplastic syndromes of all cancers. These are summarized in Table 8.4.

Table 8.4 Paraneoplastic syndromes associated with small cell lung cancer

Syndrome	Frequency of syndrome
SIADH (syndrome of inappropriate antidiuretic hormone secretion)	15–40%
Lambert-Eaton syndrome	3%
Cushing's syndrome	2–5%
Limbic encephalitis and encephalomyelitis	<1%
Paraneoplastic cerebellar degeneration	<1%

Hypercalcaemia and hypertrophic pulmonary osteoarthropathy are rare in SCLC, occurring much more commonly with non-small cell lung cancer: most commonly, in squamous cell carcinoma and adenocarcinoma, respectively. Note that paraneoplastic syndromes may pre-date the diagnosis of SCLC, sometimes by years (particularly Lambert-Eaton syndrome). The endocrine paraneoplastic syndromes generally improve together with treatment for the underlying cancer, while the neurological syndromes do not. Plasmapheresis and immunoglobulin infusions have been used with limited success to treat these.

Staging of SCLC has recently changed to the TNM staging system similar to NSCLC, but in practical terms the definitions of limited and extensive stage disease are still used to determine treatment options. Curative disease remains that which can be encompassed within a radiation field; the presence of distant metastatic disease, or extensive disease within the chest, which is beyond that which can be treated with a curative dose of radiation, is defined as incurable. The most common sites of metastatic disease are liver, brain, adrenal, and bone.

The survival of SCLC without treatment is generally very short (usually less than 12 weeks), with more than two thirds of patients presenting with metastatic disease. Staging is generally based on CT scanning (including brain CT, as many patients will have metastatic disease in the brain at diagnosis). Treatment is either curative intent, if disease is localized, or palliative if disease is extensive. Curative intent consists of concurrent chemotherapy (platinum based) and radiation treatment; and requires relatively fit patients with adequate lung and renal function to withstand the treatment. The standard comorbidities of current, or ex-heavy smokers, however, mean that few patients with limited stage small cell lung cancer are well enough to be treated with curative intent. The five-year survival of those treated with curative intent chemo/irradiation remains low at 10–15% usually due to recurrence of distant metastatic disease, or death from other co-morbidities. Those who are treated with curative intent should receive prophylactic cranial irradiation, which has been shown to increase survival. Without this, 50% of patients will develop brain metastases.

Those with extensive disease may be treated with palliative radiation for local symptoms (such as superior vena cava syndrome, occlusion of a bronchus, or brain metastases), or palliative chemotherapy. Palliative chemotherapy for those with extensive disease can work rapidly, even in patients with significant symptoms, resulting in a significant improvement in both quality and quantity of life. Those with bulky disease are at risk of tumour lysis syndrome when treated with standard chemotherapy (cisplatin or carboplatin +/− etoposide). The average survival of those who receive palliative chemotherapy is around 12–18 months.

Further Reading

Van Meerbeeck J, Fennell D, Ruysscher D, et al. (2011). Small-cell lung cancer. *Lancet* 378: 1741–1755.

168. **D)** Her previous radiation will affect her ability to have adjuvant radiation treatment to the chest wall

This question is examining the long-term effects of previous treatment. The correct answer is that her previous radiation will limit the potential for further therapy, as each area of the body has a lifetime maximum limit of radiation it can withstand. She will have had significant exposure on the chest with her previous mantle radiation, therefore leaving no room for further radiation treatment. Her previous treatment may also have affected her cardiac function, which could impact on your choice of chemotherapy for her, but will not affect her response to hormone treatment. Previous chemotherapy does not affect the radiation treatment however—had she not already had radiation to the area, this would be fine. She should undergo surgery, which will likely be a mastectomy. A wide local excision (or breast conserving surgery) would ideally be accompanied by adjuvant radiation treatment.

Tutorial

The risk of second cancers following previous treatment with radiation and chemotherapy is one of the most significant long-term toxicities for those treated with curative intent. It is well known that childhood cancer survivors experience more cancers in adulthood than age-matched individuals who have not previously had cancer.

The risk of developing second cancers depends on the original tumour, the treatment received, and the presence of other risk factors, such as germline gene mutations. Large cohort trials of those treated for Hodgkin's lymphoma are most at risk for the following malignancies (in decreasing order of risk):

- Breast
- Thyroid tumours
- Sarcoma
- Leukaemia
- Non-Hodgkin's lymphoma
- GI carcinoma
- Melanoma
- CNS tumour
- Lung (if a smoker)

Some of these tumours will be related to previous radiation treatment (i.e. radiation induced) such as breast, thyroid, and sarcomas; others, such as haematological malignancies, are due to chemotherapy. In general, most second malignancies will be multifactorial and can include things like co-existing viral infections, genetic abnormalities, diet, and even smoking. Higher rates of second cancers have also been noted in patients who have had radiation treatment as part of curative treatment for breast, testicular, cervical, and other childhood cancers. These patients are most likely to survive their first cancer, and live long enough to develop a second, with the additional risk factors from their previous treatment including radiation and chemotherapy.

Radiation induces tumours in irradiated tissue by damaging the DNA. Tumours which develop in previously irradiated areas are often more resistant to chemotherapy, and may also be slow to heal after surgery due to altered blood flow in the area. It is hoped that more modern techniques, with more precise targeting of the tumour, and overall lower doses will reduce the risk. Chemotherapy has been linked with the risk of developing both solid tumours and haematological malignancy. Two different families of drugs are commonly implicated: alkylating agents such as cyclophosphamide, chlorambucil, and platinum agents; and topoisomerase II inhibitors, such as etoposide. Those with haematological malignancies (leukaemias, myelodysplasias) as a result of alkylating chemotherapy have a much worse prognosis than those with *de novo* haematological malignancy, and are also less likely to withstand transplants due to co-morbidity from previous treatments. Solid tumours that have been linked to alkylating agents include bladder carcinoma (following cyclophosphamide use), sarcomas, and non-Hodgkin's lymphoma.

Further Reading

Meadows A, Friedman D, Neglia, J, et al. (2009). Second neoplasms in survivors of childhood cancer: findings from the childhood cancer survivor study cohort. *Journal of Clinical Oncology* 27: 2356–2362.

169. C) The median survival for those with completely resected pancreatic tumours is 36–48 months

Pancreatic cancer has an underlying inherited gene mutation in up to 10% of patients—one of the most common is BRCA2. This should be considered in anyone with a family history of other BRCA-related cancers, such as ovary and breast. At presentation, around 25% of patients have diabetes, and up to 40% will have impaired glucose tolerance. The use of adjuvant chemotherapy with either 5-FU or gemcitabine has been shown to add 3–5 months to overall survival, which averages 20–22 months in those with completely resected disease.

Tutorial

Pancreatic cancer is the fourth highest cause of death from cancer, despite being one of the less common malignancies. It has poor survival rates: even in those treated with curative intent, less than 20% of patients presenting with localized disease and less than 5% of all patients are still alive five years after diagnosis.

The presentation of pancreatic cancer is generally either with new onset painless jaundice, new onset diabetes (up to 25% of patients), malabsorption, or vague systemic symptoms such as back pain, weight loss, nausea, and vomiting. Risk factors include smoking, alcohol intake, chronic pancreatitis, diabetes, increasing age, and male gender.

Patients presenting with suspected pancreatic cancer should be worked up with blood tests including liver function tests, glucose, renal function, and CA19-9. The latter is a tumour marker, which is not particularly useful in diagnosis due to its low specificity, but can be useful in following treatment response, and estimating prognosis for patients in whom it is elevated. Patients should also have a CT scan to assess for metastatic disease. Formal staging which is based on the standard TNM (tumour, nodes, metastases) system, does not correlate well with outcome. Therefore generally categorization is resectable, locally advanced, or metastatic. Patients who present with jaundice should undergo ERCP (endoscopic retrograde cholangio-pancreatography) and stenting or dilation to relieve the jaundice. Brushings of any visible mass, or of the malignant stricture may also give a histological diagnosis.

Surgical resection with pancreaticoduodenectomy is the only curative treatment for pancreatic cancer, in those with localized disease. The use of adjuvant chemotherapy, with either 5-fluoroucil or gemcitabine, doubles the chance of disease free survival at two years. Locally advanced disease includes tumours which are invading other local structures, or invading more than a 180 degree extent of the surrounding blood vessels, therefore making it impossible to get a clear margin with surgical resection. Trials have investigated using multi-agent neoadjuvant chemotherapy to downstage the disease, prior to considering surgical resection in those who respond well.

They have shown response rates in up to 40% of patients subsequently able to undergo surgical resection, but with significant toxicity from the treatment. Those who have metastatic disease at presentation may undergo palliative chemotherapy with gemcitabine and/or 5-FU analogues such as capecitabine, or alternatively may have palliative radiation for symptomatic relief. While radiological response rates to palliative chemotherapy are low (generally less than 10%), the clinical benefit rate of symptomatic improvement was approximately 40%.

Up to 10% of affected patients will have a family history of pancreatic cancer in first-degree relatives. The risk is highest in those with young onset disease (<50 years), with germline BRCA2 mutations as the most common underlying mutation. There are six main genetic syndromes associated with pancreatic carcinoma:

1 BRCA2—hereditary breast and ovarian cancer syndrome.
2 Hereditary pancreatitis—patients develop pancreatitis in childhood/adolescence, and have a risk of pancreatic cancer 50 times that of the general population.
3 HNPCC associated with a germline mutation in a DNA mismatch repair gene (MLH1, MSH1, etc.).
4 Peutz-Jeghers syndrome—associated with haematomas of the mucosal membranes and GI tract.
5 Ataxia-telangiectasia syndrome—also associated with an increased risk of breast, ovarian, gastric, biliary tree tumours, leukaemia, and lymphoma.
6 Familial atypical multiple mole melanoma.

Compared stage for stage, most of those patients with underlying genetic mutations generally have a better outcome than those patients without genetic mutations. It is likely that future drug development will target these mutations for therapeutic benefit, such as the PARP inhibitor drugs, which have shown significant promise in breast and ovarian cancer patients with BRCA mutations.

Further Reading

Hidalgo M (2010). Pancreatic cancer. *New England Journal of Medicine* 253: 1605–1617.

170. A) Commence hormone manipulation with a GnRH agonist such as goserelin

This patient has asymptomatic metastatic prostate cancer, as demonstrated by his elevated PSA and positive bone scan. Traditional hormone treatment was with an oestrogen analogue, but this has now been surpassed by GnRH analogues such as goserelin, and non-steroidal treatments such as bicalutamide. Hormonal manipulation with progesterones is occasionally used, but both this and the oestrogen analogues carry a higher risk of thromboembolic disease. Radiation to metastatic deposits can be useful for pain or complications such as spinal cord compression, but he currently has no symptoms, so this is not indicated. Observation may be an option, but there has been shown to be a survival advantage in early treatment, so the best option would be hormone manipulation with a GnRH agonist. He could also have undergone a bilateral orchidectomy if he was open to further surgery.

Tutorial

Advanced prostate cancer has been a rapidly moving area over the last few years. Traditionally treated with surgery, hormones, and occasional radiation until the disease became hormone resistant, there have been a range of new treatments for hormone resistant patients in the last few years, with chemotherapy, androgen therapy, and immunotherapy all showing good response rates. The commonest site of metastases is bone (85–90%), then pelvic soft tissue disease (20–40%). Visceral metastases such as liver and lung occur late and much less commonly (5–10%). Therefore, the primary staging investigation is a radionuclide bone scan. Bone marrow infiltration is also well recognized, and can complicate the use of treatments such as chemotherapy due to profound myelosuppression. Most patients will produce PSA with progressive disease, which may be followed to assess response to treatment, and detect relapse.

The mainstay of initial treatment for patients with metastatic prostate cancer is hormone treatment, aiming to reduce the testosterone level to less than 50 ng/dL. This can be achieved by surgery, with bilateral orchidectomy, or hormonal treatment. There are two main classes: GnRH agonists and anti-androgens. The most commonly used GnRH agonists, goserelin and triptorelin, are administered as depot injections on a monthly or three-monthly basis. Anti-androgen agents, such as flutamide and bicalutamide bind to the androgen receptor on cells, and, used in isolation, can increase testosterone levels. They are most commonly used in combination with GnRH agonists. Anti-androgen treatment is generally well tolerated, but the side effects can include cardiovascular side effects such as increased risk of MI, osteoporosis, hot flushes, myalgias, oedema, weight gain, gynaecomastia, and mood changes (in many ways, similar to menopausal symptoms).

A survival advantage in favour of early androgen suppression, even in asymptomatic patients, has been shown, at one-, two-, and five-year follow-up. Patients were shown to have delayed progression and fewer complications in the early treatment group. This is not the most cost-effective strategy, however. It is cheaper to commence treatment at the onset of symptoms, and this strategy is still followed in some countries.

The type of androgen blockade—whether combination blockade with a GnRH antagonist and non-steroidal anti-androgen, single blockade with one of the above, or an orchidectomy—did not seem to alter the benefit seen. Patients who have painful metastases who are started on LH agonists such as goserelin alone often experience a flare of pain due to activation of the feedback mechanism, but this can be prevented by the concurrent use of non-steroidal anti-androgens. The onset of pain can happen in those started on goserelin with previously asymptomatic disease, but is generally less severe. Most patients will be well controlled on hormone treatment, but will eventually become hormone resistant, in which case chemotherapy can be considered.

Further Reading

Kunath F, Jensen K, Pinart M, et al. (2019). Early versus deferred androgen suppression in the treatment of advanced hormone sensitive prostate cancer. *Cochrane Database of Systematic Reviews* 6: CD003506.

171. E) The vaccine is most effective in those who have not been exposed to HPV and therefore she should be vaccinated now

The original trials testing the bivalent HPV vaccine were performed in women aged 15–25 years, but the decision to vaccinate at an earlier age was made as the vaccine is most effective in those who have not been exposed to the HPV virus, and therefore widespread vaccination programmes were planned for girls at an age prior to most becoming sexually active. Catch-up programmes were arranged for those up to 18 years old after vaccination first started, but it is thought to be less effective in those older due to a higher risk of having been exposed to HPV. The quadrivalent vaccine includes the two HPV strains most strongly associated with the risk of anogenital warts, but not the bivalent vaccine.

Tutorial

Cervical cancer is the second most common malignancy in females worldwide, although the disease burden is disproportionately higher in the developing world. This is due to a range of factors, including lack of screening facilities and treatment of pre-malignant precursor conditions such as cervical intraepithelial neoplasia (CIN) and higher rates of other risk factors such as smoking.

Squamous cell carcinoma accounts for two thirds of cases, with the remainder adenocarcinoma or mixed histology (adenosquamous). In the metastatic setting, it is an aggressive cancer with an average life expectancy of 6–12 months.

There is a well-recognized progression of cervical lesions from atypia, through CIN to invasive squamous cell carcinoma, which makes this ideally suited to a screening programme (Figure 8.1). The pre-malignant lesions can be detected and treated before they become malignant. Though the numbers of invasive squamous cell cervical carcinoma has decreased in screened populations, those at highest risk tend to be those in populations where screening is unavailable.

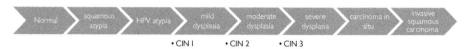

| | • CIN I | • CIN 2 | • CIN 3 | |

Figure 8.1 Natural history of progression from normal epithelia to invasive cancer.

The most common presenting symptom of cervical carcinoma is abnormal vaginal bleeding (often post-coital), with other symptoms such as vaginal discharge and pelvic pain (due to direct invasion of pelvic structures or hydronephrosis) also frequent. The disease generally spreads first to the local regional lymph nodes, and secondarily via haematogenous spread. The most common sites of metastatic disease are therefore other pelvic organs (such as the bladder or bowel), followed by the lungs, liver, extra-pelvic lymph nodes, and bones.

Invasive cervical carcinoma is staged based on the FIGO (International Federation of Gynaecology and Obstetrics) staging system. This has four basic stages, with subdivisions within each stage, and is described further in Table 8.5.

Table 8.5 Stages of cervical cancer

Stage	Description
I	Carcinoma is strictly confined to the cervix
II	Carcinoma extends beyond the cervix, but not to the pelvic wall, and does not extend to the lower third of the vagina
III	Extension onto the pelvic wall but not beyond the true pelvis
IV	Spread to adjacent or distant organs

Reproduced with permission from N Bhatla, Revised FIGO staging for carcinoma of the cervix uteri, *International Journal of Gynecology & Obstetrics*, 145, 1, pp. 129–135. © 2019 International Federation of Gynecology and Obstetrics.

Early stage disease is treated with radiation and/or surgery, whilst later stages are generally treated with a combination of chemotherapy and radiation. Metastatic disease is generally treated with chemotherapy and palliative radiation for symptom control (bleeding, pain). Oncogenic HPV types 16 and 18 cause around 70% of cases of cervical cancer worldwide, although up to 18 strains altogether have been implicated. This knowledge led to the development of both bivalent vaccines (covering types 16 and 18), and quadrivalent vaccines (currently used in the USA), which also cover types 6 and 11, the most common strains found in anogenital warts.

The vaccination is given as a course of three injections over six months (0, 1 and 6 months), with over 99.5% of patients seroconverting after completing the vaccinations. The injections were well tolerated, with the most common side effects reported being transient local injection symptoms, headache, and myalgia. The new onset of chronic disease and autoimmune disease was essentially the same in the treatment and control groups.

The trials showed that the vaccine was very effective in preventing HPV infection, and thus the rates of CIN and invasive carcinoma were significantly lower in the vaccinated groups. However, those who had already been infected with HPV at the time of vaccination did not gain protection from progression of CIN, nor did it seem to improve the rates of clearance of HPV. Therefore, it was recommended that large-scale vaccination target 11–12-year-olds, where it was most likely to be effective.

Further Reading

FUTURE II study group (2007). Quadrivalent vaccine against human papillomavirus to prevent high-grade cervical lesions. *New England Journal of Medicine* 356: 1915–1927.

Paavonen J, Jenkins D, Bosch X, et al. (2007). Efficacy of a prophylactic adjuvanted bivalent L1 virus-like-particle vaccine against infection with human papillomavirus types 16 and 18 in young women: an interim analysis of a phase III double-blind, randomised controlled trial. *Lancet* 369: 2161–2170.

172. A) Continue paracetamol and add in diclofenac EC 50 mg TDS

Bony pain often responds very well to non-steroidal anti-inflammatory drugs (NSAIDs), and should be used as part of the analgesic regimen if there is no contraindication such as impaired renal function or a history of gastric ulceration. An alternative, if there is inadequate renal function, is to use a short course of steroids, such as dexamethasone, especially as a bridge while awaiting radiation treatment. Another alternative would be to use long acting morphine, but this pain has not been particularly opioid responsive, which may mean inadequate dosing or poor patient compliance. There is nothing in the stem to suggest a neuropathic element to the pain, for which amitriptyline might be useful. As her analgesic requirements are not stable, a fentanyl patch is not appropriate either.

Tutorial

NSAIDs have demonstrated efficacy in all types of cancer pain and, used appropriately, may be opioid sparing for some patients. For others, they delay the requirement to start opioid analgesia, and the subsequent associated side effects.

There are few good trials looking at the use of NSAIDs specifically in patients with bony pain, despite this being widespread practice. Three small trials have shown improvements in pain measurement scores when patients are treated with NSAIDs or steroids for the bony pain. This is thought to be effective due to the potential of the bony lesions to cause a significant inflammatory response, partially (or mostly) through the release of pro-inflammatory cytokines. Reducing these levels through the use of NSAIDs or steroids seems to improve pain, particularly nocturnal bony pain, more efficaciously than using opioid analgesia.

A recent meta-analysis by the Cochrane Collaboration looked at a number of studies comparing NSAIDs with other analgesia in cancer patients. However, few of the studies were in patients with bony pain, and they included diverse situations such as post-operative pain. Most showed an improvement in pain when both an opioid and NSAID were used together in moderate to severe pain, irrespective of the cause of pain.

There is no good evidence for one NSAID over another in the control of bony pain, but enteric coated and slow release forms are generally preferred. This is mostly due to the more favourable side effect profile. The most common side effects of regular NSAID use include nausea, gastric irritation/ulceration, diarrhoea, fluid retention, and renal impairment. The risk of gastric side effects with NSAIDs is not insignificant, and most patients receive concurrent proton pump inhibitors, such as omeprazole or lansoprazole, to minimize these symptoms. This risk of more significant gastrointestinal toxicity is higher in those aged greater than 60 years, smokers, those treated with concurrent steroids/anticoagulants/selective serotonin reuptake inhibitors, and patients with underlying renal or hepatic impairment. In those treated with regular NSAIDs for two months, there is a 1:1200 risk of death from gastrointestinal haemorrhage.

Cyclo-oxygenase 2 (COX-2) inhibitors were initially designed as an alternative to standard NSAIDs with less gastrointestinal toxicity. They work by inhibiting the enzyme (COX-2) that acts as a catalyst for the formation of the prostaglandins, which are thought to be responsible for the GI toxicity. They appear to have analgesic benefits comparable to standard NSAIDs, and were widely used until an increased risk of myocardial infarction and stroke was noted amongst users. Analysis confirmed a link, and most COX-2 inhibitors have now been removed from the market. This also prompted retrospective analysis of patients treated with non-selective NSAIDs to assess their cardiovascular risk. There appeared to be less of a link in NSAIDs than with COX-2 inhibitors; however, they should be used with caution in those with underlying cardiovascular or cerebrovascular disease, as there is a small increased risk of thrombotic events (such as myocardial infarction or stroke) with long-term regular use of NSAIDs.

Further Reading

McNicol E, Strassels S, Goudas L, Lau J, Carr D (2015). NSAIDs or paracetamol, alone or combined with opioids, for cancer pain (Review). *Cochrane Database of Systematic Reviews* 1: CD005180.

173. E) Octreotide by continuous subcutaneous infusion

In bowel obstruction oral medications will not always be absorbed, hence parenteral medications should be used. Octreotide helps stimulate water and electrolyte reabsorption, and reduces secretions into the small bowel, and therefore may be useful to reduce her distension and large volume secretions.

Chlorpromazine may be helpful for intractable hiccups, often caused by phrenic nerve irritation, but is not useful in this situation, and may be very sedating. Metoclopramide is avoided in complete obstruction as it will worsen colicky pain; however, it can sometimes be used in patients with functional or incomplete obstruction. The effect of starting metoclopramide should be observed and it should be discontinued if it is ineffective or if there is any increase in gut colic. Levomepromazine is a very useful antiemetic for intractable nausea; but this patient's nausea is well controlled with cyclizine, therefore she is unlikely to gain anything other than side effects with this addition. Ketamine is a powerful drug that is often used for those with severe pain on large doses of opioids, but is generally given for short courses only, under specialist supervision. It would not help this woman's symptoms.

Tutorial

Malignant bowel obstruction is a common presentation for patients with a variety of intra-abdominal malignancies, particularly those with multiple peritoneal deposits, such as ovarian, colorectal, or lobular breast cancer, and peritoneal mesothelioma. Many patients will have episodes of subacute obstruction first, or episodes of obstruction which settle quickly with conservative management. However, this can progress, and bowel obstruction is a terminal event for many patients with intra-abdominal malignancy. Bowel obstruction may occur because of disease progression (peritoneal/serosal/bowel disease), previous surgery (adhesions), or previous radiation treatment. Although it is most commonly caused by disease, up to 10% of patients with active cancer will have a benign cause for obstruction, usually adhesions. Severe constipation, as a result of drugs such as anti-cholinergics and opioid analgesics, may mimic obstruction.

Typically, bowel obstruction occurs due to extrinsic occlusion of the bowel lumen, from disease pressing on or infiltrating the serosal surface, although it may also be secondary to intraluminal occlusion due to obstructing colorectal primaries (which may be the first presentation of malignancy). Those with disseminated peritoneal disease will often have multiple levels of obstruction, which may involve both the small and large bowel.

In obstruction, the bowel becomes distended, both from the bowel contents, and from the additional accumulation of non-absorbed bowel secretions. As the bowel becomes increasingly distended, it stimulates increased secretion of intestinal fluid. This then stimulates an inflammatory response in the bowel, which may involve release of prostaglandins and vasoactive intestinal peptide (VIP), causing further bowel wall oedema. Patients may develop 'third-spacing' loss of fluids due to fluid build-up in the abdomen; this may cause relative hypotension, particularly if they are not receiving intravenous hydration.

Patients with unresolving bowel obstruction are at risk of complications such as electrolyte imbalance, acid/base disturbance, and (rarely, but most seriously) perforation. This is an often fatal complication, with the risk increasing as the degree of bowel distension increases. Those with a single level of obstruction and a reasonable life expectancy otherwise may benefit from surgery to create a stoma above the level of obstruction. Surgery should also be performed in those for whom a benign cause (such as adhesions) is suspected, although it should be noted that disseminated small volume peritoneal disease might be missed on CT scans.

For palliative patients being treated conservatively, particularly when the obstruction is distal (i.e. distal small intestine and large intestine), parenteral medications can generally relieve symptoms without the need for a nasogastric tube and intravenous fluids. For more proximal obstructions, a nasogastric tube can be inserted to drain the stomach and decompress the bowel, and is generally effective in reducing the vomiting. Most patients will have some degree of pain and nausea, and should be given medications by the subcutaneous route by preference, to ensure absorption. This is often done using a 24-hour infusion by syringe driver, with agents such as morphine, diamorphine, or oxycodone for pain, together with an antiemetic such as haloperidol or cyclizine. Levomepromazine can be helpful in intractable nausea, but is sedating. Despite a negligible evidence base, dexamethasone is often used to reduce bowel oedema, but can increase the risk of bowel perforation, so should be used with caution. A trial of high dose dexamethasone (e.g. 12 mg) subcutaneously or intravenously (given as a single dose in the morning, or as a divided dose at morning and lunchtime) can be given for seven days. It can then be stopped if there has been no benefit, or weaned gradually if it has helped. Anti-muscarinic agents such as hyoscine hydrobromide, or hyoscine butylbromide, can reduce bowel colic and volume of secretions.

Those treated conservatively whose symptoms do not resolve within a week are unlikely to have spontaneous resolution of their obstruction. Selected patients (otherwise reasonable condition, chemotherapy naive, or those who have a high chance of responding to chemotherapy) may be considered for chemotherapy to resolve the obstruction, but this is not common. A venting gastrostomy may be considered for symptomatic relief in highly selected patients with problematic abdominal distension and vomiting; however, this is rarely necessary or appropriate in advanced cancer.

Further Reading

Twycross R, Wilcock A, Stark Toller C (2009). *Symptom Management in Advanced Cancer*, Fourth Edition. Palliativedrugs.com Ltd, Nottingham.

174. B) Morphine sulphate 90 mg plus metoclopramide 30 mg

The correct conversion from oral to parenteral (intravenous or subcutaneous) morphine is 0.5. This man has been taking an average of 180 mg per day (140 mg plus 40 mg top up), hence the appropriate dose would be 180/2 = 90 mg. This leaves B or C as the right answer. Lansoprazole is not given subcutaneously, therefore the correct answer is B.

Tutorial

Converting the dose of oral to parenteral morphine is required in patients who are going to be nil by mouth for significant lengths of time, those who cannot absorb oral medications, or those with intractable vomiting who cannot keep such medications down. Of the two parenteral routes, subcutaneous is preferred: it is comfortable; there is good absorption; it does not require intravenous access; and it can be used long term. Some drugs can cause skin irritation, so it is important to monitor the sites, and rotate the site of the subcutaneous needle. Drug syringes are generally changed once a day by district nurses when in the community.

Syringe drivers can be used for analgesics, antiemetics, or combinations. Not all drugs are compatible, so thought needs to be given to the most appropriate therapeutic combination (e.g. cyclizine tends to precipitate in combination with many other drugs).

Patients may have variable absorption of oral morphine, and therefore may require less or more parenteral morphine. The conversion factor of 0.5 is a guide, but individuals may differ. Diamorphine may be used in syringe drivers for those on large doses of opioids as it is much more soluble than morphine, and therefore smaller volumes are needed than the equivalent dose of morphine.

Further Reading

BMJ (2016). Prescribing in palliative care (2020). In *British National Formulary*. Seventy-Ninth Edition. BMJ Group and Pharmaceutical Press, London. Available at: https://bnf.nice.org.uk/guidance/prescribing-in-palliative-care.html

175. A) Alfentanil subcutaneous infusion

This patient requires an opioid which does not have predominantly renally excreted metabolites, given her renal impairment and described opioid toxicity. Although oxycodone has predominant hepatic clearance, it still has renally excreted metabolites and therefore this is not the best option. Intravenous pethidine will not give good analgesic coverage as it has a very short half-life; in addition, its metabolites are also renally excreted. Ketamine will not help her sedation or replace her opioid, so is not appropriate. A fentanyl patch would have been a good alternative if her pain had been stable and well controlled, but her pain has been problematic, and the long duration (changed every 72 hours) makes titration more difficult. Alfentanil is a good choice as it can be given as a subcutaneous infusion, therefore providing constant analgesia, and is predominantly hepatically cleared.

Tutorial

Approximately 20% of cancer patients have a baseline creatinine clearance of <60 ml/min, and many others will have fluctuating renal impairment as a result of hydronephrosis/ureteric blockage, post chemotherapy with nephrotoxic agents, or dehydration with significant vomiting or diarrhoea. A number of opioids and their metabolites can accumulate and cause toxicity, and therefore renal function should always be considered when choosing analgesia.

Meta-analyses have shown that those with a creatinine less than 1.5 × upper limit of normal did not have any increased risk of severe toxicity with morphine, although they may be more at risk of associated nausea and vomiting. Above this creatinine level, there was a much higher risk of accumulation, but there is little data on these patients as most were treated with alternative analgesics. The main toxicity in those with more significant renal failure was neurological: they experienced myoclonus, decreased levels of consciousness, and depressed respiratory function. Opiate toxicity responds well to naloxone treatment but the duration may need to be prolonged as the drug will take a long time to clear the body.

Alfentanil is a good alternative to morphine, and several small studies have shown patients with renal impairment who developed toxicity on morphine were able to be switched to alfentanil with resolution of both pain and toxicity. Half of these patients who were later switched back to oral opioids developed recurrent opioid toxicity within 48 hours.

Fentanyl is another useful alternative, but its short half-life means that repeated injections are required. It can be used as a transdermal patch for stable pain, but titration can be more difficult than with other opioids due to prolonged duration and limited variability of patch sizes. A small study showed that almost 60% of patients with low GFRs (median of 25 ml/min) who switched to fentanyl due to opioid-induced toxicity had resolution of their symptoms.

Oxycodone has less renal clearance than morphine, but can still accumulate in significant renal impairment, as can its metabolites noroxycodone and oxymorphone. A prospective trial of a small number of patients with a creatinine clearance of <60 ml/min who switched from morphine to oxycodone achieved adequate pain control with the latter, and fewer (but not none) reported opiate toxicity. The main toxicities noted were confusion, nausea, and increased sedation.

Pethidine itself is not renally cleared, but its metabolite norpethidine is, and therefore accumulates in renal impairment. The adverse effects of this accumulation can include myoclonus, confusion, seizures, and death. The CNS toxicity does not respond well to naloxone reversal.

Further Reading

King S, Forbes K, Hanks G, Ferro C, Chambers E, et al. (2011). A systematic review of the use of opioid medication for those with moderate to severe cancer pain and renal impairment: a European Palliative Care Research Collaborative opioid guidelines project. *Palliative Medicine* 25: 525–552.

176. B) Oxycontin 30 mg bd and OxyNorm 10 mg PRN

The appropriate conversion factor from morphine to oxycodone is 0.5: that is, 10 mg morphine is equivalent to 5 mg of oxycodone, therefore the correct answer is 0.5 × 60 mg = 30 mg bd.

The breakthrough dose remains one sixth of the total daily dose: that is, 30 + 30 mg = 60 mg and ⅙ of this is 10 mg; therefore the appropriate answer is 30 mg bd plus 10 mg PRN.

Importantly, it is worth noting that conversion ratios are never more than an approximate guide because of a number of factors, including the wide variation in opioid pharmacokinetics between individuals. Many sources recommend commencing the new opioid at the equianalgesic dose based on the accepted conversion factor as described above. However, other sources recommend routinely reducing the calculated equivalent dose of the new opioid by 25–50%, then modifying that reduction by taking various patient factors into account, such that the reduction can be removed (e.g. young patient, no undesirable effects, in severe pain, switching at low dose) or increased further (e.g. older patient, delirium, switching at high dose). In the above example, the patient has had intolerable side effects from morphine, hence a dose reduction could be considered; however, he is relatively young, and has had problems with pain when his morphine has been reduced, hence switching opioids without a dose reduction is reasonable.

Tutorial

Each patient will respond slightly differently to a change in opioids, but Table 8.6 is a *guide* to conversion factors for opioids. Note that renal function or metastatic disease in the liver should always be taken into account when choosing alternative opioids, especially in the face of intolerable side effects. When re-titrating patients who have been changed to long-acting preparations, remember that it will take time for the appropriate steady-state concentration in the blood to be reached, and therefore do not change the long-acting dose more often than every 2–3 days.

Table 8.6 Approximate conversions between various opiates

Opioid	Conversion from oral morphine	Approximately equivalent dose to 30 mg oral morphine/24 hours
Alfentanil (S/C)	Divide by 30	1 mg/24 hours
Diamorphine (IV/SC)	Divide by 3	10 mg/24 hours
Codeine	Multiply by 10	300 mg/24 hours (> max daily dose)
Fentanyl (transdermal)	*	25 mcg/hour every 72 hours
Morphine IV/SC	Divide by 2	15 mg/24 hours
Oxycodone PO	Divide by 2	15 mg/24 hours
Oxycodone IV/SC	Divide by 4	7.5 mg/24 hours

*There exists a wide consensus on the exact equivalents between oral morphine and transdermal fentanyl. Specialist advice is often suggested when making these changes.

Further Reading

Mercadante S, Caraceni A (2011). Conversion ratios for opioid switching in the treatment of cancer pain: a systematic review. *Palliative Medicine* 25: 504–515.

Twycross R, Wilcock A (eds) (2011). *PCF4—Palliative Care Formulary*, Fourth Edition. Palliativedrugs. com Ltd, Nottingham.

177. An 83-year-old man was seen for a routine follow-up in the heart failure clinic. He had suffered a **NSTEMI** a year previously, which was managed medically. He was stable clinically and had no further anginal symptoms but reported that he felt he was 'growing breasts'. His past medical history included gout, eczema, and diabetes. His medication included metformin, allopurinol, bisoprolol, ramipril, furosemide, isosorbide mononitrate, spironolactone, simvastatin, and aspirin. On examination he had gynaecomastia. He had no loss of hair and his testicles were of normal size.

```
Investigations:
    Hb                      136 g/L
    WCC                     7.6 × 10⁹/L
    Creatinine              86 µmol/L
    Urea                    8.3 mmol/L
    Sodium                  133 mmol/L
    Potassium               4.5 mmol/L
    AST                     67 iU/L
    ALT                     57 iU/L
    ALP                     57 iU/L
    Bilirubin               7 µmol/L
    Albumin                 44 g/L
    Protein                 66 g/l
    ECG:                    left ventricular hypertrophy
```

What is the most likely cause of his gynaecomastia?

A. Bisoprolol

B. Furosemide

C. Liver cirrhosis

D. Ramipril

E. Spironolactone

178. **A 45-year-old woman of African origin was admitted to hospital with a two-day history of watery diarrhoea and vomiting. She had a past medical history of depression, hepatitis B, type II diabetes, and HIV. Her CD4+ count in clinic a week before admission was 450. On examination she had a blood pressure of 85/60 mmHg, pulse rate of 120, respiratory rate of 28, and a temperature of 37.4°C. Her JVP was not visible. Her abdomen was soft with hyperactive bowel sounds, and a PR revealed no blood in the rectum. She was managed conservatively and fluid resuscitated. No organisms were grown from stool cultures and viral PCR was also negative.**

Her condition improved significantly and by the fourth day she was euvolaemic and haemodynamically stable with a pulse rate of 74 beats per minute, blood pressure of 125/85 mmHg, a respiratory rate of 22, and a temperature of 36.5°C. A diagnosis of resolved viral gastroenteritis was made. Her bloods were reviewed prior to discharge.

Investigations:
These are shown in Table 9.1.

Table 9.1 Investigations

	Admission	Day 4
Hb	104 g/L	107 g/L
WCC	10.1 ($\times$ 10^9/L)	8.44 $\times$ 10^9/L
Platelets	260 ($\times$ 10^9/L)	310 $\times$ 10^9/L
CRP	44 mg/L	4 mg/L
Creatinine	179 µmol/L	108 µmol/L
Urea	12.4 mmol/L	4.9 mmol/L
Sodium	148 mmol/L	135 mmol/L
Potassium	2.6 mmol/L	3.1 mmol/L
Blood glucose	4.8 mmol/L	7.1 mmol/L
Corrected calcium	2.26 mmol/L	1.93 mmol/L
Phosphate	0.7 mmol/L	0.65 mmol/L
Venous blood gas		
pH	7.24	7.31
Lactate	3.1 mmol/L	0.4 mmol/L
Bicarbonate	12 mmol/L	16 mmol/L
Chloride	120 mmol/L	112 mmol/L
Urine dipstick		
Glucose	++	++
Ketones	—	—
WCC	—	—
RBC	—	—
Nitrites	—	—
Protein	+	+

What is the underlying cause of the patient's biochemical abnormalities on discharge?

A. DKA

B. HAART

C. Myeloma

D. Refeeding syndrome

E. Resolving dehydration

179. **A 13-year-old boy was brought to A&E collapsed and hypotensive having been found in his room by his mother drowsy and confused. There was vomit over his sheets, along with both urine and diarrhoea. He had no past medical history and was fine earlier in the day having spent it playing with his friends in fields near his house. His observations revealed a pulse of 45 beats per minute, blood pressure of 85/55 mmHg, a respiratory rate of 8 breaths per minute, and saturations of 88% on room air. On examination he was unresponsive to voice and only grunted in response to pain, though he was drooling excessively. His pupils were small, constricted, and non-responsive to light. He was not moving his limbs but fasciculations were noted. Auscultation of his chest revealed a widespread wheeze. He was cardiovascularly resuscitated.**

```
Investigations:
Arterial blood gas on room air
   pO2                      9.4 kPa
   pCO2                     5.5 kPa
   pH                       7.33
   Sodium                   134 mmol/L
   Potassium                3.8 mmol/L
   HCO3-                    21 mmol/L
   Glucose                  18 mmol/L
   ECG:                     sinus rhythm, rate 45 beats per minute
```

Given the likely diagnosis, which one of these options is the *least* appropriate management option?

A. Give IV adrenaline

B. Give IV atropine

C. Make attempts to contact and check up on the boy's friend who he was playing with

D. Prompt anaesthetic review for consideration of invasive ventilation

E. Remove all clothing and clean skin with water and soap

180. An 84-year-old man was admitted to hospital from a nursing home with increasing confusion and agitation. On admission he was pyrexial, hypotensive, and had pyuria. Blood tests revealed a raised white cell count and CRP. He was treated empirically for urosepsis with intravenous fluids and co-amoxiclav, and his long-term urinary catheter was replaced. His past medical history included COPD, ischaemic heart disease, stroke, benign prostatic hyperplasia, depression, and vascular dementia. His regular medications were clopidogrel, mirtazapine, simvastatin, and salbutamol inhaler. During admission, whilst his observations and inflammatory markers were settling, he remained agitated and confused. He often wandered the ward and was also quite aggressive, particularly at night, when he was given intramuscular sedation on numerous occasions.

A few days later he was a found lying flat in bed covered in sweat. His observations showed a pulse rate of 100 beats per minute, a blood pressure of 180/95 mmHg, a respiratory rate of 24, saturations of 99% on room air, and a temperature of 38.7°C. His eyes were open and followed staff as they moved around his bed, but when speaking he was only able to utter a few incomprehensible words. He was also noted to be very difficult to move into any position, with movements being slow globally and uncoordinated. His reflexes were normal. His heart sounds were normal, his chest was clear, and his abdomen was soft.

```
Investigations:
   Hb                      137 g/L
   WCC                     12.3 × 10⁹/L
   Creatinine              105 µmol/L
   Urea                    10.4 mmol/L
   Sodium                  139 mmol/L
   Potassium               3.9 mmol/L
   Blood glucose           8.8 mmol/L
   Creatinine kinase       755 iU/L
```

Admission urine and blood cultures: *E. coli* resistant to trimethoprim and amoxicillin. Intermediate sensitivity to co-amoxiclav. Sensitive to nitrofurantoin.

What is the most likely cause of his current clinical situation?

A. Encephalitis

B. Neuroleptic malignant syndrome

C. Serotonin syndrome

D. Subdural haemorrhage

E. Worsening of urosepsis

181. A 19-year-old woman was admitted to hospital following ingestion of over 35 paracetamol tablets the previous day. Despite treatment with N-acetylcysteine and intravenous fluids, her liver function and renal function continued to deteriorate and she required transfer to critical care.

With regards to transplantation in liver failure associated with paracetamol overdose, which one of the following statements is *not true*?

A. A dose of paracetamol less than 150 mg/kg is unlike to cause hepatotoxicity
B. A patient should be listed for transplantation if after fluid resuscitation the pH is less than 7.3 or lactate is >3.0 mmol/L
C. If a patient is listed for transplantation, it is common practice to continue NAC infusion until PT returns to normal or until transplantation has occurred
D. If within the same 24-hour period the patient has a PT of more than 100 seconds (or INR of >6.5) and a creatinine of more than 300 mmol/L, the patient should be listed for liver transplant
E. Prothrombin time is the earliest indicator of hepatic impairment in paracetamol toxicity

182. A 64-year-old man was reviewed following admission to hospital two weeks previously with a severe chest infection and acute kidney injury. He had a past medical history of hypertension, hypercholesterolaemia, and 40-pack year smoking history. During the admission, he was treated with intravenous antibiotics and fluids but then developed signs of fluid overload. A chest X-ray showed cardiomegaly and an ECG showed left bundle branch block. A diagnosis of underlying heart failure was made and the patient was started on appropriate treatment and cardiology follow-up arranged. Since discharge, the patient reported that whilst his breathing and cough had improved he felt extremely fatigued, more so than when he left hospital. On examination he was haemodynamically stable but had pitting oedema to his mid shins.

```
Investigations:
  Hb                    120 g/L
  MCV                   89 fL
  WCC                   9.1 × 10⁹/L
  Creatinine            96 µmol/L
  Urea                  6.8 mmol/L
  Sodium                141 mmol/L
  Potassium             4.8 mmol/L
  TSH                   0.3 mu/L (0.4–5.0 mU/L)
  Serum freeT4          9 pmol/L (10–22 pmol/L)
  HbA1c                 40 mmol/mol (20–42 mmol/mol)
```

What is the most likely explanation for the patient's fatigue?

A. Anaemia
B. Heart failure
C. Hypothyroidism
D. Side effect of medication
E. Silent myocardial infarction

183. A 54-year-old man of Southeast Asian origin presented with severe pain in his right big toe. The pain had come on in the preceding days and was throbbing in nature. He reported the pain was worse at night and even a touch from the bed sheets was excruciating. His past medical history, for which he took medication, included hypertension, diabetes, chronic kidney disease, pulmonary tuberculosis, for which he had started treatment over a month previously, asthma, and osteoarthritis. His big toe on his right foot was grossly swollen, erythematous, and very tender to touch.

Investigations:

Hb	115 g/L
MCV	65 fL
WCC	4.4 × 10⁹/L
Platelets	660 × 10⁹/L
Sodium	141 mmol/L
Potassium	4.9 mmol/L
Urea	7.1 mmol/L
Creatinine	155 µmol/L
AST	85 iU/L
ALT	107 iU/L
ALP	114 iU/L
Bilirubin	15 µmol/L
Albumin	41 g/L
CRP	27 mg/L
Urate	880 µmol/L
HbA1c	66 mmol/mol (20–42 mmol/mol)

Given the likely diagnosis, what is the most likely precipitant?

A. Ethambutol

B. Hepatitis

C. Myeloproliferative disorder

D. Pyrazinamide

E. Thiazide diuretics

184. **A 68-year-old male was brought to casualty having been found
collapsed at home by a neighbour. He had recently been diagnosed
with stage IV lung cancer with bony metastases. His past medical
history included COPD, ischaemic heart disease, hypertension,
chronic kidney disease, depression, and benign prostate hyperplasia.
His medication included a salbutamol inhaler, a Seretide inhaler,
amlodipine, ramipril, aspirin, amitriptyline, paracetamol, tramadol,
and tamsulosin.**

On examination he was unresponsive to voice or pain. He had a regular
pulse of 120 beats per minute, a blood pressure of 85/55 mmHg, a
temperature of 38.2°C, a respiratory rate of eight breaths per minute,
and saturations on room air of 92%. He was peripherally warm. His
pupils were dilated and responded sluggishly to light. Heart sounds
were normal and his chest was clear on auscultation. His abdomen was
soft but bowel sounds were absent and there was a palpable bladder.
Catherization revealed a residual of 1.5 litres of urine.

```
Investigations:
    Hb                       110 g/L
    WCC                      12.6 × 10⁹/L
    Platelets                540 × 10⁹/L
    Sodium                   139 mmol/L
    Potassium                3.1 mmol/L
    Urea                     8.9 mmol/L
    Creatinine               137 µmol/L
    ALT                      24 iU/L
    ALP                      84 iU/L
    Bilirubin                17 µmol/L
    Albumin                  32 g/L
    CRP                      46 mg/L
    CK                       765 iU/L
Arterial blood gas:
    pO₂                      7.6 kPa
    pCO₂                     6.4 kPa
    pH                       7.22
    HCO₃⁻                    8 mmol/L
    Lactate                  5.1 mmol/L
    Urine dipstick           blood ++ protein + leucocytes ++
```

**The patient was resuscitated as per advanced life support protocol and
was given oxygen and IV fluids.**

Given the likely diagnosis, what is the best next management?

A. Intravenous antibiotics

B. Intravenous sodium bicarbonate infusion

C. Naloxone

D. Non-invasive ventilation

E. Withdraw treatment as the patient has stage IV lung cancer

185. **A 66-year-old man was referred to the endocrine clinic with suspected thyroid disease. His only symptom was of weight loss. He reported no recent illnesses. His past medical history included ischaemic heart disease and atrial fibrillation for which he was started on amiodarone a few months previously. His other medications included ramipril, aspirin, and simvastatin. The only significant findings on examination were a pulse rate of 100 beats per minute and that he was very slim. He had no neck swelling and no signs of thyroid eye disease.**

```
Investigations:
    Serum free T4          34 pmol/L (10-22 pmol/L)
    Serum free T3          3.3 pmol/L (3-7 pmol/L)
    TSH                    0.3 mu/L (0.4-3.6 mu/L)
    Anti-TPO               negative
    Anti-TSH               negative
```

What is the next step for managing the abnormal thyroid function?

A. Carbimazole

B. Prednisolone

C. Repeat thyroid function test in six months

D. Stop amiodarone

E. Sub-total thyroidectomy

186. A 44-year-old man who was known to suffer from alcoholic liver cirrhosis was admitted to hospital with decompensated liver disease. On examination he was jaundiced, had extensive bruising on his arms, signs of gross fluid overloaded with pitting oedema up to his nipples, ascites, and bilateral pleural effusions. Whilst agitated and a little confused he was still able to communicate and follow instructions. He reported significant pain due to gross scrotal oedema and had thus far received no analgesia.

```
Investigations:
    Hb                        104 g/L
    WCC                       7.3 × 10⁹/L
    Platelets                 44 × 10⁹/L
    Sodium                    125 mmol/L
    Potassium                 4.4 mmol/L
    Urea                      2.4 mmol/L
    Creatinine                88 µmol/L
    ALT                       70 iU/L
    ALP                       212 iU/L
    Bilirubin                 65 µmol/L
    Albumin                   22 g/L
    CRP                       12 mg/L
    Corrected calcium         2.31 mmol/L
    INR                       1.6
```

What is the initial safest course of action with regards to the patient's pain?

A. Hold prescription of any analgesia as risks outweigh benefits and provide a scrotal brace

B. PRN codeine—30 mg qds PO

C. PRN ibuprofen—300 mg tds PO

D. PRN paracetamol—1 g tds PO/IV

E. PRN—short acting oral morphine sulphate solution 5 mg four hourly

187. **A 78-year-old man was referred to the memory clinic because his wife noticed a worsening of his memory in the preceding few months. She reported that he often got lost at the supermarket when out shopping and frequently forgot meeting people or having already done things earlier in the day. The patient was otherwise healthy and had a past medical history of osteoarthritis and psoriasis for which he took occasional analgesia and used regular emollients. On examination he had no focal neurology but had an MMSE of 18/30. Investigations showed no reversible causes of cognitive impairment and following a detailed clinical assessment, a diagnosis of Alzheimer's dementia was made.**

With regards to treatment in dementia, which of the following statements is true?

A. A patient's MMSE should be 10–20 in order for them to be started on an acetylcholinesterase inhibitor

B. Currently, only four acetylcholinesterase inhibitors (donepezil, galantamine, memantine, and rivastigmine) are recommended for use in Alzheimer's dementia

C. In cases where there are co-existing pathologies accounting for the dementia, treatment should take into account, and be aimed at, all causes

D. Normal CT imaging of the head rules out vascular dementia

E. Patients with vascular dementia should only be started on acetylcholinesterase inhibitors if their cognitive impairment is mild

188. **A 66-year-old man presented with melaena. His past medical history included diabetes, atrial fibrillation, osteoarthritis, and eczema for which he took warfarin, gliclazide, and metformin, with occasional paracetamol and NSAID use. He was also penicillin allergic. He reported being generally well but unfortunately had developed a skin infection for which his GP prescribed him an oral antibiotic after creams failed to work. On examination he was haemodynamically stable and the only examination finding of note was melaena on digital rectal examination.**

Investigations:

Hb	94 g/L
WCC	12.1 × 10⁹/L
Platelets	355 × 10⁹/L
Sodium	134 mmol/L
Potassium	4.2 mmol/L
Urea	22 mmol/L
Creatinine	134 μmol/L
ALT	72 iU/L
AST	58 iU/L
ALP	254 iU/L
Bilirubin	12 μmol/L
Albumin	44 g/L
INR	7.4

What is the likely cause of his raised INR?

A. Acute liver failure

B. Ciprofloxacin

C. Erythromycin

D. Fluconazole

E. Metronidazole

189. A 52-year-old female was referred with polydipsia and polyuria. She reported passing up to five litres of fluid a day. Her past medical history included hypertension and bipolar disorder for which she took lithium.

```
Investigations:
    Sodium                    146 mmol/L
    Potassium                 3.9 mmol/L
    Urea                      2.4 mmol/L
    Creatinine                89 µmol/L
    Blood glucose             12 mmol/L
    Corrected calcium         2.36 mmol/L
    Urine dipstick            glucose—ketones—protein +
Water deprivation test and desmopressin challenge is shown in
Table 9.2.
```

Table 9.2 Water deprivation test and desmopressin challenge

	At 0 minutes	At 360 minutes	Eight hours post-desmopressin
Plasma osmolality (mOsm/L)	302	325	320
Urine osmolality (mOsm/L)	185	186	264

What is the most appropriate management strategy?

A. Fluid restriction

B. Start amiloride

C. Start DDAVP nasal spray

D. Stop lithium

E. Start oral hypoglycaemic agents

190. A 74-year-old lady with a past medical history of hypertension, diabetes, and gastritis was admitted to hospital with a pneumonia and a swollen leg. She was treated with antibiotics but was also found to have a **DVT** and subsequently treated with subcutaneous **LMWH**: tinzaparin (175 units/kg) with a view to converting to warfarin in the community. Two days later, a few hours after she had her tinzaparin injection, she had a large volume of frank haematemesis and became haemodynamically unstable. A gastric ulcer was suspected. She was cardiovascularly resuscitated with blood transfusions and prepared her for emergency endoscopy.

```
Investigations:
   Hb                      102 g/L
   WCC                     16.1 × 10⁹/L
   Platelets               170 × 10⁹/L
   CRP                     123 mg/L
   Sodium                  136 mmol/L
   Potassium               4.1 mmol/L
   Urea                    25.4 mmol/L
   Creatinine              160 µmol/L
   INR                     1.5
   PT                      19 seconds
   APTT                    56 seconds
```

What is the best management of her coagulopathy?

A. Conservative management and allow clearance of LMWH

B. Fresh frozen plasma only

C. Intravenous phytonadione

D. Intravenous protamine sulphate

E. Prothrombin complex concentrate

191. A 63-year-old man presented with fatigue following a primary **PCI** for acute **ST-elevation myocardial infarction** six weeks previously. He reported that whilst pain free, he was struggling to return to his normal activities. On further assessment he revealed that he felt persistently low in mood and motivation, with a reduced interest in his previous hobbies. He felt quite hopeless about the future and had developed persistent negative thoughts about himself. He denied any suicidal ideation or thoughts of self-harm. He also stated that he was sleeping poorly.

What is the most appropriate treatment option?

A. Citalopram

B. Imipramine

C. Selegiline

D. Sertraline

E. Venlafaxine

192. A 28-year-old woman presented to A&E with thoughts of harming her children. She said she had been having a recurring and disturbing thought that she might kill her youngest child. The thoughts were associated with feelings of anxiety and palpitations. She felt that she would never harm her children and that she would rather harm herself than see them come to harm. She got the thought every few days. When she got this thought she asked her partner for reassurance that she was not a bad person. She said that her mood had been affected by these thoughts and at times she felt low. She denied any other psychiatric symptoms. On examination, she was noted to be fidgety and the skin on her hands appeared cracked and red.

What would be the most appropriate form of psychological treatment for this condition?

A. Cognitive analytic therapy
B. Cognitive behaviour therapy with behavioural activation
C. Dialectic behaviour therapy
D. Exposure and response prevention
E. Psychodynamic psychotherapy

193. A 54-year-old man with stage I Huntington's disease was seen in A&E following an overdose of paracetamol. He said that for the last four weeks he had been feeling increasingly depressed. He described a lack of enjoyment in his life and a lack of energy. He felt that his situation was hopeless and saw no point in living. He also described a lack of motivation to get things done at home and had not been attending to his self-care. He said that he felt that his mood had deteriorated recently but couldn't understand why. He had experienced some falls over the eight weeks prior to his presentation and was seen by a neurologist and started on medication to manage his motor symptoms. On examination, there was mild psychomotor slowing and minimal chorea.

Which medication is most likely to be associated with this presentation?

A. Citalopram
B. Haloperidol
C. Mirtazapine
D. Risperidone
E. Tetrabenazine

194. A 24-year-old woman presented with a feeling of palpitations, muscle cramps, and fatigue. She had been feeling this way for several months, but symptoms had worsened recently. When asked about her appetite she reported being careful with her food as she didn't like putting on weight. She admitted having difficulty controlling how much she ate on occasions, and that she had worked out ways of dealing with these episodes. On examination her pulse was irregular and on neurological examination there was generalized symmetrical muscle weakness. Her BMI was 27 and she had calluses on the knuckles of her right hand.

What is the most appropriate pharmacological treatment this patient's psychiatric diagnosis?

A. Citalopram
B. Fluoxetine
C. Mirtazapine
D. Olanzapine
E. Venlafaxine

195. A 26-year-old woman was brought to A&E by her family who were concerned about her mental state. In the preceding two weeks she had been acting bizarrely and not sleeping. The patient reported feeling very good. She said that she simply had too many ideas and she spent most of the night writing them down. She also felt full of energy and regularly ran long distances to burn off some of her energy. She said that many of her ideas came directly from God with whom she believed that she had a unique relationship. She described hearing God speak directly to her at night. She had difficulty accepting that her experiences might be due to any form of illness. With some encouragement from her family she agreed to take some medication but was adamant that she did not want to put on weight.

Which medication would be most appropriate in this case for long-term management of her symptoms?

A. Aripiprazole
B. Diazepam
C. Lithium
D. Olanzapine
E. Sodium Valproate

177. E) Spironolactone

Spironolactone is commonly associated with gynaecomastia, with some studies reporting a prevalence of nearly 10%. Spironolactone has been postulated to cause gynaecomastia in a multitude of ways: by competing for binding site and displacing oestradiol from sex hormone-binding globulin, by decreasing testosterone production, and increasing peripheral conversion of testosterone to oestradiol. These effects are unsurprising given that spironolactone is a mineralocorticoid and is structurally related to sex steroids such 17-hydroxyprogesterone. Eplerenone is a newer more selective mineralocorticoid receptor antagonist that has a different structure to spironolactone and other androgens. Unsurprisingly, it has fewer anti-androgynous side effects and thus is often used when patients suffer from side effects of spironolactone. Ramipril could also potentially cause gynaecomastia though this is less common. Liver cirrhosis, whilst a known cause of gynaecomastia due to impaired metabolism of oestrogens, is not the cause here. The patient has a mild transaminitis but no evidence of liver cirrhosis. Furosemide and bisoprolol are not known to cause gynaecomastia.

Tutorial

Many drugs are attributed to causing gynaecomastia in a dose dependent manner, the mechanisms of which are not always understood. These are summarized in Table 9.3.

Table 9.3 Summary of drugs that are attributed to causing gynaecomastia

Anti-hypertensive medication: • Potassium sparing diuretics, for example. spironolactone. • ACE inhibitors, for example enalapril and captopril. • Calcium channel antagonists, for example nifedipine, amlodipine, verapamil, and diltiazem. • Alpha blockers, for example. doxazosin and prazosin.	Drugs which interfere with testosterone metabolism/action: • Alpha-reductase inhibitors used in BPH, for example finasteride and dutasteride. • Androgen receptor blockers. • Chemotherapy drugs. • Inhibitors of testosterone production: for example metronidazole, ketoconazole. • Heavy cannabis use.
Exposure to excess oestrogens: • Exogenous steroid use, for example body builder. • Digitalis (mechanism poorly understood). • Oestrogen containing cosmetics.	By stimulating prolactin secretion: • Tricyclic antidepressants. • Opiates. • H2 antagonists, for example cimetidine, ranitidine. • Dopamine receptor blockers: atypical antipsychotics, for example risperidone, pro-kinetics, for example metoclopramide.

Further Reading

Niewoehner C, Schorer A (2008). Gynaecomastia and breast cancer in men. *British Medical Journal* 29(336) (March): 709–713.

178. B) HAART

The patient's initial biochemical profile is very much in keeping with a normal anion gap metabolic acidosis caused partly by lactic acidosis and renal impairment, both likely due to dehydration caused by the diarrhoea and vomiting.

The patient's bloods on day four illustrate a normal anion gap acidosis with hypophosphataemia, hypokalaemia, hypocalcaemia, and evidence of proteinuria and glycosuria. These findings are the hallmarks of proximal renal tubular dysfunction, sometimes called Fanconi's syndrome. The proximal tubule is the main site of absorption of many ions and molecules in the kidney, impairment of this apparatus thus leads to increased loss of sodium, bicarbonate, amino acids, glucose, and phosphate. Whilst impaired potassium absorption does occur at the proximal tubule, the main reason for hypokalaemia is preferential absorption of the excess sodium in the distal nephron at the expense of potassium.

The patient's bloods on day four could represent residual dehydration but the patient's euvolaemic status clinically, normal lactate, and normal creatinine and urea argue against this. Refeeding syndrome is very unlikely to occur in someone who has not eaten for so few days and there is no history of prior starvation. Whilst the patient is acidotic and has glucose in her urine, she has no history of diabetes, does not have ketones in her urine, has normal blood sugars, and lastly has a normal anion gap; DKA causes a raised anion gap.

Myeloma can potentially also cause Fanconi's syndrome due to light chain deposition in the proximal tubule causing subsequent toxicity. However, there a few factors that point against this. First, the patient's age is a bit young for myeloma. Second, the patient has a low calcium and you might expect this to be raised (or at least normal if there was indeed co-existing proximal tubule dysfunction) due to lytic bone lesions. Lastly, the patient has a normal renal function which you would not expect in myeloma with renal involvement. It should be noted that whilst the urine dipstick is negative, this does not exclude myeloma because of the low sensitivity in detecting urinary light chains. Indeed a negative dipstick can still be accompanied by a urinary protein in myeloma. Serum electrophoresis and serum free light chains would be the definitive tests to exclude multiple myeloma in this case. Urinary Bence-Jones protein has a low sensitivity.

Tutorial

There are various causes of proximal tubule syndrome ('Fanconi's syndrome) which are summarized in Table 9.4 Congenital causes present much earlier and you would expect a larger degree of clinical manifestations mainly due to ongoing hypophosphataemia, namely rickets. Whilst the exact metabolic abnormalities can vary between specific causes and the way in which they affect the proximal tubule, the condition does have some hallmark clinical and biochemical findings. These are summarized in Table 9.5

Table 9.4 Causes of Fanconi's syndrome

Acquired	Congenital
• Heavy metals—lead, mercury • Drugs—chemotherapy agents, for example HAART (tenofovir in particular seems to most frequently cause tubular dysfunction), tetracyclines, • Protein deposition: light chains deposition, for example myeloma, or amyloidosis • Interstitial nephritis • Sjögren's syndrome (though more commonly causes distal tubular dysfunction)	• Idiopathic • Cystinosis • Galactosaemia • Wilson's disease • Tyrosinaemia • Lowe's syndrome

Table 9.5 Clinical and biochemical features of Fanconi's syndrome

Clinical features	Biochemical features
• Polyuria • Polydipsia • Growth failure • Hypophosphataemic rickets/osteomalacia • Fractures (secondary to above) • Recurrent episodes of dehydration	Serum: • Hypophosphataemia • Hyperchloremic acidosis • Hypokalaemia Urine: • Hyperphosphaturia • Glycosuria • Amino-aciduria • Hyperuricosuria

Further Reading

Kurtzman N (2000). Renal tubular acidosis syndromes. *Southern Medical Journal* 93(11): 1042–1052.

179. A) Give IV adrenaline

The onset of this scenario is highly suggestive of an acute process, possibly a severe infection, anaphylaxis, or poisoning. Given the cardinal signs of parasympathetic over activity (pinpoint pupils, respiratory depression, excessive secretion, diarrhoea, and urinary incontinence), combined with the fact that he has been playing in fields near his house, organophosphate poisoning is the most likely diagnosis here.

Given this boy's critical state, prompt critical care review should be sought as intubation and ventilation is likely to be required. Treatment consists of removal of poison which can be absorbed through the skin (thus the rationale for removal of clothing and washing skin), fluid resuscitation, and treatment with anti-cholinergic drugs. Note, clinical staff should take great care to avoid contaminating themselves and personal protective equipment should be worn. Atropine, a muscarinic antagonist, is usually given every ten minutes at a dose of 20 µg/kg in children until there is evidence that peripheral perfusion has returned and bradycardia has begun to resolve. Drug therapy should not be titrated to pupil response which is not thought to be as sensitive as assessment of cardiovascular status.

In cases of moderate to severe poisoning pralidoxime chloride, a cholinesterase activator, can also be given on the advice of a clinical toxicologist. This is particularly important where there is respiratory compromise as atropine, a muscarinic receptor antagonist, will have no effect on nicotinic receptors. Intubation may still be necessary as these receptors may have desensitized as they have been overstimulated for a prolonged period. Adrenaline may help to increase heart rate and blood pressure, but is unlikely to overcome the remaining cholinergic effects or mask the clinical response to atropine and is likely to increase the risk of tachyarrhythmias.

Tutorial

Symptoms of organophosphate poisoning occur due to over activation of the parasympathetic system. This occurs due to direct inhibition of anti-cholinesterase enzymes by the organophosphates which normally break down acetylcholine at synapses. It is worth noting, that sarin ('nerve gas') which is used in chemical warfare is an organophosphorus compound and also a very potent inhibitor of acetylcholinesterase. Symptoms can vary depending on exposure but include:

Mild

• Excess secretions: lacrimation/salivation
• Headache/nausea

- Mild muscle weakness/localized twitching
- Mild agitation
- Blurry vision
- Constricted/pinpoint pupils

Moderate

- Excess secretions: lacrimation/salivation
- Coughing/wheezing
- Dyspnoea
- Pinpoint pupils
- Dizziness/confusion
- Vomiting
- Urinary incontinence
- Diarrhoea
- Marked weakness with muscle twitching

Severe

- Copious excess secretions
- Respiratory depression or respiratory arrest
- Pinpoint pupils
- Confusion and agitation
- Collapse/coma
- Flaccid paralysis
- Seizures (can be masked due to flaccid paralysis and can be unmasked with treatment)
- Cardiac arrhythmias
- Death

A good mnemonic to remember is DUMBELLS (Diarrhoea, Urination, Miosis, Bronchospasm, Emesis, Lethargy, Lacrimation, and Seizures).

Further Reading

BMJ Group (2016). Emergency treatments of poisoning. *British National Formulary*, Seventieth Edition. BMJ Group and Pharmaceutical Press, London.

Roberts D, Aaron C (2007). Clinical review: management of acute organophosphorus pesticide poisoning. *British Medical Journal* 334: 629–634.

180. B) Neuroleptic malignant syndrome

This scenario, a septic confused patient receiving sedation whilst aggressive at night, is all too common in hospitals. The patient's initial presentation is quite clearly due to severe urosepsis which is evident by the patient's clinical symptoms of shock, raised inflammatory markers, and acute kidney injury. Delirium, however, can persist long after the infection has improved, especially in patients with known dementia.

On the day of review, the patient's delirium has switched from hyperactive to hypoactive. He exhibits hyperthermia, tachycardia, hypertension, profuse sweating, rigidity on examination, a raised white blood cell count, and rising creatinine kinase (CK). In the context of repeated administration of sedation, likely haloperidol, neuroleptic malignant syndrome (NMS) is the most likely cause. Serotonin syndrome is a strong differential for NMS and presents similarly but is unlikely given the short timescale and the fact that there is no indication that the mirtazapine is new. Furthermore, serotonin syndrome is associated with nausea and vomiting, shivering, and neurologically, whilst rigidity is present, there is invariably some degree of ataxia and clonus which are not present here.

The causative organism shows intermediate resistance to co-amoxiclav which in the context of worsening of delirium and pyrexia may suggest worsening of urosepsis, a septic patient on ineffective antibiotics therapy would have continued low blood pressure and rising inflammatory markers. The rising CK would also not occur and so option B is unlikely. Encephalitis is very unlikely given the presentation but is important to consider. It can cause confusion, agitation, pyrexia, and tachycardia; it can be present with very little systemic markers of inflammation. Tonic-clonic seizures might also be causing rhabdomyolysis which may explain the raised CK. However, one would hope that seizures would have come to the attention of the ward's clinical staff. A subdural haemorrhage could account for some of the features seen here. The raised CK may have occurred if a patient has fallen and been on the floor for some time. However, given the patient is in hospital and is known to be confused, it is unlikely a fall would go unnoticed and even less likely the patient would have been left on the floor long enough to cause a rhabdomyolysis. Furthermore, a subdural haemorrhage would not account for the pyrexia, making option D unlikely.

In reality, it is always possible that there are multiple aetiological causes for such a presentation, for example worsening sepsis and a subdural. However, given the timing of symptoms following haloperidol administration, NMS must be considered the single most likely explanation here.

Tutorial

Neuroleptic malignant syndrome can be a life-threatening condition characterized by four cardinal clinical features: cognitive change, pyrexia (can be very high), muscle rigidity, and autonomic instability (tachycardia, excess sweating, hypertension). The presentation usually manifests within a few days of starting a causative agent, though delayed reactions can also occur. A raised CK is commonly seen and reflects a degree of rhabdomyolysis, which if severe enough can even cause acute renal failure due to acute tubular necrosis. Other features include a raised white blood cell count, a metabolic acidosis, and electrolyte imbalances.

The syndrome is also invariably associated with neuroleptic agents/dopaminergic antagonists. These include:

- 'Typical' antipsychotics (perhaps most common cause); haloperidol, chlorpromazine, fluphenazine
- 'Atypical' antipsychotics (less commonly); clozapine, olanzapine, quetiapine risperidone
- Cessation of Parkinson's medication
- Anti-emetics (anti-dopaminergic); metoclopramide/promethazine

Other drugs which do not appear to directly affect the dopaminergic pathways have also been implicated, which include lithium, tetrabenazine, and anticholinergics.

The exact mechanism for the symptoms behind NMS are unclear, but inhibition of the cerebral dopaminergic pathways, either due to drug antagonists or depletion of neurotransmitter, appears to be central to the syndrome.

Patients particularly at risk of NMS are those with Parkinson's disease or Lewy body dementia, or those taking antipsychotics over a longer time. Age or race does not seem to determine whether someone is affected but generally more males are affected than females.

Treatment is usually supportive, with withdrawal of the causative agent. Antipyretics help reduce the temperature and IV fluids can help reduce the risk of precipitating renal injury if there is rhabdomyolysis. Active treatment is seldom indicated but high dose benzodiazepines can be used. Other drugs have mostly been trialled from experience but can include: dantrolene, a potent muscle relaxant which can help reduce muscle rigidity and reduce pyrexia; bromocriptine, a dopaminergic agonist; amantadine, a dopamine agonist which is also an anticholinergic; or electroconvulsive therapy in patients who remain severely catatonic.

Further Reading

Strawn J, Keck P Jr, Caroff S (2007). Neuroleptic malignant syndrome. *American Journal of Psychiatry* 164(6): 870–876.

181. D) If within the same 24-hour period the patient has a PT of more than 100 seconds (or INR of >6.5) and a creatinine of more than 300 mmol/L, the patient should be listed for liver transplant

King's College Hospital have published what is considered to be the most widely accepted criteria for listing a patient with paracetamol overdose, which was modified once again in 2002:

- An arterial pH <7.3 or arterial lactate >3.0 mmol/L after adequate fluid resuscitation, *or*
- If *all* of the following occur with the same 24-hour period:
- Creatinine >300 µmol/L
- PT >100 seconds (INR >6.5)
- Grade III/IV encephalopathy

Reprinted from *The Lancet*, 359, Bernal W, et al. Blood lactate as an early predictor of outcome in paracetamol-induced acute liver failure: a cohort study, pp. 558–563, Copyright 2002, with permission from Elsevier.

Note: transplantation should strongly be considered if arterial lactate >3.5 mmol/L after early fluid resuscitation (with exclusion of other causes of lactic acidosis).

Answer D is the untrue option here because it does not account for the patient needing to also have developed grade III or IV encephalopathy within the 24-hour window.

Tutorial

Paracetamol-induced liver failure is now thankfully uncommon due to good treatment guidelines in emergency departments. It is a common presentation and it is thus worth being familiar with the treatment and its rationale. Paracetamol (also known by its drug name of acetaminophen) is absorbed quickly in the stomach with a peak serum concentration within 1–2 hours. It is then broken down by the liver, with a half-life of approximately two hours. This can be dramatically increased in those with pre-existing hepatic impairment. Paracetamol is usually metabolized in the liver mainly by glucuronidation (addition of glucuronic acid) but also various other conjugation reactions producing non-toxic metabolites. In paracetamol overdoses, the amount of substrate far exceeds the normal and 'safe' metabolic pathways and there is flux in an alternate P450 metabolic pathway in which a toxic metabolite N-acetyl-p-benzoquinoneimine (NAPQI) accumulates and causes hepatic necrosis. This metabolite can be inactivated by conjugation with glutathione, but the doses in toxicity exceed glutathione reserves. The dose required to cause hepatotoxicity varies with individuals and is of course lower in individuals with pre-existing liver disorders, chronic alcoholics or those taking medications which cause hepatic enzyme induction. Acetylcysteine (NAC) is a drug that can be given intravenously that will help maintain or replete the livers stores of glutathione allowing ongoing safe metabolism of NAPQI. The figures often quoted for adults are a dose below 150 mg/kg of paracetamol is unlikely to cause liver damage, whereas above 250 mg/kg is likely to cause it.

Treatment aims to prevent hepatotoxicity in the first place rather than cause recovery from it. Activated charcoal may be of some benefit if given within an hour of ingestion but is unlikely to be of great significance thereafter due to rapid absorption of paracetamol. The mainstay of treatment is then NAC infusion, its administration depending upon on the patient's serum paracetamol levels. Treatment is indicated if levels are above the line on the paracetamol overdose treatment nomogram (Figure 9.1). It is worth noting, that if a patient has had a staggered overdose or the timing of their overdose is unknown, clinical practice is to err on the side of caution and treat as per the usual protocol with NAC.

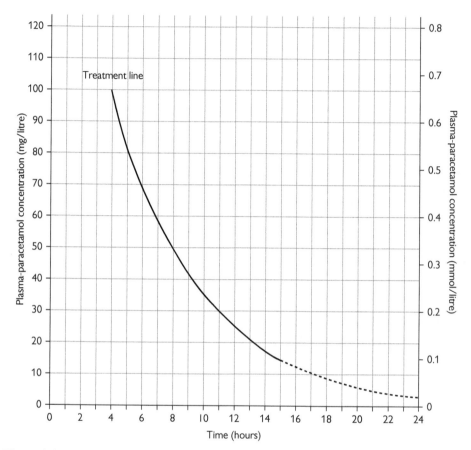

Figure 9.1 Revised paracetamol overdose treatment nomogram.

Reproduced from Medicines and Healthcare products Regulatory Agency (2014). Treating paracetamol overdose with intravenous acetylcysteine: new guidance. *Drug Safety Update.* Contains public sector information licensed under the Open Government Licence v3.0. https://www.gov.uk/.

A venous blood gas, liver function, renal function, and INR should be taken at baseline and be repeated shortly after finishing the third NAC infusion to determine the patient's improvement. Features such as a deranged INR (>1.3) or doubling of transaminases compared to admission might warrant further NAC infusions at 50 mg/kg over 16 hours and further clinical and biochemical monitoring. If started early, especially within the first eight hours of paracetamol overdose, NAC usually prevents any liver damage. Whilst most guidelines only include what to do for the first 24 hours, the overwhelming consensus is to repeat blood tests after finishing NAC infusion and if there is still evidence of hepatic impairment, for example high INR, or high ALTs, to continue NAC infusions until biochemical improvement is seen. In a patient waiting for a transplant, this would certainly be the case to try and retard the progression to liver failure.

In worse case scenarios, a patient may progress onto fulminant liver failure. Advice should always be sought from a liver specialist as these patients may benefit from transfer to a specialist unit for further management or liver transplant.

These guidelines pertain only to the parameters that warrant referral early on in the patient's clinical course. If the patient shows poor response to NAC and generally poor recovery, a hepatology opinion should always be sought.

Further Reading

Buckley N, Dawson A, Ibister G (2016). Treatments for paracetamol poisoning. *British Medical Journal* 353(May): i2579.

Dargan P, Jones A (2002). Acetaminophen poisoning: an update for the intensivist. *Critical Care* 6(2): 108–110.

Toxbase (2020). Clinical guidelines on paracetamol overdose. Available at: www.toxbase.org

182. D) Side effect of medication

This question relies on candidates to know the management of congestive heart failure. There a number of potential explanations for the patient's fatigue but considering the timing of symptoms, a side effect of the newly started bisoprolol for the patient's heart failure is most likely. The patient is indeed anaemic, but this is very mild so unlikely to be causing symptoms. Considering he is likely to have also been started on aspirin, he should be questioned for any GI blood loss. Haematinics and iron studies should also be done as iron deficiency in a male over 60 years old would prompt investigation looking for malignancy. A silent MI could account for increased fatigue but is unlikely in a non-diabetic, especially if not accompanied by decreased exercise tolerance. Similarly, heart failure can also cause fatigue but will also be coupled with decreased exercise tolerance and should not have occurred in just two weeks. The patient has a deranged thyroid function but it is worth noting that the patient has both low TSH and T4, a pattern seen in central hypothyroidism which is extremely uncommon. More likely it represents a sick euthyroid picture following the recent episode of sepsis. The test should be repeated in 6–12 weeks.

Tutorial

Side effects to cardiac medications are common and can frequently result in poor adherence from patients. Patients are often started on a cocktail of drugs for heart failure (ACEi, spironolactone, beta blocker) or after a myocardial infarction (aspirin, statin, beta blocker, and ACEi) due to prognostic benefits. Knowing the common side effects is very useful not just for MCQs but also for clinical practice. The specific side effects associated with commonly prescribed cardiac drugs, which are usually predictable due to mechanism of action, are listed in Table 9.6.

Table 9.6 Side effects of commonly used medications to treat ischaemic heart disease

Drug	Common side effects
ACEi	• Dry paroxysmal cough • Acute kidney injury
Beta blockers	• Fatigue • Postural hypotension/dizziness • Cold peripheries • Shortness of breath (in asthmatics) • Erectile dysfunction

Table 9.6 Continued

Drug	Common side effects
Calcium channel antagonists	• Ankle oedema • Headaches • Postural hypotension/dizziness • Acid reflux • Flushing
Spironolactone	• Postural hypotension/dizziness • Gynaecomastia (in males) • Hyperkalaemia
Statins	• Muscle aches—rhabdomyolysis is rare
Aspirin	• Bruising • Indigestion/dyspepsia
Nitrates (note—no prognostic benefit in CHF or post-MI)	• Postural hypotension/dizziness • Headache • Flushing

Given that patients are likely to be started on a multiple of these drugs at the same time, caution needs to be taken with regards to starting dose, periodicity of up titration, and intervals of follow-up. A mantra often used is 'start low and go slow' to ensure patients don't end up getting too many side effects which can lead to reluctance for treatment adherence in the future.

Further Reading

Joint Formulary Committee (2016). *British National Formulary*, Seventieth Edition. BMJ Group and Pharmaceutical Press, London.

National Institute for Clinical Excellence (2018). Chronic heart failure in adults: diagnosis and management [NG106]. September 2018. Available at: http://www.nice.org.uk/guidance/ng106

183. D) Pyrazinamide

This patient is suffering from gout. The answer to this question requires knowledge of the side effects of anti-TB medication. Pyrazinamide can cause a flare of gout due to decreased renal excretion of uric acid, which in this patient is probably already diminished due to his co-existing CKD. Ethambutol's pharmacokinetics is the most renal sensitive of the standard TB regime (rifampicin, isoniazid, pyrazinamide, and ethambutol), but does not cause gout. Whilst myeloproliferative disorders and lymphoproliferative disorders can cause hyperuricaemia due to increased cell turn over, there is no indication that this patient has either of these conditions. His microcytic anaemia is most likely due to thalassaemia which is prevalent in Southeast Asia. This patient has a transaminitis not hepatitis. Neither causes gout. To note, the derangement in liver function is again likely due to his TB medication (rifampicin and pyrazinamide) which may actually need dose reduction or tapering.

Thiazide diuretics are known to precipitate gout by interfering with renal excretion of uric acid, and are thus prescribed with caution in patients with known gout and CKD. They can also worsen glycaemic control in diabetic patients. It would no doubt have contributed to this patient developing gout but there is no suggestion it is newly started. Pyrazinamide, has just been started and thus remains the most likely explanation. In clinical practice, one would most likely stop the thiazide and consider another anti-hypertensive given the efficacy and relative safety of pyrazinamide compared to his other medications.

Tutorial

Basic treatment for TB consists of starting four agents: rifampicin, isoniazid, pyrazinamide, and ethambutol. The first two antibiotics are continued for six months, and the latter two are stopped after two months. However, if sensitivities show drug resistance treatment may be changed and prolonged. It is worth noting that whilst a strain of TB may be resistant to many antibiotics, especially first- or second-generation agents, the term: 'multi-drug resistant TB' is only applied if the strain is resistant to both rifampicin and isoniazid.

Patients starting on TB medication should have blood tests prior to commencing treatment, including liver function tests, full blood count, renal function tests, and urate levels. Dosing should be changed in patients with impaired kidney function. Blood tests should be repeated early on in treatment but only regularly thereafter if there is evidence of liver impairment on initial blood tests, the patient has pre-existing liver disease, or there is clinical suspicion of side effects (e.g. jaundice, easy bruising, etc.).

For common side effects of anti-TB treatment, see Table 9.7.

Table 9.7 Common side effects of anti-TB treatment

Drug	Common side effects
Rifampicin	• Mild rash • Urticaria (common) • Hepatitis (stop if ALT > × 5 ULN/patient symptomatic) • Liver enzyme induction • Red/orange bodily fluids • Decreases efficacy of corticosteroids
Isoniazid	• Peripheral neuropathy (due to vitamin B6 depletion), thus pyridoxine is given to many patients empirically • Agranulocytosis • Decrease dose in CKD • Hepatitis (stop if ALT > × 5/patient symptomatic)
Pyrazinamide	• Arthralgia • Gout (hyperuricaemia) • Hepatitis (stop if ALT > × 5 ULN/patient symptomatic).
Ethambutol	• Optic neuritis.

Note: all drugs need dose reduction in CKD.

Further Reading

National Institute for Clinical Excellence. Tuberculosis [NG23]. January 2016, updated September 2019. Available at: https://www.nice.org.uk/guidance/ng33

Van der Werf M, Langendam M, Huitric E, et al. (2012). Knowledge of tuberculosis treatment prescription of health workers a systematic review. *European Respiratory Journal* 39(5): 1248–1255.

184. B) Intravenous sodium bicarbonate infusion

This a complex case where multiple aetiologies could be responsible, but given the story of a patient who lives alone and has recently been diagnosed with stage IV cancer, a suicide attempt should at least be considered. The patient exhibits many cardinal signs of tricyclic antidepressant (TCA) overdose, and this is the only diagnosis that accounts for all of the symptoms. Sodium bicarbonate is the correct answer because it is considered an antidote in TCA overdose.

Opiate overdose, either deliberate or accidental (especially in view of chronic renal impairment and possible tramadol use to control pain), may present in a similar manner and account for the respiratory depression and hypotension. However, the tachycardia and dilated, not constricted, pupils go against opiate toxicity. This patient is in type II respiratory failure and has a low GCS so is in danger of going into respiratory arrest. However, NIV requires a patient to be awake and co-operative, thus making it inappropriate in this case. If a decision for ventilatory support was made, it would have to be intubation. Given the patient's diagnosis of stage IV lung cancer, escalation to ITU may not necessarily be in his best interests. However, as overdose is a reversible cause, this may still be considered depending on his performance status and baseline function. For the same reason, withdrawing treatment at this stage is not appropriate as, given supportive measures, the patient may yet recover to baseline.

It is conceivable that the patient is septic and treating empirically with antibiotics is a course many would take. However, the absence of any infective focus, dilated pupils, and respiratory depression all go against a diagnosis of sepsis. The relative discrepancy between severity of clinical signs and relatively poor inflammatory response is also a clue that points against sepsis, but it's worth noting this can occur in the elderly and immunosuppressed.

Tutorial

TACs principally act as serotonin-norepinephrine re-uptake inhibitors centrally. However, they also have broad direct antagonistic effects on many other receptors, including dopaminergic, histaminergic, alpha-adrenergic, and muscarinic, as well as direct effect on sodium and potassium channels. The side effects are thus a combination of interference of both the central and peripheral nervous systems. Symptoms can be divided into three broad categories:

- CNS symptoms: respiratory depression, seizures, rigidity, extra-pyramidal symptoms, drowsiness, and coma.
- (Peripheral) anti-cholinergic symptoms: dry skin, dry mouth, blurred vision, dilated pupils, urinary retention, and tachycardia.
- Cardiovascular (mixture of causes): vasodilation, hypotension, prolonged QT intervals, widening of QRS complex, ST changes, ventricular fibrillation, ventricular tachycardia, and asystole.

Acidosis, whilst a common feature of TCA overdose, does not occur directly due to the drug but is thought to occur due to respiratory depression and hypotension induced tissue hypoperfusion, causing respiratory and metabolic acidosis, respectively.

Overdoses from this class of drug are now less common because they are no longer first line for depression. However, they are still often used for depressed patients who cannot tolerate SSRIs, who have been on antidepressants for a while, and those with anxiety and agitation. In addition, they are used in patients who have neuropathic pain (which may encompass cancer patients) and migraines.

TCAs are rapidly absorbed from the GI tract, thus giving a very narrow window in which gastric lavage (no longer recommended in most hospitals due to risk of aspiration) or activated charcoal may be administered. The drug is then principally bound to protein but also has a large volume of distribution, giving it a relatively long half-life of over 24 hours.

Treatment is first supportive to ensure the airway and circulation is maintained. Intubation and admission to ITU should be considered in severe cases. Sodium bicarbonate is the main form of treatment for TCA overdose because the drug is principally bound to protein in the circulation. Acidosis results in competition from protons to binding sites on proteins thus increasing the concentration of free unbound drug. It has been suggested that sodium bicarbonate may be beneficial even in patients with normal or mildly alkalotic pH to free up further binding sites on proteins. An additional mechanism may be due to direct effect on cardiac sodium channels preventing prolongation of QT intervals and the occurrence of arrhythmias.

Other treatments that are mentioned in the literature are usually specific to treating cardiac arrhythmias. Some studies have suggested that hypertonic saline may be as, if not more, effective than sodium bicarbonate in stabilizing cardiac membranes. Lidocaine has been suggested for frequent ventricular ectopics and magnesium sulphate for ventricular tachycardia or torsade de pointes. Intralipid, a 20% fat emulsion that is administered intravenously, can also be used, usually on the advice of a clinical toxicologist, although the mechanism is incompletely understood.

Further Reading

Blackman K, Brown S, Wilkes G (2001). Plasma alkalinization for tricyclic antidepressant toxicity: a systematic review. *Emergency Medicine* (Fremantle) 13(2): 204–210.

Kerr G, McGuffie A, Wilkie S (2001). Tricyclic antidepressant overdose: a review. *Emergency Medicine Journal* 18(4): 236–241.

185. C) Repeat thyroid function test in six months

The potential answers in this question correspond to different diagnoses: a) Grave's disease; b) amiodarone induced thyrotoxicosis type II (destructive thyrotoxicosis); c) normal physiological changes seen with amiodarone treatment; d) amiodarone induced thyrotoxicosis type I (Jod-Basedow effect); and e) hot thyroid nodule.

The patient's thyroid function results show a slightly raised serum free T4, low serum free T3, and a low-normal TSH. Whilst it may seem that the patient has hyperthyroidism or possible subclinical hyperthyroidism the fact that fT3 (the metabolically active form of the hormone) is low means this is not the case. Therefore, none of the other options are correct. In fact, these test results are not unexpected given the effects amiodarone has on thyroid function result in a patient who has newly started treatment (discussed further in the tutorial).

Clinically, the only symptom this patient has of thyroid disease is weight loss. The atrial fibrillation preceded his mild thyroid abnormality. Of concern here with a symptom of weight loss is the fact that the 66-year-old male patient also has anaemia. A GI source should be sought, especially if he has also been started on warfarin (his CHADS-Vasc score is 2).

Tutorial

Amiodarone has varying and complex effects on thyroid function. It can cause overt disease, unmask pre-existing disease, or cause biochemical abnormality without any clinical features. The effects can be either due to the drug itself, or due its high iodine content—amiodarone contains approximately 35% iodine which can be around 100 times the daily requirement in a normal dose of the drug.

Physiological effects of amiodarone on thyroid hormone synthesis and metabolism

Amiodarone inhibits the peripheral 1-5` deiodinase enzyme which decreases peripheral conversion of T4 to the active form T3, and usually breaks down reverse T3. The result is increased levels of T4 (up to 40%) and rT3 and decreased levels of T3 (around 25%). There is also inhibition of the 2-5` deiodinase enzyme centrally which results in decreased T3 mediated inhibition of TSH secretion in the pituitary, initially causing high TSH levels (so if thyroid function tests were done early on in treatment, it may give the false worry of a pituitary adenoma). Over 12–16 weeks, TSH levels begin to drop, likely due to a rise in peripheral T4 levels and other metabolic changes. The result is normalizing of results, with basal TSH levels being low or low-normal, T4 remaining slightly raised, and T3 remaining slightly low. Whilst the thyroid function results may not fall within 'normal' limits, if the patient is euthyroid no treatment is necessary except observation in case progression to disease does occur.

Amiodarone induced hypothyroidism—Wolff-Chaikoff effect

Physiologically, any person given an excess of iodine (either as an ion in itself or as amiodarone) will have transient decrease in thyroxine production—the Wolff-Chaikoff effect. This is thought to be a physiological mechanism by which large amounts of ingested iodine would prevent a surge in thyroxine production. After around ten days the gland 'escapes' this effect and thyroid function returns to normal. However, in some cases, especially those with latent (or pre-existing) auto-immune hypothyroidism, there is inability to escape from the Wolff-Chaikoff phenomenon and they will become hypothyroid. Blood tests would show raised TSH and low serum free T4 and T3. Treatment with thyroxine replacement depends on clinical symptoms, cardiac risk factors, or extent of rise in TSH.

Amiodarone induced thyrotoxicosis type I—Jod-Basedow effect

Type I amiodarone induced thyrotoxicosis is caused by the high iodine content of the drug. It usually occurs in patients with pre-existing thyroid disease such as Graves' disease, subclinical Graves' or multi-nodular goitre (especially those caused by iodine deficiency). The result is an excess production of thyroxine. TSH will be low and T4 and T3 will be raised. Thyroid antibodies may also be present but would indicate pre-existing disease rather than being a result of the thyrotoxicosis itself. The clinical manifestation of hyperthyroidism is usually quite severe and difficult to treat due to the long half-life of amiodarone and hyperthyroidism may persist for up to eight months. Discontinuation of the drug is usually indicated unless very mild disease has occurred and the benefits of treatment outweigh the risks. High doses of thionamides are usually indicated.

Amiodarone induced thyrotoxicosis type II—destructive thyroiditis

This form of thyroiditis appears to affect patients with otherwise normal thyroid glands and occurs spontaneously. The exact mechanism is unknown but is thought to be due to direct cytotoxic effect of amiodarone and/or its metabolites causing an inflammatory and destructive thyrotoxicosis. On examination the thyroid gland is usually tender. Thionamides are of no use here because the hyperthyroidism is due to release of pre-formed hormone rather than excess production. Instead, high dose glucocorticoids have been shown to be of benefit.

Differentiation between type I and type II thyrotoxicosis may be difficult and a mixed picture may occur. However, it is important due to the different treatment regimens. Imaging of the glands, using ultrasound doppler to measure blood flow or radio-iodine uptake studies, can help to differentiate with the two entities.

Further Reading

Padmanabhan H (2010). Amiodarone and thyroid dysfunction. *Southern Medical Journal* 103(9): 922–930.

Wiersinga W, Trip M (1986). Amiodarone and thyroid hormone metabolism. *Postgraduate Medical Journal* 62(732): 909–914.

186. D) PRN paracetamol—1 g tds PO/IV

There are a few clinically important things to consider when prescribing drugs for patients with decompensated liver disease. First, though not explicitly mentioned, one should suspect portal hypertension and likely gastric and oesophageal varices given the fact that the platelet count is 44×10^9/L (this likely reflects splenomegaly and platelet sequestration). Second, the patient also has gross oedema and a sodium of 125 mmol/L which represents renal hypoperfusion due to intravascular hypovolemia activating the renin-angiotensin-aldosterone system as well as ADH release. This axis is subject to gross interference, as discussed in more detail in the tutorial, by the use of NSAIDs. Third, though the creatinine may be in the 'normal' range, cirrhotic patients have very little muscle mass and thus creatinine is an underestimate of their true GFR. Similarly, the low urea should not be reassuring because of protein metabolism and thus urea is usually low in liver cirrhosis. Lastly, whilst able to speak, the patient does appear agitated and confused. This may represent mild hepatic encephalopathy. In any case, there is a serious risk of precipitating hepatic encephalopathy in this patient by using opiates. Of all the options listed, paracetamol is the safest option to start with, and is indicated in patients with liver failure at a lower dose of 1 g tds daily. Scrotal support would be a good idea, but will not alleviate the patient's pain and may take some time to procure.

Tutorial

NSAIDs should be avoided in cirrhotic patients, and especially those with liver failure, bleeding dyscrasias, renal impairment, and portal hypertension. NSAIDs are principally protein bound in the circulation, so the low albumin state of cirrhotic patients means a higher circulating drug concentration. NSAIDs are also metabolized by the liver and thus in cirrhosis and acute failure, they will have a longer half-life. The risks they pose are two-fold. First, the risk of GI bleeding due to gastric erosion, especially if there is thrombocytopaenia. Second, due to excess dilation of the splanchnic circulation and imbalances between endothelin and nitrates, cirrhotic patients can have decreased renal perfusion which activates the renin-angiotensin-aldosterone system. This is reflected clinically by fluid retention and also hyponatraemia if there is co-existing activation of the ADH system—the 'under filled' theory. NSAIDs inhibit the production of prostaglandins in the kidney which usually dilate the afferent arteriole. Their use upsets the balance and decreases renal perfusion, causing or worsening renal failure.

Nearly all opiates are metabolized by the liver and thus their pharmacokinetics are affected in cirrhosis and liver failure. For some drugs such as codeine, which require activation in the liver, it means the drug's efficacy is difficult to predict. However, the greater risk is the increased half-life and serum concentrations of the drug. This is of particular concern as it can precipitate or worsen hepatic encephalopathy.

Paracetamol is of course also metabolized by the liver. Whilst the non-toxic metabolite producing pathway may well be impaired in cirrhotic patients, studies have shown that glutathione levels are not reduced in cirrhotic patients. Therefore, the toxic metabolite NAPQI which builds up in paracetamol overdose, is not accumulated. The BNF advises that a maximum of 3 g of paracetamol may be given in patients with hepatic impairment, providing their weight is over 50 kg.

Further Reading

Chandok N, Watt K (2010). Pain management in the cirrhotic patient: the clinical challenge. *Mayo Clinic Proceedings* 85(5): 451–458.

187. A) A patient's MMSE should be 10–20 in order for them to be started on an acetylcholinesterase inhibitor

NICE recommends that acetylcholinesterase inhibitors should only be started by specialists in patients with a diagnosis of moderate dementia, that is, an MMSE between 10 and 20. However, as with any clinical test, there exist other factors which may skew the sensitivity of the MMSE and these should also be taken into account. These include but are not limited to patients:

- With linguistic difficulties or other pre-morbid disabilities (e.g. visual impairment).
- For whom English (or language in which the MMSE is carried out) is not their first language.
- With learning disabilities.
- Who despite having an MMSE of over 20, still have significant impairment in behavioural, social, and personal function.

Option B is incorrect because memantine is an NMDA receptor antagonist. It is indicated only if acetylcholinesterase inhibitors, the first-line drugs, are not tolerated, or the patient has severe dementia. Although option C seems sensible, NICE guidance is that when multiple aetiologies for dementia co-exist, which they often do, treatment should be aimed at controlling the most common aetiology of the cognitive impairment. If after specialist review it is felt that the primary cause is vascular dementia (this may be suggested by atherosclerotic risk factors, presence of ischaemic damage in other organs, changes on CT imaging), acetylcholinesterase would not be indicated as it would have no benefit on symptoms and may only cause unwanted and potentially fatal side effects. Thus, as acetylcholinesterase has no benefit in vascular dementia, option E is also incorrect. Lastly, option D is incorrect because whilst a normal imaging of the brain does allude to an alternative aetiology to vascular dementia, MRI imaging is the preferred modality and early cognitive impairment may occur before any discernible radiological change.

Tutorial

Alzheimer's disease is the most common cause of cognitive impairment in the elderly, with figures of around 60% of all cases of dementia being attributed to it. Alzheimer's disease typically has an indolent presentation with short- term memory being affected first. Later, long-term memory and high order cognitive impairments occur. Sensorimotor deficit is not common and occurs only at the very end of the disease's natural progression—this is in contrast to the other common causes of dementia. It is worth noting that patients can also have mixed dementias. For example, both vascular dementia and Alzheimer's may co-exist. See Table 9.8 for features of common dementia syndromes.

Table 9.8 Features of common dementia syndromes

	Alzheimer's	**Vascular dementia**	**Lewy body dementia***	**Frontotemporal dementia (Pick's disease)**
Onset of deficits	Slow and indolent	Step-wise deficits Progressions can be acute	Fluctuating cognitive impairment	Gradual
Early features	Short-term memory loss	Varied presentation depending site of ischaemia	Deficits in attention and executive function	Changes in personality, disinhibition.
Defining features	In addition to above, also requires: language dysfunction, apraxia, agnosia, visuospatial disorder, as well as executive dysfunction	Focal neurological deficits often present	Visual hallucinations, autonomic dysfunction, and parkinsonism (which can fluctuate)	Not obviously demented Often seem like personality disorders
Episodic memory	Affected early, short-term deficit prior to long-term memory	Usually impaired	Memory usually preserved till later in disease	Episodic and spatial orientation often preserved till later on
Sensori-motor impairment	Absent until very late in disease progression	Present early on	Present—usually truncal rigidity and ataxia; other PD features less common (only in 25% of cases)	Usually absent though incontinence often present
Other features	CT imaging shows global atrophy.	Atherosclerotic disease often co-exists CT imaging shows small vessel disease	Poor response to L-Dopa.	Disproportionate atrophy of frontal-temporal lobe on CT

* Parkinson's dementia (PD) and Lewy body dementia (LBD) are two separate clinical entities though the term Lewy body dementia is often used for both. The difference between the two conditions is the onset of motor symptoms. In PD, motor symptoms precede cognitive decline by at least a year. In LBD, cognitive decline usually comes before motor symptoms or can come within one year of onset of motor symptoms. Furthermore, tremor and good (though declining) response to L-DOPA is more common in PD dementia, whereas truncal rigidity, bilateral symptoms, and poor-response to L-DOPA is more a feature of LBD.

Management of dementia requires first, exclusion of any reversible causes: for example B12/folate deficiency, hypothyroidism, anaemia, or other systemic but reversible conditions. It also requires stopping any medication that may be worsening symptoms of the disease or cognitive impairment such as anticholinergics, opiates, benzodiazepines, TCA, H2-receptor antagonists, or certain antipsychotics. Once a formal diagnosis of dementia is made, which usually requires input from a specialist, a holistic approach towards the patient's care from various members of the multidisciplinary team is needed. The aim should be to support patients and their families to continue to live as independent and normal of a life as possible by providing support and care tailored to an individual's need.

Currently, pharmacological treatment for cognitive impairment is reserved for Alzheimer's disease, and even then only in cases of 'moderate' deficit (usually quoted as an MMSE of 10–20). Studies have shown a global decrease in levels of acetylcholine in the brain, and though not fully understood, this deficit is thought to underlie the cognitive impairments in the disease. Treatment thus aims to increase levels and currently three cholinesterase inhibitors (donepezil, galantamine, and rivastigmine) are recommended as first line by NICE for treatment. Memantine, an NMDA receptor antagonist, is indicated if first-line drugs aren't tolerated, or for severe dementia.

Further Reading

Muangpaisan W (2007). Clinical differences among four common dementia syndromes. *Geriatrics and Aging* 10(7): 425–429.

National Institute for Clinical Excellence (2016). Donepezil, galantamine, rivastigmine and memantine for the treatment of Alzheimer's disease [TA217]. March 2011, updated May 2016. Available at: https://www.nice.org.uk/guidance/TA217

National Institute for Clinical Excellence (2018). Dementia: assessment, management and support for people living with dementia and their carers [NG97]. July 2018. Available at: http://www.nice.org.uk/guidance/ng97

188. D) Fluconazole

Whilst erythromycin, ciprofloxacin, and metronidazole all inhibit warfarin metabolism leading to a raised INR, it is very unlikely that the patient was given these agents for a skin infection. Skin infections are usually due to Gram positive cocci, usually *Staphylococcus aureus* or *Streptococcus pyogenes*, or due to yeast. The fact that creams were trialled first suggests a fungal infection. The patient has a mild transaminitis which may be due to his diabetes but this is unlikely to be related to the patient's current problem.

Tutorial

A large number of drugs are metabolized by a group of liver enzymes known collectively as cytochrome P450 enzymes. Certain drugs will induce/inhibit only certain P450 enzymes, and thus they won't necessarily affect the concentrations of drugs that are metabolized by the different enzymes of the family. The individual enzymes and their specific inhibitors, inducers, and substrates are not included here. However, Table 9.9 shows a comprehensive list of the common enzyme inhibitors and inducers, as well as drugs commonly affected.

Table 9.9 Common CYP450 enzyme inducers and inhibitors

Enzyme inducers	Enzyme inhibitors	Drugs commonly affected
Carbamazepine	Sodium valproate	OCP
Rifampicin	Isoniazid	Warfarin
Alcohol (chronic)	Cimetidine	Opiates
Phenytoin	Erythromycin	Ciclosporin
Phenobarbital	Ketoconazole	Tacrolimus
Sulphonylureas	Fluconazole	Simvastatin
St John's Wort	Diltiazem	Amiodarone
	Verapamil	Diazepam
	Ciprofloxacin	
	Citalopram	
	Fluoxetine	
	Alcohol (acute) Grapefruit juice	

Note: CYP450 enzymes are a group of enzymes and thus not all of the drugs listed in the inducers and inhibitors columns will necessarily interact with those listed in the third column.

Further Reading

A more comprehensive list of inducers, inhibitors as well as individual enzymes and substrates can be found at: http://www.resourcepharm.com/pre-reg-articles/substrates-inhibitors-and-inducers-of-the-major-CYP450-enzyme.pdf

189. B) Start amiloride

This patient has nephrogenic diabetes insipidus secondary to lithium. This is clearly demonstrated by the inability to concentrate urine after a six-hour water deprivation test, and her inability to respond appropriately to exogenous desmopressin; urine osmolality should increase to over 750. Fluid restriction would be indicated if the results suggested a psychogenic polydipsia. If this was the case, the patient's urine osmolality would appropriately increase during the water deprivation test as the kidney concentrates the urine.

The patient does have a slightly raised blood sugar, but this is a random sample not fasting and whilst a diagnosis of diabetes mellitus may be present, it cannot be made from these results alone. The absence of glycosuria also makes it unlikely that diabetes mellitus is the cause of her polyuria. Patients who are on lithium should not have their medication stopped for nephrogenic diabetes insipidus as relapse of their psychiatric condition is far more serious. Starting synthetic DDAVP® (desmopressin) is not appropriate here due to the patient's resistance to the drug. Amiloride has been shown in randomized control trials to reduce the effect of lithium's downstream inhibition of ADH, and improve clinical symptoms.

Tutorial

Lithium induced nephrogenic diabetes insipidus is not an uncommon side effect and may affect up to 10% of patients on the drug. It is worth noting that the polyuria is mostly driven by polydipsia itself caused by relative hypernatraemia, and not the kidney's inability to concentrate urine. Patients are thus euvolaemic and can function well for some time.

Whilst the exact cellular mechanisms of how lithium induces nephrogenic diabetes insipidus are not fully understood, accumulation of the ion in principal cells of the collecting duct inhibits translocation of aquaporin 2 (AQP2) channels to cellular membrane, thus rendering the nephrons resistant to the downstream effects of ADH and impairing the kidneys' ability to concentrate urine. Lithium accumulates in the collecting duct because sodium channels (ENaC) on the apical membrane are selective to both sodium and Li^+. However, the basolateral membrane is poorly permeable to Li^+ resulting in accumulation of the ion. Amiloride, which blocks EnaC, reduces the concentrations of lithium in the principal cells, reducing the inhibition on AQP2 translocation and thus improving the sensitivity of the collecting duct to ADH.

Further Reading

Bedford J, Weggery S, Ellis G, et al. (2008). Lithium-induced nephrogenic diabetes insipidus: renal effects of amiloride. *Clinical Journal of the American Society of Nephrology* 3(5): 1324–1331.

190. D) Intravenous protamine sulphate

LMWHs work by binding to antithrombin (AT), a serine protease which cleaves multiple clotting factors including X and II, and changing its confirmation thereby increasing its cleaving efficacy of activated factor Xa. Thus, it effectively acts as an indirect inhibitor of factor X. Once the LMWH has activated one AT protein, it is not 'consumed' but rather can dissociate and bind to further AT proteins and activate them too. Unlike unfractionated heparin, which increases ATs' cleaving efficacy of both factor Xa and IIa, LWMHs only antagonize factor X. As they effectively result in the inhibition of factor X, both the prothrombin time (PT) and activated partial thromboplastin time (APTT) are often raised but these *cannot* be used to assess the anticoagulation effect of LMWH. Instead, an anti-factor Xa assay must be done. LMWHs usually have a half-life of around 2–4 hours, and so in most cases of minor bleeding do not actually need any reversal. However, in cases of renal impairment—as in this case—the half-life can increase, and it is for this reason most manufacturers advise a dose reduction in renal impairment. Even so, in acute kidney injury, whilst serum creatinine is rising, it is not possible to calculate eGFR accurately. So, even 'corrected' doses of LMWH can accumulate and cause a supra-therapeutic blockade of factor X activation.

Even in cases where renal impairment or potential overdosing of LMWH isn't an issue, if the patient is experiencing a significant haemorrhage, for example one that causes haemodynamic compromise, guidelines advise that the effects of LMWH should be pharmacologically reversed if the bleed has occurred within 12 hours of a treatment dose (NB: prophylactic LMWH given for venous thromboprophylaxis does not need reversal). For this reason, conservative management is not appropriate here. Phytonadione is the name for vitamin K, the antidote for warfarin and so is not appropriate here. Fresh frozen plasma will contain all the clotting factors. Whereas prothrombin complex concentrate contains the vitamin K dependent clotting factors (X, IX, VII, and II) and is thus more specific to reverse the effects of warfarin in a bleeding patient. Both agents are likely to be of limited help with reversing the effects of LMWH if given alone. However, the drug is still circulating in the patient and will continue to result in the breakdown of new factor Xa. Protamine sulphate is a polypeptide with a high positive charge that binds to and neutralizes heparin and LMWH molecules, which are negatively charged. This complex then forms a permanent ionic bond which is later removed by the reticuloendothelial system.

In clinical practice, haematologists will often still advise to give fresh frozen plasma (FFP) in cases of massive haemorrhage where LMWH has been used, as by providing enough 'substrate' the effects of the factor Xa inhibition may at least be partially overcome through dilution. Especially if it is also being given with protamine sulphate which will neutralize the LMWH.

Tutorial

Anticoagulant drugs are increasingly being used to reduce the risk of thromboembolic complications of atrial fibrillation. Additionally, newer non-vitamin K antagonist oral anticoagulants (NOACs): rivaroxaban, apixaban, and dabigatran are being used. They have been shown in a number of studies to be as efficacious as warfarin (though long-term follow-up studies are yet to be completed) and may, according to a few studies, even have a smaller risk of intra-cranial haemorrhage. Their main shortfalls from the limited available studies include: contraindication with renal impairment, poor efficacy for metallic heart valves (in actual fact, studies have shown an increased thrombosis risk with dabigatran compared to warfarin), lack of efficacy in acute coronary syndromes, lack of data for use in pregnancy, and lastly lack of antidote or effective reversibility in most cases.

Reversing anticoagulation is not an uncommon scenario for medical patients and is thus often a source for questions in the MRCP exam. It is thus worth familiarizing oneself with the mechanisms of actions of anticoagulants, as well as their shortfalls and ways to reverse their effects. These are summarized in Box 9.1.

Box 9.1 Commonly used anticoagulants: their mechanisms of action, half-life, advantages, disadvantages and reversal treatments. NB: half-lives correspond to patients with normal renal function without any co-existing condition causing metabolic derangement, for example infection, cancer, sepsis.

Warfarin

- Impairs vitamin K dependent synthesis of clotting factors II, VII, IX, and X.
- Is very cheap (though monitoring drug levels in clinics can be expensive).
- Half-life of ~40 hours.
- Requires regular monitoring of INR which can easily fluctuate due to other drug interactions or acute illnesses.
- Reversed by either omitting drug, use of oral or parenteral vitamin K or PCC in cases of severe bleeding,

LMWH, for example tinzaparin

- Binds to and activates anti-thrombin increasing its inhibition of factor Xa (note, LMWH does not cause anti-thombin to inhibit thrombin (factor II) like heparins do.
- Half-life 4–7 hours depending on drug. Effect of inhibition lasts ~12 hours. Dosing can thus be split in cases of high risk.
- Relatively short half-life. Not effected by metabolic derangements such as sepsis or cancer. Requires less (or no) monitoring than unfractionated heparin and less likely to cause heparin induced thrombocytopaenia.
- Relatively expensive and requires subcutaneous administration which again incurs cost.
- In cases of large haemorrhage, protamine can be used as an antidote.

Apixaban (Pfizer)

- Reversibly binds to and inhibits factor Xa.
- ~12-hour half-life.
- Relatively short half-life. Doesn't require drug level or coagulation effect monitoring. Not affected by metabolic derangements. Can be used in CKD stage IV and above (eGFR >15 ml/minute).
- Relatively expensive (though cost arguably offset by lack of need to monitor drug levels; no antidote).
- In case of large haemorrhage, PCC (or FPP) can be used to 'dilute' and partially overcome the inhibition of the drug. Tranexamic acid is also often advised. If administered within two hours (six hours in one study), activated charcoal can be used to diminish exposure to apixaban.

Dabigatran

- Reversibly inhibits thrombin (factor II).
- Has 8–12-hour half-life. Dosing can thus be split.
- Relatively short half-life. Doesn't require drug level or coagulation effect monitoring. Not affected by metabolic derangements. Can be dialysed.
- Relatively expensive (though cost arguably offset by lack of need to monitor drug levels). No antidote. Contraindicated in CKD IV and below (eGFR<30 ml/min).
- In case of large haemorrhage, idarucizumab—a monoclonal antibody to dabigatran which has been licensed for use by NICE in 2017 can be used. Tranexamic acid is also often advised. Dialysis may also be an option to remove the drug. If administered within two hours, activated charcoal can be used to diminish exposure to dabigatran.

Rivaroxaban (Bayer)

- Reversibly binds to and inhibits factor Xa.
- Has ~5–9-hour half-life. Dosing can thus be split.
- Relatively short half-life. Doesn't require drug level or coagulation effect monitoring. Not effected by metabolic derangements. Can be used in CKD stage IV and above (eGFR >15 ml/minute).
- Relatively expensive (though cost arguably offset by lack of need to monitor drug levels). No antidote. Can't be dialysed.
- In case of large haemorrhage, PCC (and FPP) can be used to 'dilute' and partially overcome the inhibition of the drug. Tranexamic acid is also often advised. If administered within 2–4 hours, (eight hours in one study) activated charcoal can be used to diminish exposure to rivaroxaban.

Further Reading

Dentali F, Riva N, Crowther M, et al. (2010). Efficacy and safety of the novel oral anticoagulants in atrial fibrillation: a systematic review and meta-analysis of the literature. *Circulation* 126: 2381.

Lubetsky A, Yonath H, Olchovsky D, Loebstein R, Halkin H, Ezra D (2003). Comparison of oral vs intravenous phytonadione (vitamin K1) in patients with excessive anticoagulation: a prospective randomized controlled study. *Archives of Internal Medicine* 163(20): 2469.

Siegal D, Crowther M (2013). Acute management of bleeding in patients on novel oral anticoagulants. *European Heart Journal* 34: 489.

191. D) Sertraline

Depression is very common following an acute MI and is associated higher morbidity and mortality. When choosing an antidepressant in this setting cardiac side effects will determine choice. Monoamine oxidase inhibitors such as selegiline are associated with a range of cardiac side effects including bradycardia, postural hypotension, increased risk of arrhythmia, and hypertensive crisis, if taken with tyramine containing foods. TCAs such as imipramine are associated with tachycardia, postural hypotension, prolonged QTc interval, and increased risk of arrhythmia and are also not indicated in this scenario. Venlafaxine is a serotonin and noradrenaline reuptake inhibitor (SNRI) which can cause a dose dependent increase in blood pressure and should not be considered post-MI.

Both citalopram and sertraline are SSRI medications with evidence of safety in cardiovascular disease. However, sertraline is considered to be the drug of choice in this scenario. Clinical trials, such as SADHART, have shown that post-MI sertraline is safe and effective for the management of depression. Although citalopram is considered safe, there is evidence to suggest a dose-related QTc prolonging effect and therefore in this scenario, sertraline would be preferred.

Tutorial

Depression is a common sequalae of many common medical conditions including MI, stroke, neurological disease, and renal disease. Depression in medical populations adversely affects long-term medical outcomes and has a direct impact on the patient's quality of life.

The three core symptoms of depression are low mood, low energy, and lack of enjoyment. Depression also disrupts sleep, sexual drive, and appetite and patients report multiple negative cognitions including low self-esteem, loss of hope, and thoughts of ending their lives. Anergia, disrupted sleep, altered appetite and libido are commonly seen in many medical conditions. However, concomitant features of low mood and depressive cognitions may indicate comorbid depression. The Hospital Anxiety and Depression Scale (HADS) was developed to aid the detection of depression in the medical setting and concentrates on symptoms less likely to be confounded by physical illness.

SSRI medications show good efficacy with a narrower range of side effects than older classes of antidepressants and are typically first-line treatments for unipolar depression in medical populations.

Further Reading

Glassman A, O'Connor C, Califf R, et al. (2002). Sertraline treatment of major depression in patients with acute MI or unstable angina. *Journal of American Medical Association* 288(6): 701–709.

Lichtman J, Dawood N, Vaccarino V, et al. (2008). Depression and coronary heart disease. *Circulation* 118: 1768–1775.

NICE Clinical Knowledge Summary. Depression. (2015). Available at: https://cks.nice.org.uk/depression

192. D) Exposure and response prevention

This patient is reporting obsessions which are intrusive anxiety provoking thoughts and are a symptom of obsessive compulsive disorder (OCD), an anxiety disorder. Obsessions, as in this case, may be violent in nature. However, critically, these thoughts are not associated with any desire to commit violent actions. They are also intrusive and associated with significant anxiety symptoms. Reassurance seeking, cleaning, hand washing, and checking are common compulsions. These are actions, or 'neutralizing thoughts', that the patient takes to reduce the feelings of anxiety associated with the obsessional thoughts. The degree to which compulsions reduce anxiety following obsessions reduces with time, often leading to increased time spent doing compulsions which can become very disruptive and disabling.

Cognitive behaviour therapy with exposure and response prevention is the recommended psychological treatment for OCD. Exposure and response prevention focuses on breaking the connection between obsession and compulsion with the eventual aim of reducing the anxiety provoking nature of the obsession itself. SSRI medications are also indicated for OCD.

Tutorial

Psychological treatments such as cognitive behavioural therapy (CBT) have proven efficacy for psychiatric conditions such as affective and anxiety syndromes. As compared to psychodynamic approaches, CBT sessions are highly structured, and courses of CBT are limited to a defined number of sessions. CBT therapists often follow a manual to deliver standardized treatment.

The focus of CBT is understanding the link between abnormal or unhelpful cognitions, mood, and behaviour. Patients learn to record and critically appraise dysfunctional cognitions and beliefs that may be contributing to their current symptoms. They also learn to adapt their behaviour based on behavioural experiments that they design with their therapist. These include exposure and response prevention in OCD as described above or by encouraging patients to engage in enjoyable activities in depression ('behavioural activation'). Patients play an active role in CBT therapy and will be asked to complete 'homework' between sessions, which include assessment of thinking patterns or behavioural experiments.

Dialectic behaviour therapy (DBT) is a specialized form of CBT designed for use in personality disorder and in patients with chronic suicidality. In addition to the principles of CBT described above, DBT includes emotion regulation, mindfulness training, and tolerance of distress.

Further Reading

Stein G, Wilkinson G (2007). *Seminars in General Adult Psychiatry* (College Seminar Series), Second Edition. Royal College of Psychiatrists, London.

NICE Clinical Knowledge Summary (2015). Obsessive-compulsive disorder. Available at: https://cks.nice.org.uk/obsessive-compulsive-disorder

193. E) Tetrabenazine

Tetrabenazine is a reversible vesicular monoamine transporter type II inhibitor used for the symptomatic treatment of chorea in HD. It causes reversible monoamine depletion and is associated with an increased risk of depression and suicide in patients with HD. Although depression is common in HD, and antidepressants are commonly used, in this scenario it seems likely the tetrabenazine was started to manage chorea and caused severe depression. The correct course of action would be to stop the tetrabenazine and manage movements with an alternative medication such as an antipsychotic medication like risperidone. Haloperidol is rarely used in HD due to the risk of dystonia. Citalopram and mirtazapine are antidepressants commonly used in the management of HD. However, these are not likely to be the cause of this patient's presentation.

Tutorial

Huntington's disease is an autosomal dominant triplet repeat expansion disorder of the *huntington* gene on the short arm of chromosome 4 (4p16.3). Expansion of the CAG triplet repeat to greater than 40 repeats leads to full penetrance. Lower than 26 repeats are considered normal. Intermediate repeat lengths are associated with partial penetrance and increased risk to offspring. HD causes an adult onset neurodegenerative condition characterized by a movement disorder, cognitive impairment, and psychiatric features.

Depression, obsessional thinking, apathy, and irritability are common psychiatric features of HD. These patients are also at higher risk of committing suicide. SSRI medications are the preferred treatment for depression and anxiety in HD due to lower side effect profiles. Atypical antipsychotics are often used for the management of irritability and aggression, especially if there is co-morbid chorea. Apathy in HD is difficult to treat and is associated with functional decline.

Further Reading

Mestre T, Ferreira J, Coelho, M, Rosa M, Sampaio C (2009). Therapeutic interventions for symptomatic treatment in Huntington's disease. *Cochrane Database of Systematic Reviews* (3): CD006456.

Walker F (2007). Huntington's disease. *Lancet* 369(9557): 218–228.

Zielonka D, Mielcarek M, Landwehrmeyer G (2015). Update on Huntington's disease: advances in care and emerging therapeutic options. *Parkinsonism and Related Disorders* 21(3): 169–178.

194. B) Fluoxetine

This patient is most probably suffering from bulimia nervosa. This condition is characterized by bouts of overeating and pre-occupation with controlling body weight. Attempts to counteract weight gain may include self-induced vomiting, periods of starvation, or the inappropriate use of medications such as diuretics or laxatives. In this case, repeated self-induced vomiting has led to hypokalaemia resulting in physical symptoms and findings on examination. Calluses on the knuckles are a sign of self-induced vomiting and are known as 'Russell's sign'.

The first-line pharmacological treatment for bulimia is fluoxetine, often used at a higher dose of 60 mg/day as compared to its use in depression. Fluoxetine reduces the frequency of binge eating and purging behaviours.

Primary psychiatric differential diagnosis in this case is anorexia nervosa. Although there is considerable overlap between the conditions, typically anorexia is associated with deliberate and significant weight loss and widespread endocrine abnormalities because of low body weight. Both groups of patients are at risk of sudden death from electrolyte abnormalities.

Tutorial

Eating disorders, especially anorexia nervosa, are associated with elevated risk of mortality and morbidity. Patients with anorexia have low BMI, endocrine dysfunction (such as amenorrhea), wasting, cardiovascular abnormalities, and electrolyte imbalance. Safe weight gain and psychotherapy are the principle interventions for the management of anorexia. No specific psychiatric medication is effective in anorexia beyond those used to encourage weight gain and treat co-morbid psychiatric conditions.

Patients with bulimia nervosa classically restrict their food intake, binge on large volumes of food and then engage in some form of purging behaviour. Purging includes using laxatives, inducing vomiting, or extreme exercising to limit weight gain. Patients with bulimia are typically of normal weight. They may also suffer from electrolyte disturbances especially because of purging behaviour. Fluoxetine at higher doses (60 mg per day) has been shown to be effective in bulimia nervosa by reducing binge and purging behaviour frequency. Psychological interventions are also effective in the management of bulimia.

Further Reading

Mehler P, Krantz M, Sachs K (2015). Treatments of medical complications of anorexia nervosa and bulimia nervosa. *Journal of Eating Disorders* 3: 15.

NICE Clinical Knowledge Summary. Eating disorders. (2014). Available at: https://cks.nice.org.uk/eating-disorders

Stein G, Wilkinson G (2007). *Seminars in General Adult Psychiatry*, Second Edition. Royal College of Psychiatrists, London.

195. A) Aripiprazole

This patient is suffering from an episode of acute mania. Antipsychotic medications, mood stabilizers (like valproate), and lithium are all effective for the treatment of mania. However, in this case aripiprazole is likely to be the best tolerated agent. Although effective, caution should be used when prescribing lithium or sodium valproate to women of child-bearing age due to concerns around teratogenicity. Diazepam and other benzodiazepines may be useful in the short-term management of agitation during acute manic phases; however, they are not recommended for long-term treatment. As compared to aripiprazole, olanzapine is more effective for the management of acute mania but is associated with a high degree of weight gain and sedation. Given the patient's preference not to gain weight aripiprazole is preferred in this scenario. It has a proven efficacy in acute mania and is not associated with significant weight gain or sedation. Aripiprazole is, however, associated with akathisia, a feeling of restlessness, which some patients find distressing.

Tutorial

Bipolar affective disorder (BPAD) is characterized by mood fluctuation at both poles of the mood spectrum, with both depressive and elated episodes. Periods of elated mood result in feelings of elevated mood, increased self-esteem with racing or pressured thoughts. Patients typically have reduced need for sleep, with increased involvement in pleasurable activities and goal-directed behaviour. Patients with BPAD may also be irritable and agitated. In severe cases, increased self-esteem results in grandiose thinking and mood congruent delusions and hallucinations.

Mood stabilizers such as lithium, antiepileptic, and antipsychotic medications can be used for the treatment of manic episodes. Choice of medication should be guided by medication side effect profile and monitoring requirements. In women of childbearing age, both lithium and antileptics (such as valproate and carbamazepine) are not advised. In the depressive phase of the illness, there is an elevated risk of suicide as compared to unipolar depression. Depression in BPAD is best managed with combined treatment of antipsychotic and SSRI medication especially olanzapine and fluoxetine. Use of antidepressants in isolation risk a switch to manic phase.

Further Reading

Brown R, Taylor M, Geddes J (2013). Aripiprazole alone or in combination for acute mania. *Cochrane Database of Systematic Reviews* 12: CD005000.

Cipriani A, Barbui C, Salanti G, et al. (2011). Comparative efficacy and acceptability of antimanic drugs in acute mania: a multiple-treatments meta-analysis. *Lancet* 378(9799): 1306–1315.

NICE guidelines (2016). Bipolar Disorder. Available at: https://www.nice.org.uk/guidance/conditions-and-diseases/mental-health-and-behavioural-conditions/bipolar-disorder

196. A 36-year-old man was referred for investigations for deranged renal function. His past medical history included recurrent episodes of labyrinthitis treated by the GP with vestibular sedatives, and an episode of arthritis following a diarrhoeal illness five years previously. His maternal uncle had previously been diagnosed with chronic kidney disease but was not currently on dialysis. On examination, the patient was noted to be hypertensive, with a blood pressure of 170/95 mmHg, but he was euvolaemic and the remainder of his physical examination was unremarkable.

```
Investigations:
    Sodium                      136 mmol/L
    Potassium                   4.8 mmol/L
    Urea                        18 mmol/L
    Creatinine                  210 µmol/L
    Urine dipstick              blood + protein +++
    24-hour urine protein       4 g/24hrs
      quantification
    Serum IgA                   normal
    Renal biopsy                light microscopy showed
                                mesangial cell proliferation
                                and increased mesangial matrix;
                                immunofluorescence showed
                                mesangial IgA and C3 deposition.
```

Which one of the following is true about this patient's ongoing medical treatment?

A. He has a low risk of reaching end-stage renal disease

B. He should be treated with cyclophosphamide and prednisolone

C. He should not be offered a renal transplant if he reaches end-stage renal disease

D. His renal disease has a significant chance of recurring after renal transplantation

E. His underlying disease can also cause sensorineural hearing loss

197. **A 38-year-old man presented to A&E with colicky left-sided abdominal pain radiating from his loin to his groin. He experienced severe nausea with this pain and had also noted an episode of visible haematuria. He was receiving antiviral therapy for HIV infection but was unable to recall all the medications he was taking. He had no other past medical history. He had no allergies, but reported claustrophobia during a CT scan he had had as a volunteer for a research project.**

On examination, the patient had a blood pressure of 160/80 mmHg and normal heart sounds and respiratory examination. Abdominal examination revealed renal angle tenderness on the left and his urine dipstick was strongly positive for blood but was otherwise normal.

```
Investigations:
   Hb                      120 g/L
   MCV                     88 fL
   WCC                     4 × 10⁹/L
   Platelets               630 × 10⁹/L
   Sodium                  142 mmol/L
   Potassium               5.2 mmol/L
   Urea                    4.8 mmol/L
   Creatinine              71 µmol/L
   Bilirubin               12 µmol/L
   Albumin                 38 g/L
   ALP                     162 iu/L
   AST                     38 iu/L
   ALT                     61 iu/L
```

Plain urinary tract radiograph: normal, no calculi seen

He was reviewed by the surgical team who felt his history and examination were strongly suggestive of a renal calculus and asked for further imaging to rule this out before agreeing to accept the patient for further management.

Which is the next appropriate investigation?

A. A 24-hour urine collection for 'stone screen'
B. Give pain relief and wait for a calculus to pass in the patient's urine and then send for biochemical analysis
C. Intravenous urography
D. Serum uric acid level
E. Unenhanced CT scan renal tract

198. A 64-year-old man presented to the medical admissions unit with lethargy, vomiting, and back pain. His past medical history consisted of benign prostatic hypertrophy. His only medication was tamsulosin.

On examination he had dry mucous membranes, a lying blood pressure of 110/75 mmHg, and a standing blood pressure of 90/60 mmHg with a low JVP.

```
Investigations:
    Hb                        90 g/L
    MCV                       88 fL
    White cell count          9 × 10⁹/L
    Platelets                 150 × 10⁹/L
    Sodium                    138 mmol/L
    Potassium                 5.1 mmol/L
    Urea                      35 mmol/L
    Creatinine                430 µmol/L
    Corrected calcium         3.2 mmol/L
    Magnesium                 1.20 mmol/L
```

Protein electrophoresis: M band with serum concentration of 38 g/L

Plain spinal radiographs: compression fracture of T12

Bone marrow aspirate: 60% clonal plasma cells

Which of the following would be the most likely histopathological finding on renal biopsy?

A. Abnormal angular and fractured cast deposition in the distal tubules

B. Deposits in the mesangium and capillaries which are birefringent under polarized light on Congo red stain

C. Fibrillary glomerulonephritis

D. Membranoproliferative glomerulonephritis

E. Thin glomerular basement membrane

199. **A 68-year-old man presented to his GP with lethargy. He had no past medical history and was on no medications. He had a blood pressure of 140/90 mmHg, with normal heart sounds on auscultation. Respiratory and abdominal examinations were normal and his weight was 76 kg, with a height of 1.78 m. Routine blood tests were performed.**

```
Investigations:
   Hb                      98 g/L
   MCV                     82 fL
   White cell count        11 × 10⁹/L
   Platelets               430 × 10⁹/L
   Sodium                  139 mmol/L
   Potassium               7.2 mmol/L
   Urea                    71 mmol/L
   Creatinine              1500 µmol/L
```

He was immediately sent to the emergency department where his ECG showed tenting of his T waves. He was given calcium gluconate followed by insulin and dextrose. His potassium decreased to 6.5 mmol/L, but rapidly rose back to 7 mmol/L after six hours.

A temporary haemodialysis catheter was inserted into his right internal jugular vein and haemodialysis commenced for five hours at a blood flow of 300 ml/min. Towards the end of this dialysis session he complained of headache and blurred vision. His GCS then fell from 15 to 10 and he developed asterixis. Dialysis was stopped at this point and his blood tests re-checked urgently.

```
   Sodium                  140 mmol/L
   Potassium               4.5 mmol/L
   Urea                    28 mmol/L
   Creatinine              810 µmol/L
   Glucose                 9.1 mmol/L
```

A bolus of naloxone was given but his GCS did not improve. He subsequently underwent a head CT scan head which was normal. He was transferred to the intensive care unit for supportive management and improved steadily over the next 24 hours.

Which patients are at increased risk of this syndrome?

A. Patients commenced on haemodialysis with a slower blood flow
B. Patients who are commenced on peritoneal dialysis compared to haemodialysis
C. Patients whose first haemodialysis session is five hours compared to two hours
D. Patients with a urea less than 30 mmol/L
E. Patients with no history of head injury or stroke

200. **A 44-year-old woman with a background history of diffuse scleroderma presented with a severe headache and blurred vision. On examination she had a GCS of 15/15 but was drowsy. Her blood pressure was 245/140 mmHg. Heart sounds revealed a gallop rhythm and chest examination revealed course crackles bibasally with oxygen saturations of 92% on room air and a respiratory rate of 28 per minute. Abdominal and neurological examinations were normal, as was fundoscopy.**

```
Investigations:
   Hb                        89 g/L
   MCV                       98 fL
   WCC                       11 × 10⁹/L
   Platelets                 300 × 10⁹/L
   Sodium                    143 mmol/L
   Potassium                 5.9 mmol/L
   Urea                      30 mmol/L
   Creatinine                580 µmol/L
Chest radio graph: bilateral pleural effusions, batwing
   appearance and fluid in the horizontal fissure
   CT head:                  unremarkable
```

She was admitted to the intensive care unit where an arterial line was placed for close blood pressure monitoring. She was commenced on captopril at a dose of 12.5 mg tds which was gradually titrated up. Her blood pressure dropped by 10–15 mmHg each day over the following week and she required haemofiltration to treat her peripheral and pulmonary oedema. A renal biopsy was performed which showed fibrinoid necrosis and 'onion-skin' intimal thickening.

Which of the following factors is predictive of a scleroderma renal crisis in a patient with scleroderma?

A. Abnormal urinalysis

B. Anti-centromere antibodies

C. Limited cutaneous scleroderma

D. New pericardial effusion

E. Previous renal impairment

201. A 45-year-old woman was visiting the UK on holiday and presented with low back pain radiating to her buttocks and thighs. She spoke no English and an interpreter was not immediately available. Her blood tests showed the following:

```
Investigations:
   Hb                            86 g/L
   White cell count              11 × 10⁹/L
   MCV                           75 fL
   Platelets                     300 × 10⁹/L
   Sodium                        146 mmol/L
   Potassium                     5.2 mmol/L
   Urea                          32 mmol/L
   Creatinine                    341 µmol/L
   Urinalysis                    blood 4+, protein +
Lumbar spine radiograph: significant calcified cysts in liver
   and kidneys
```

Which of the following is true about this patient's condition?

A. Alpha fetoprotein levels should be checked

B. Lactulose is likely to be the most effective treatment

C. Magnetic resonance angiography of her intracranial vessels should be performed

D. MRI of her spine should be performed

E. She has about a 55% chance of a mutation on chromosome 16

202. **A 21-year-old woman presented to the eye clinic with visual impairment. She also complained of weight loss and pyrexia. At the eye clinic she was diagnosed with uveitis and she had the following blood test results.**

```
Investigations:
   Hb                            110 g/L
   MCV                           90 fL
   WCC                           10 × 10⁹/L
   Platelets                     300 × 10⁹/L
   Sodium                        146 mmol/L
   Potassium                     4.8 mmol/L
   Urea                          18 mmol/L
   Creatinine                    300 µmol/L
```

She went on to have a renal biopsy which showed normal glomeruli but an intense inflammatory infiltrate of lymphocytes and monocytes in the interstitium.

What is the most likely diagnosis?

A. Acute tubulointerstitial nephritis (ATIN)

B. Alport's syndrome

C. IgA nephropathy

D. Sarcoidosis

E. TINU syndrome

203. **A 62-year-old man presented with intermittent claudication of his right leg. He was booked for an angiogram of his leg. His blood tests showed chronic kidney disease with a creatinine of 190 μmo/l and an eGFR of 38 ml/min.**

His medication included lisinopril, aspirin, and frusemide. As well as stopping his lisinopril and frusemide before and after his angiogram, which of the following is most likely to prevent radio contrast media induced nephropathy (RCN)?

A. 0.9% NaCl 1 ml/kg/hr for 12 hours pre and 12 hours post procedure

B. Three hours of dialysis directly after the angiogram

C. Adenosine A1 receptor antagonists

D. Low dose dopamine

E. N-acetylcysteine 600–1200 mg PO bd for 24 hours pre and post procedure

204. **A 24-year-old male presented with an episode of visible haematuria. He had no other symptoms. His father also had persistent non-visible haematuria. His blood tests, including U + Es, were all normal; he had 0.18 g/l protein in his urine and a normal renal ultrasound. He went on to have a renal biopsy: light microscopy and immunofluorescence were normal. The electron microscopy showed a glomerular basement membrane diameter of 184 nm.**

What is the most likely diagnosis?

A. Acute tubular necrosis

B. Alport's syndrome

C. Autosomal recessive polycystic kidney disease

D. C1q nephropathy

E. Thin membrane disease

205. **A 27-year-old woman presented with weakness, muscle aches, and cramps. Her past medical history included depression, anorexia diagnosed in her teens, and HIV which was well controlled. Her medication included tenofovir, emtricitabine, and ritonavir. Her only family history was of hypertension. On examination she appeared dehydrated with dry mucous membranes and a blood pressure of 85/55 mmHg systolic. Her jugular venous pressure was not visible. She was noted to have a short stature and her BMI was 17. The remainder of her examination was unremarkable.**

```
Investigations:
   Haemoglobin              132 g/L
   MCV                      98 fL
   White cell count         12 × 10⁹/L
   CD4 count                550 cells/µL
   HIV viral load           undetectable
   Bilirubin                14 umol/L
   Albumin                  28 g/L
   ALT                      28 iu/L
   ALP                      180 iu/L
   Sodium                   131 mmol/
   Potassium                2.1 mmol/L
   Urea                     14.1 mmol/L
   Creatinine               98 umol/l
   HCO₃⁻                    34 mmol/l
   Cl⁻                      86 mmol/l
   Magnesium                0.64 mmol/L
   Corrected calcium        2.01 mmol/L
   Phosphate                0.5 mmol/L
   Urinary sodium           44 mmol/L
She was admitted to hospital and given intravenous
   rehydration.
```

Which of the following statements is most likely to be true?

A. Her antiretroviral treatment is most likely responsible for the biochemical abnormalities

B. Not all family members will be affected as her condition is autosomal recessive

C. She would benefit from amiloride therapy

D. She will require lifelong sodium and potassium supplementation

E. Urinary sodium excretion will decrease during admission whilst on intravenous rehydration

206. **A 55-year-old woman presented with increasing peripheral oedema and nausea. She had a long-standing history of joint pains and stiffness but these had improved over the previous three years. She had never seen a doctor with regard to these pains but found relief using over the counter analgesics.**

On examination she had significant pitting peripheral oedema to the lower thighs, a blood pressure of 145/95 mmHg, and normal heart sounds. Abdominal examination revealed shifting dullness and respiratory examination was normal. She had ulnar deviation and Boutonnière's deformity of her hands.

```
Investigations:
    Hb                      95 g/L
    MCV                     87 fL
    WCC                     13 × 10⁹/L
    Platelets               400 × 10⁹/L
    Sodium                  136 mmol/L
    Potassium               4.6 mmol/L
    Urea                    15.6/L
    Creatinine              315 umol/L
    Bilirubin               12 µmol/L
    Albumin                 15 g/L
    ALP                     150 iu/L
    AST                     55 iu/L
    ALT                     69 iu/L
Urine dipstick blood - protein +++
24-hour urine protein: 4.3 g
```

Renal biopsy: amorphous deposits of pale hyaline material in the mesangium and capillary loops demonstrating green birefringence under polarized light. Immunofluorescence for light chains negative. Electron microscopy: fibrils seen.

The protein making up these fibril deposits is produced in which organ?

A. Heart

B. Kidneys

C. Liver

D. T cells

E. Thymus

207. **A 38-year-old man with a long history of intravenous drug use and known hepatitis C infection presented with increased lethargy and arthralgia. On examination he had a palpable purpuric rash on his legs. He had a blood pressure of 145/90 mmHg with normal heart sounds. Abdominal examination revealed splenomegaly. Neurological examination revealed a glove and stocking sensory loss to light touch.**

```
Investigations:
    Hb                      105 g/L
    MCV                     97 fL
    WCC                     11 × 10⁹/L
    Platelets               570 × 10⁹/L
    Sodium                  138 mmol/L
    Potassium               3.6 mmol/L
    Urea                    12.6/L
    Creatinine              240 umol/L
    Urine dipstick:         blood +++ protein +++
```

Renal biopsy: diffuse mesangial hypercellularity and double contour appearance of glomerular basement membrane

Which of the following would be consistent with the underlying pathology?

A. ANCA positivity

B. Cryoglobulins precipitating after five days

C. Cryoglobulins precipitating in the first 24 hours

D. Decreased serum C3 and increased C4

E. Negative rheumatoid factor

208. A 48-year-old woman presented with a four-week history of fevers, lethargy, and painless oral ulcers. On examination she had a malar rash and a temperature of 37.8°C. Heart sounds were normal and blood pressure was 150/85 mmHg. Respiratory, abdominal, and neurological examinations were normal. She underwent the following investigations:

```
Investigations:
   Hb                        95 g/L
   MCV                       85 fL
   WCC                       15 × 10⁹/L
   Platelets                 610 × 10⁹/L
   Sodium                    142 mmol/L
   Potassium                 4.9 mmol/L
   Urea                      17.6/L
   Creatinine                390 µmol/L
   CRP                       14 mg/L
   ANA                       positive
   Anti-ds DNA antibodies    positive 89 IU/ml
   ESR                       80 mm in first hour
   C3                        0.7 g/L (0.8-1.6 g/L)
   C4                        0.1 g/L (0.16-0.48 g/L)
Urine dipstick blood ++ protein ++
Chest radiograph normal cardiac size and no pleural effusion
```

A renal biopsy was subsequently performed which showed: Active focal glomerulonephritis involving <50% of all glomeruli. Subendothelial and mesangial immune deposits positive for IgG and C3 and C1q.

Which of the following is true?

A. As her 24-hour protein is less than 1 g, no treatment should be given at present but should be closely monitored with monthly urinary dipsticks and U + Es

B. She has class II lupus nephritis

C. She has class III lupus nephritis

D. The decreased complement indicates quiescent lupus

E. The normal CRP indicates quiescent lupus

209. **A 54-year-old woman presented with confusion and seizures. Her husband reported that she had suffered from one week of intermittent numbness and tingling followed by two seizures in the space of two days, with increasing confusion. He had noticed bruise-like lesions on her skin and she had become more tired. On examination she had a GCS of 15 out of 15 but an AMT score of 4 out of 10. She had a temperature of 36.9°C and her blood pressure was 125/80 mmHg. Her neurological examination was otherwise entirely normal. Purpuric lesions were identified on her arms, legs, and trunk.**

```
Investigations:
   Hb                        85 g/L
   MCV                       91 fL
   WCC                       9 × 10⁹/L
   Platelets                 18 × 10⁹/L
   Sodium                    138 mmol/L
   Potassium                 3.6 mmol/L
   Urea                      6.4/L
   Creatinine                98 µmol/L
   LDH                       310 U/L (100-190 U/L)
   Haptoglobins              0.2 g/L (0.7-3.2 g/l)
   D-Dimer                   410 ng/mL
   Fibrinogen                2 g/L (1.9-4.3 g/L)
   Blood film:               red cell fragments
```

Which of the following statements is correct?

A. A decrease in factor IX would be seen

B. A decrease in factor VIII would be seen

C. ADAMTS13 activity 2% of normal is diagnostic

D. The pathology is due to an increase in factor H

E. The pathology is due to decreased von Willebrand factor

210. **A 45-year-old man on treatment for acute myeloid leukaemia (AML)
with daunorubicin and arabinosylcytosine presented with a three-day
history of nausea, vomiting, malaise, and decreased urine output.
He had a past medical history of epilepsy, chronic kidney disease of
unknown aetiology (with a baseline creatinine of 220 µmol/L), G6PD
deficiency, hypertension, and type II diabetes mellitus. On examination
he appeared dehydrated, with a blood pressure of 90/40 mmHg. He
had not passed urine in nearly 24 hours and a bladder scan showed only
30 ml of urine.**

```
Investigations:
   Hb                          120 g/L
   MCV                         88 fL
   WCC                         31 × 10⁹/L
   Platelets                   350 × 10⁹/L
   Sodium                      138 mmol/L
   Potassium                   5.8 mmol/L
   Urea                        31/L
   Creatinine                  760 µmol/L
   Corrected calcium           1.9 mmol/L
   Phosphate                   2.1 mmol/L
   Uric acid                   750 µmol/L
```

Which of the following should *not* be undertaken?

A. Aggressive intravenous hydration aiming for a urine output >100 ml/hour

B. Allopurinol 100 mg three times/week

C. Close monitoring of fluid balance and urea and electrolytes

D. Imaging of the renal tract to rule out obstruction

E. Rasburicase 200 mg/kg/day IV

211. **A 22-year-old student presented with severe diffuse muscle pain and
cramps following her first rowing training session. She had experienced
a previous, less severe episode two weeks prior when she had gone
for a short jog in preparation for her rowing training. She had not
experienced such symptoms previously, but did recall muscle aches
when she was eight years old. Her parents reported being told by the
doctor at the time that they were 'growing pains'. She had no other
past medical history and was not on any medications. She denied
taking any recreational drugs and never drank alcohol. She had not
travelled abroad in the previous five years.**

**On examination she had significant diffuse muscle tenderness. There
were no skin lesions. Heart sounds were normal, as were respiratory
and abdominal examinations. No neurological deficit was seen on
examination. Her urine was dark.**

```
Investigations:
   Hb                      140 g/L
   MCV                     98 fL
   WCC                     9 × 10⁹/L
   Platelets               280 × 10⁹/L
   Sodium                  141 mmol/L
   Potassium               5.8 mmol/L
   Urea                    28 mmol/L
   Creatinine              330 µmol/L
   Phosphate               2.1 mmol/L
   Corrected calcium       1.8 mmol/L
   CK                      65000 iu/L
   Urinalysis:             blood 3+, protein +, leucocytes -,
                           nitrites -
                           Urine sediment: normal
                           Urine microscopy: no red cells
```

**She was treated with vigorous IV hydration and pain relief and the
symptoms resolved. Her CK decreased but did not return to baseline.
She went on to have a muscle biopsy.**

**Muscle biopsy: deposits of subsarcolemmal PAS positive glycogen
deposits at the periphery of myofibres. Enzyme histochemistry
reveals absence of myophosphorylase but presence of acid maltase,
debranching enzyme, and phosphofructokinase.**

**Which of the following is the underlying cause of rhabdomyolysis in this
patient?**

A. Cori disease

B. McArdle's disease

C. Pompe disease

D. Tarui disease

E. von Gierke disease

212. **A 38-year-old man presented with a one-week history of persistent cough. He brought up about half a cup of frank haemoptysis each day. Over the previous two days he had become very nauseated and experienced cramps. He was a smoker but had no other past medical history and was not on any regular medication.**

On examination he was tachypnoeic and had oxygen saturations of 85% on air. Heart sounds were normal, and he had a blood pressure of 130/ 80 mmHg. Auscultation of his chest revealed widespread crackles.

```
Investigations:
    Haemoglobin              74 g/dL
    MCV                      84 fL
    White cell count         7 × 10⁹/L
    Platelets                380 × 10⁹/L
    Sodium                   136 mmol/L
    Potassium                6.8 mmol/L
    Urea                     65 mmol/L
    Creatinine               1480 µmol/L
    c-ANCA (PR3) positive:   84
    anti-GBM titre positive: 160
```

He underwent urgent haemodialysis and renal biopsy was then performed which showed segmental necrosis and crescent formation, with immunofluorescence showing linear staining for anti-GBM.

Which of the following statements is true?

A. Double positivity for c-ANCA and anti-GBM means the patient has granulomatosis with polyangiitis and anti-GBM disease

B. Double positivity for c-ANCA and anti-GBM means the patient has granulomatosis with polyangiitis only

C. If the patient does not recover renal function, renal transplantation is possible in the long term

D. If the patient progresses to end-stage renal failure and undergoes renal transplantation Alport's syndrome may occur within the transplanted kidney

E. Plasma exchange should not be offered as the patient is unlikely to gain any renal benefit

213. **A 45-year-old man presented with increasing leg swelling and nausea. He had noticed that his legs had gradually increased in size over the previous four months, and that over that time his urine had become increasingly frothy. His blood pressure was 115/80 mmHg and he had pitting oedema to his thighs, along with shifting dullness on abdominal examination. He was admitted to hospital and investigated further.**

```
Investigations:
   Haemoglobin                    121 g/dL
   MCV                            99 fL
   WCC                            9 × 10⁹/L
   Platelets                      160 × 10⁹/L
   Sodium                         146 mmol/L
   Potassium                      4.7 mmol/L
   Urea                           7.5 mmol/L
   Creatinine                     95 µmol/L
   Albumin                        10 g/L
   Urine dipstick                 blood - protein +++
   24-hour urinary protein 8.2 g/day
```

Renal biopsy: thickening and 'spikes' of GBM extending around subepithelial deposits. Loss of podocyte foot processes. Immunofluorescence: granular IgG deposits.

He is managed with intravenous furosemide to improve his peripheral oedema.

Which of the following is true regarding membranous glomerulonephritis (MGN)?

A. Eighty-five per cent of cases of MGN are secondary to infections, drugs, infections, etc.

B. An M type phospholipase A2 receptor antibody can be identified in 70% of cases of primary idiopathic MGN

C. MGN is more common in patients of Afro-Caribbean origin

D. Serum C3 levels are often elevated in MGN

E. Two thirds of patients undergo spontaneous remission if untreated

214. A 32-year-old woman was referred to clinic with increasing ankle swelling over the preceding weeks. On respiratory examination she had stony dull percussion note at both bases. Cardiovascular and abdominal examination was normal. She had pitting oedema to her thighs. Her blood pressure was 155/90 mmHg.

```
Investigations:
    Hb                        110 g/L
    MCV                       95 fL
    WCC                       11 × 10⁹/L
    Platelets                 210 × 10⁹/L
    Sodium                    149 mmol/L
    Potassium                 5.1 mmol/L
    Urea                      9.5 mmol/L
    Creatinine                145 μmol/L
    Albumin                   21 g/L
    Urinalysis:               protein 4+, blood -, leucocytes -,
                              nitrites -
                              24-hour urinary protein 9.4 g/day
    CXR:                      small bilateral effusions
    Renal US:                 normal size kidneys with no signs
                              of obstruction
```

She then had the following tests performed to screen for a secondary cause of nephrotic syndrome: ANA, dsDNA, IgG, C3/C4, serum paraprotein, serum/urine free light chains, hepatitis B/C, and HIV. All of these were negative. It was therefore decided to perform a renal biopsy.

Renal biopsy: areas of glomerular sclerosis and tuft collapse affecting segments of some but not all glomeruli. Three areas of segmental sclerosis are affecting the outer tip of the glomerulus alongside the proximal tubule. Immunostaining is positive for IgM and C3. There is loss of podocyte foot process effacement.

Which of the following is correct?

A. The patient has focal and segmental sclerosis and the collapsing variant indicates a better prognosis

B. The patient has focal and segmental sclerosis and the glomerular tip lesion indicates a better prognosis

C. The patient has membranous nephropathy

D. The patient has minimal change nephropathy

E. The patient would not experience recurrence of the renal pathology after renal transplant

215. **A 27-year-old intravenous drug user was found to have deranged renal function tests and referred for further investigation. On examination his blood pressure was 160/88 mmHg, he had normal heart sounds with no audible murmurs, a clear chest on auscultation, and a soft abdomen. He had no rashes on examination and had no signs of pitting oedema.**

```
Investigations:
   Hb                                104 g/L
   MCV                               82 fL
   WCC                               7.8 × 10⁹/L
   Platelets                         453 × 10⁹/L
   Sodium                            135 mmol/L
   Potassium                         4.2 mmol/L
   Urea                              17.5 mmol/L
   Creatinine                        163 µmol/L
   Albumin                           34 g/L
   C3                                0.5 g/L (0.8-1.6 g/L)
   C4                                0.05 g/L (0.16-0.48 g/L)
   Urinalysis:                       protein +, blood +
   Urine protein:creatinine ratio:   145 mg/mmol
```

A renal biopsy was performed which showed changes consistent with a membranoproliferative glomerulonephritis. There was granular deposition of IgM, C3, and both kappa and lambda light chains. IgG was present, and C1q was negative.

What is the most likely underlying cause for this patient's renal impairment?

A. Bacterial endocarditis

B. Cellulitis

C. Hepatitis C

D. HIV

E. Syphilis

216. A 67-year-old gentleman presented to A&E with a two-day history of abdominal pain. He had end-stage kidney disease secondary to diabetic nephropathy and had been established on peritoneal dialysis two years previously.

On examination he was pyrexial with a temperature of 38.1°C but was haemodynamically stable. His abdomen demonstrated generalized tenderness but no guarding or signs of peritonism. His peritoneal dialysis (PD) catheter exit site was clean; however, the effluent in the PD bag was cloudy.

Analysis of the fluid revealed WCC 650 with 60% neutrophils and he was commenced on intra-peritoneal vancomycin and gentamicin as per the local protocol.

What is the most likely causative organism for PD peritonitis?

A. *Escherichia coli*
B. *Klebsiella pneumoniae*
C. *Pseudomonas aeruginosa*
D. *Staphylococcus aureus*
E. *Staphylococcus epidermidis*

217. A 30-year-old lady attended her GP for advice regarding commencing the oral contraceptive pill. She was well within herself. However, she was found to have a pulse of 74 beats per minute and a blood pressure of 180/100 mmHg. Her chest was clear on auscultation and both heart sounds were normal with no added sounds. There were no pitting oedema.

```
Investigations:
  Hb                         111 g/L
  WCC                        7.8 × 10⁹/L
  Platelets                  453 × 10⁹/L
  Sodium                     135 mmol/L
  Potassium                  3.2 mmol/L
  Urea                       6.8 mmol/L
  Creatinine                 86 µmol/L
  9 am cortisol              380 nmol/L
  Renin                      6.1 ng/ml/hr    (0.65–5.0 ng/ml/hr)
  Aldosterone                181 ng/dL       (<21 ng/dL)
  Aldosteron:renin ratio     30
```

What is the most likely underlying aetiology of this lady's hypertension?

A. Cushing's syndrome
B. Essential hypertension
C. Phaeochromocytoma
D. Primary hyperaldosteronism
E. Renal artery stenosis

218. **A 56-year-old female with nephrotic syndrome attended her follow-up appointment in clinic. She had been feeling more fatigued than usual and felt her oedema had worsened. Blood tests revealed an acute decline in renal function. Urinalysis showed blood 2+, protein 3+. Her urinary protein:creatinine ratio was 995 mg/mmol, comparable to 550 mg/mmol when seen in clinic three months previously.**

    A CT scan was done which revealed a renal vein thrombosis.

    What underlying nephropathy is most commonly associated with RVT in patients with nephrotic syndrome?

    A. Focal segmental glomerulosclerosis
    B. Membranoproliferative glomerulonephritis
    C. Membranous nephropathy
    D. Minimal change disease
    E. Rapidly progressive glomerulonephritis

219. **A 46-year-old man with end-stage renal disease had routine dialysis bloods performed.**

    He had a history of congenital dysplastic kidneys and developed end-stage renal disease at the age of 11. He underwent renal transplantation, but unfortunately the transplant was rejected due to poor compliance with immunosuppressive medication. He was established on haemodialysis but compliance with medications remained variable.

    ```
    Investigations:
      Hb                    89 g/L
      WCC                   7.2 × 10⁹/L
      Platelets             279 × 10⁹/L
      Sodium                139 mmol/L
      Potassium             3.7 mmol/L
      Urea                  4.8 mmol/L
      Creatinine            289 µmol/L
      Phosphate             2.1 mmol/L
      Corrected calcium     2.02 mmol/L
      ALP                   1200 iU/L
      PTH                   240 pmol/L
    ```

    Which of the following statements is true regarding patient with CKD stage 5?

    A. Bone-derived turnover markers of collagen synthesis (procollagen type I C-terminal propeptide) and breakdown (such as type I collagen cross-linked telopeptide, cross-laps, pyridinoline, or deoxypyridinoline) should be measured
    B. A lateral abdominal radiograph can be used to detect the presence or absence of vascular calcification
    C. Levels of FGF23 are decreased
    D. PTH levels should be brought to normal levels using both or either phosphate binders and vitamin D supplements
    E. Serum calcium, phosphate, and PTH should be checked six-monthly

220. A 58-year-old female presented with right-sided loin pain. In the past she had suffered from three urinary tract infections and haematuria. An abdominal X-ray was performed which showed a small cluster of 2–3 mm opacified lesions in keeping with renal caluli on the right side.

A subsequent CT urogram was reported as showing: 'multiple papillary calcifications accompanied by a brushwork of dilated ducts that fill with contrast material'.

Which of the following is most in keeping with the underlying disorder?

A. Dent's disease
B. Diabetic nephropathy
C. Medullary sponge kidney
D. Renal cell carcinoma
E. Renal dysgenesis

221. A 36-year-old patient attended renal low clearance clinic for review. He suffered from polycystic kidney disease and had had a gradual decline in renal duration over the preceding seven years. His eGFR was 15 mL/min/1.73 m2 and he had been listed for renal transplantation.

Following transplantation, which of the following factors would put this patient at high risk of acute rejection?

A. Aetiology of renal failure
B. Black ethnicity
C. Cold ischaemic time >4 hours
D. Older recipient
E. Prior use of immunosuppression

222. A 28-year-old pharmacist was found collapsed at work by a colleague. He had recently been suffering from low mood and was thought to have taken an overdose. He was rushed to A&E.

Which of the following medications would *not* be cleared by acute dialysis?

A. Aspirin
B. Carbamazepine
C. Levetiracetam
D. Methanol
E. Theophylline

223. **A 68-year-old lady was seen for her annual diabetic check-up. She suffered from hypertension, type II diabetes mellitus, and hyperlipidaemia. She had undergone laser photocoagulation for diabetic retinopathy in the previous year and also attended the GP surgery on four occasions for treatment of urinary tract infections. On examination, the patient's blood pressure was 150/85 mmHg and her BMI was 28. She had mild pitting oedema to her mid-shin. Her urine dipstick testing revealed only 2+ of protein and was negative for blood, glucose, or ketones. Quantified, she had an albumin:creatinine ratio of 250 µg/mg.**

    What is the most likely underlying cause for this patient's renal pathology?

    A. Amyloidosis
    B. Kimmelstiel-Wilson glomerulosclerosis
    C. Membranous nephropathy
    D. Minimal change disease
    E. Renal papillary necrosis

224. **A 46-year-old man with type II diabetes mellitus was referred to the diabetic renal clinic after routine blood tests revealed a decline in renal function. His diabetes was generally poorly controlled with his latest Hba1c being measured at 68 mmol/mol.**

    ```
    Investigations:
       Hb                            92 g/L
       MCV                           78 fL
       WCC                           5 × 10⁹/L
       Platelets                     210 × 10⁹/L
       Sodium                        134 mmol/L
       Potassium                     5.6 mmol/L
       Urea                          11.6/L
       Creatinine                    160 µmol/L
       eGFR                          43ml/min
    Urine albumin:creatinine
    ratio (ACR):                     2 mg/mmol
    ```

    Renal ultrasound: right kidney 8.0 cm, left kidney 8.2 cm. Both kidneys illustrate hyperechogenicity and no evidence of hydronephrosis.

    This patient's findings are consistent with what stage of CKD?

    A. CKD G3a A1
    B. CKD G3a A2
    C. CKD G3a A3
    D. CKD G3b A1
    E. CKD G3b A2

225. **An 86-year-old lady presented to her GP with a two-month history of worsening shortness of breath. She was known to have chronic kidney disease secondary to hypertensive nephropathy. Her medication included: atorvastatin 40 mg on, aspirin 75 mg od, omeprazole 20 mg od, bisoprolol 2.5 mg od, and furosemide 80 mg bd. On examination she was dyspnoeic at rest with a respiratory rate of 22 breaths per minute. She had an elevated JVP to 8 cm and bilateral coarse crepitations in the lower zones of her lungs. She had pedal oedema to her mid-thighs. Her weight was noted to be 75 kg, it had been 70 kg four months previously.**

Investigations:

Hb	106 g/L
MCV	82 fL
WCC	7.8×10^9/L
Platelets	253×10^9/L
Sodium	133 mmol/L
Potassium	5.7 mmol/L
Urea	13.9 g/L
Creatinine	256 µmol/L

What further diuretic would be best suited to manage this patient's fluid overload?

A. Amiloride

B. Bumetanide

C. Mannitol

D. Metolazone

E. Spironolactone

196. D) His renal disease has a significant chance of recurring after renal transplantation

This question tests the ability to identify the diagnosis of IgA nephropathy. The patient is hypertensive with deranged renal function and nephrotic range proteinuria. The serum IgA is normal, which may lead one to dismiss the diagnosis, but an elevated IgA level is only seen in around 50% of patients. The key to the correct answer is recognizing the features of IgA nephropathy on renal biopsy. A confounding factor is the family history of renal disease, which may cause confusion amongst candidates who may try to link an inheritable form of renal disease. The above pattern may fit with an X-linked inheritance pattern, raising the possibility of Alport's syndrome, especially as sensorineural loss is given in the choice of answers. The history of recurrent labyrinthitis and previous episode of reactive arthritis are of no particular relevance.

Tutorial

IgA nephropathy is the most common form of primary glomerulonephritis, ranging from 5 to 40 cases per million population per year across the world, generally reflecting the difference in threshold for renal biopsy in different countries. The male:female ratio ranges from 2:1 in Japan to as high as 6:1 in northern Europe and the USA.

The disease is usually idiopathic (primary) but may also be secondary as per Table 10.1.

Table 10.1 Examples of diseases associated with IgA nephropathy

Category	Disease examples
Mucosal diseases	Coeliac disease, inflammatory bowel disease, angle-closure glaucoma, anterior uveitis, bronchial and pulmonary diseases, cystic fibrosis
Neoplasia	Bronchial carcinoma, B-cell lymphoma, cutaneous T-cell lymphoma, multiple myeloma, renal cell carcinoma, hepatocellular carcinoma
Immunological and systemic disorders	Rheumatoid arthritis, bullous pemphigoid, ankylosing spondylitis, HIV, Behçet's disease, mixed cryoglobulinaemia, myasthenia gravis
Liver disease	Alcoholic liver cirrhosis, non-cirrhotic portal fibrosis, post splenorenal shunt
Others	Myelodysplastic syndromes, Fabry's disease, leprosy, porphyria, psoriasis, diabetes mellitus, Wiskott-Aldrich syndrome

Primary IgA nephropathy is not considered to be hereditary; however, familial clustering is seen. The pathogenesis remains unclear, but is likely to involve the interplay of haematological, mucosal, and renal systems with increased IgA bearing lymphocytes and activated T helper cells, over-expression of TGF-β and IL-4 mRNA in CD4 cells, and galactosylated IgA_1 deposited in the mesangium, leading to mesangial cell proliferation and inflammatory responses causing local injury.

Histologically, segmental or diffuse mesangial hypercellularity with an increase in mesangial matrix (leading to segmental sclerosis) is seen on light microscopy. Immunostaining demonstrates deposits of IgA and C3. IgG and IgM can also be seen. Electron microscopy reveals mesangial deposits near a normal glomerular basement membrane. The only other glomerulonephritis associated with extensive glomerular IgA deposition is lupus nephritis, but IgG deposition is often more prominent and C1q is seen due to activation of the classical complement pathway, and other immune components are often also present ('full house staining').

Patients are often asymptomatic on presentation, with non-visible haematuria with or without proteinuria (only reaching nephrotic range in <15% of patients). Haematuria may be visible and timed with an upper respiratory illness (synpharyngitic haematuria). Refractory hypertension is common.

Elevated IgA levels are seen in ~50%. If associated with a skin rash (usually purpuric) a skin biopsy shows a leukocytoclastic vasculitis with IgA deposition on immunostaining. It should not be forgotten that IgA nephropathy is seen in Henoch-Schönlein purpura in which other organs (such as skin, joints, gastrointestinal tract) may be involved.

Around 5–15% of patients develop end-stage renal disease after five years, 20–50% after 20 years and Box 10.1 lists the poor prognostic features.

Box 10.1 Poor prognostic features at presentation of IgA nephropathy

1) Impaired renal function
2) Heavy proteinuria (>3 g/day)
3) Poorly controlled hypertension
4) Tubulo-interstitial fibrosis and glomerulosclerosis on biopsy
5) Rapidly progressive crescentic presentation

Those with normal renal function, episodic macroscopic haematuria, <1 g proteinuria, and normal blood pressure require yearly monitoring of blood pressure and proteinuria. Patients with >1 g proteinuria, hypertension, and increasing age should have their BP treated to a target of <125/75 mmHg and reduction of their proteinuria with an ACE inhibitor or angiotensin-II receptor blocker. The use of both agents as dual blockade may offer further benefit but this is unproven and increases risk of hyperkalaemia. Fish oils (ω-3 fatty acids) have been used to limit progression but the evidence base for this is poor.

Some authors/guidelines support a trial of steroids in cases of persistent proteinuria >1 g/24 hours with preserved renal function—despite 3–6 months of optimized supportive care with eGFR >50 ml/min. This has to be weighed up against the potential side effects and remains a topic of debate among nephrologists. Further immunosuppression with cyclophosphamide is only indicated in those presenting with crescentic disease, and can be converted to maintenance therapy on azathioprine.

IgA nephropathy recurs in about 21–58% of patients following renal transplantation, but early loss of allograft function from recurrent disease is uncommon. IgA nephropathy is therefore not a contraindication to transplantation.

Further Reading

Donadio J, Grande J (2002). IgA nephropathy. *New England Journal of Medicine* 347: 738–748.

Floege J, Feehally J (2000). IgA nephropathy, recent developments. *Journal of the American Society of Nephrology* 11(12): 2395–2403.

197. C) Intravenous urography

Imaging is required to confirm the diagnosis, locate the stone, exclude obstruction, and guide intervention to remove or break down the stone. Only calcium containing or struvite stones are radio opaque. Cystine stones are well seen on CT. All stones can cause an acoustic shadow on ultrasound. Whilst unenhanced CT is usually the best single test, other imaging modalities may be more appropriate in certain situations:

- Plain KUB radiography—provides baseline for easy follow-up monitoring of a radio opaque stone by KUB radiography.
- Ultrasound—useful when radiation needs to be minimized and will also show hydronephrosis if present. However, is less accurate for diagnosing distal ureteric stones and detecting small stones.
- Intravenous urography (IVU)—identifies the single problematic stone amongst numerous pelvic calcifications that may be seen on radiography or CT, reveals any hydronephrosis, and importantly identifies radiolucent stones by a filling defect.
- *Non-contrast CT scanning*—high sensitivity and provides anatomical view of other pathologies within the abdomen, but will not pick up radiolucent stones

In this case no radio opaque stones are seen on the plain KUB radiograph and the patient is undergoing therapy for HIV. Protease inhibitors predispose to radiolucent stones best visualized by IVU or *contrast* CT. This was seen with older agents such as indinavir and atazanavir but now with darunavir (often used in multi-drug resistant HIV). A 24-hour urine collection for 'stone screen' is described below and is used to detect metabolic disorders that predispose to recurrent stone formation rather than diagnosis and localization of a stone. A serum uric acid level will indicate if the patient has high uric acid levels which may predispose to uric acid or combined uric acid/calcium oxalate stones, but will not help in the acute diagnosis in an obstructing renal calculus. Waiting for the stone to pass is potentially dangerous as the patient may have an obstructed left renal system with infection and hydronephrosis, placing him at high risk of sepsis although the temperature and CRP are against this.

Tutorial

Renal (nephrolithiasis) and ureteric (ureterolithiasis) calculi occur in up to 15% of people, being more common in males. The five main groups of renal stones are:

1) Calcium stones (calcium oxalate, calcium phosphate)

These account for 70% of cases and are usually associated with an underlying metabolic abnormality, but may also be idiopathic. Increased calcium or oxalate delivery promote formation:

- Hypercalciuria: increased GI absorption or renal wasting due to decreased reabsorption.
- Hypercalcaemic states: particularly hyperparathyroidism.
- Hyperuricosuria: uric acid promotes calcium oxalate stone formation. Causes include a diet high in purine (fish, meat extracts, legumes, gravies), rapid cell turnover (e.g. malignancy), and uricosuric drugs.
- Hyperoxaluria: increased uptake secondary to ileal resection or Crohn's disease or increased dietary intake.
- Other: hypocitraturia, hypomagnesuria, and chronic acidosis.

2) Struvite stones (magnesium ammonium phosphate)

These account for 10% of cases. Associated with chronic Gram-negative rod urinary (*Proteus*, *Klebsiella*, and *Pseudomonas*) *E. coli* is not associated with struvite stones. Promoted by a urinary pH >7. Such stones act as a focus for continuing infection, leading to expansion of the stone to fill much of the collecting system known as staghorn calculi.

3) Uric acid stones

These account for 5% of cases. More commonly found in association with calcium oxalate stones. Promoted by a urinary pH <5.5 and hyperuricosuria.

4) Cystine stones

These account for 1–2% of cases. Caused by a mutation in renal tubular amino acid reabsorption.

5) Rarer stones

These include radiolucent stones caused by indinavir and atazanavir

General measures in the management of recurrent nephrolithiasis involve increasing oral fluid to achieve urine output greater than 2.5 litres per day, and reducing animal protein and salt intake (salt enhances calciuria). Patients with a positive family history of stones or those experiencing more than one stone per three years should be investigated to identify a treatable underlying metabolic or genetic disorder in a specialist clinic. The recommended investigations in these patients is summarized in Box 10.2.

Box 10.2 Investigations for recurrent stone formers

- Urinary pH and specific gravity
- Dipstix for haematuria
- Biochemical analysis of passed stone
- Microscopy of urine for crystals
- Urine culture for chronic infection
- U+E/urate/calcium/phosphate/ALP/PTH
- Imaging (see text)
- A 24-hour urine for 'stone screen' in acidified container, except uric acid which requires plain container

---

Further Reading

Assimos D, Krambeck, A, Miller N, et al. (2016). Surgical management of stones: American Urological Association/Endourological Society Guideline, Part I. *Journal of Urology* 196(4): 1153–1160.

Assimos D, Krambeck, A, Miller N, et al. (2016). Surgical management of stones: American Urological Association/Endourological Society Guideline, Part 2. *Journal of Urology* 196(4): 1161–1169.

Moe O (2006). Kidney stones: pathophysiology and medical management. *Lancet* 367: 333–344.

198. A) Abnormal angular and fractured cast deposition in the distal tubules

The presence of a serum M band, high bone marrow clonal plasma cell percentage, and organ damage (renal insufficiency, hypercalcaemia, and bone fracture) are consistent with a diagnosis of multiple myeloma. The patient is dehydrated and intravascularly depleted from the vomiting and hypercalcaemia. The most common histological finding in myeloma-associated renal impairment is cast nephropathy. The tubular casts are formed by filtered free immunoglobulin light chains combining with Tamm-Horsfall protein.

Congo red positive birefringent deposits would be seen with fibril formation in the mesangium in AL amyloidosis as a complication of myeloma. Tubular epithelial cell flattening and dilatation of the tubules are features seen in acute tubular necrosis which can result from decreased renal perfusion secondary to dehydration and hypercalcaemia. A thin glomerular basement membrane is seen in Alport's syndrome and thin membrane disease with a basket-weave pattern on electron microscopy diagnostic of the former.

Tutorial

A monoclonal band in serum or urine, >10% plasma cells on bone marrow testing and evidence of end organ damage ('CRAB': hyperCalcaemia, Renal impairment, Anaemia or Bone lesions) are key features of myeloma. Renal impairment occurs in around half of patients with multiple myeloma (often the first presenting feature) from the following contributing factors:

- Dehydration
- Pre-existing renal impairment
- Concomitant use of ACE inhibitors
- Hypercalcaemia (leading to renal vasoconstriction, nephrocalcinosis or direct tubular toxicity)
- Light chain burden (higher amount being more likely to cause a renal manifestation)
- Propensity for light chains to form amyloid proteins: AL Amyloidosis
- Hyperuricaemia

The most common renal manifestations of light chains in the kidney are:

- *Cast nephropathy (myeloma kidney)* occurs from obstruction of the tubules and collecting ducts when free immunoglobulin light chains (Bence Jones protein, freely filtered at the glomeruli) bind to Tamm-Horsfall protein in the tubules, forming proteinaceous casts. Whilst the casts may stain with Congo red, as well as Masson's trichrome, they are not birefringent under polarized night. The casts often show a characteristic 'fractured' appearance, and there is frequently a surrounding inflammatory reaction. Bence Jones protein can also be directly toxic to tubular cells. If free light chains are <500 mg/L then cast nephropathy is unlikely.
- *AL amyloidosis* involves the formation of amyloid fibrils from light chains (most commonly lambda) leading to the deposition sheets of amyloid in the mesangium and capillaries. This is discussed in more detail in the tutorial to question 206.
- *Light chain deposition disease* involves the deposition of light chains (usually kappa) in the capillary walls and mesangium. However, fibrils do not form and Congo red staining is negative. Light microscopy shows nodular glomerulosclerosis and light chains can be detected by immunostaining.

Management of myeloma-associated renal failure initially involves correction of hypovolaemia with intravenous rehydration and if the serum calcium remains high once euvolaemic, then bisphosphonate therapy may be administered. Allopurinol should be commenced if hyperuricaemia is present. Combination therapy with steroids and alkylating agents may be of benefit by decreasing immunoglobulin/light chain synthesis. The urgency of diagnosis is important with newer agents such as thalidomide (and derivatives) and proteasome inhibitors (such as bortezomib) gaining an increasing role (with bortezomib recommended by NICE for newly diagnosed myeloma-induced acute kidney disease). The former often require dose adjustment according to renal function. The role of plasma exchange or high cut-off dialysis to remove free light chains remains unclear.

Plasma cell dyscrasias have traditionally been classified into 'monoclonal gammopathy of undetermined significance' (MGUS—presence of paraprotein but no other adverse features), 'smouldering myeloma' (higher level paraprotein or bone marrow plasma cell burden without organ or tissue impairment—carries a higher risk of progression to myeloma), non-secretory myeloma (organ/tissue damage but with no detectable paraprotein), and full-blown myeloma. However, it is now recognized that a significant number of 'MGUS' patients have renal disease attributable to their plasma cell dyscrasia—this has been named 'monoclonal gammopathy of renal significance' (MGRS)—this includes light chain deposition disease and renal AL amyloidosis.

Further Reading

Dimopoulos M, Sonneveld P, Leung N, et al. (2016). International myeloma working group recommendations for the diagnosis and management of myeloma-related renal impairment. *Journal of Clinical Oncology* 34(13): 1544–1557.

199. C) Patients whose first haemodialysis session is five hours compared to two hours

The findings described in this scenario are consistent with dialysis disequilibrium syndrome (DDS). The patient has undergone his first dialysis for an extended time period for a first session and starting with a very high serum urea. The rapid drop in serum urea during dialysis will have made him very prone to DDS.

Other potential causes of these neurological symptoms have been excluded as evidenced by normal sodium (hyponatraemia) and normal glucose (hypoglycaemia). His CT head excludes an intracerebral bleed, although an ischaemic stroke (due to dialysis-related cerebral hypoperfusion) cannot be ruled out with this early imaging. There is no suggestion of accumulation of drugs and the lack of response to naloxone is against occult opioid toxicity.

First-time haemodialysis patients are at greater risk of DDS, particularly if they start with a urea >60 mmol/l. In such patients, a starting dialysis session would typically be for only two hours of dialysis with a slower blood flow rate (~150–200 ml/min).

Haemofiltration or peritoneal dialysis leads to a more gradual decrease in urea levels. Those who are already established on haemodialysis may become at risk if there is a significant change in their dialysis regime (e.g. increased dialysis flow rates) or if their urea rises significantly (e.g. missing dialysis sessions or following an upper gastrointestinal bleed). Patients with existing neurological disease (such as previous stroke or head injury) are also at greater risk.

Tutorial

DDS is characterized by varying degrees of neurological symptoms. Whilst uraemia itself can lead to neurological symptoms ranging from impaired concentration and hallucinations through to agitation, dialysis of uraemic patients can also lead to neurological symptoms. The pathogenesis of DDS is not fully clear but most likely results from cerebral oedema. Urea passes poorly across the blood-brain barrier, so as urea is decreased on dialysis there is a mismatch between serum and CSF osmolality with water influx into the brain leading to raised intracranial pressure.

Symptoms can occur during or after the dialysis session and include headache, disorientation, blurred vision, asterixis, and cramps. Confusion, seizures, coma, and death can also occur and it is important to recognize those at risk of DDS.

Diagnosis is one of exclusion. A low threshold for intracranial bleeding such as subdural haematomas should be taken as these patients often have coagulation disorders secondary to uraemic associated platelet dysfunction as well as the anticoagulants used on haemodialysis. Hypoglycaemia and hyponatraemia should be ruled out. Drug toxicity, particularly medications which are renally excreted should be excluded. Wernicke's encephalopathy has been reported in a few patients undergoing long-term haemodialysis due to malnourishment due to anorexia and the use of glucose containing fluids.

Treatment of DDS involves stopping dialysis and providing supportive care. The symptoms are often self-limiting. Prophylactic phenytoin may be given to prevent seizures. Intravenous mannitol is sometimes used to elevate plasma osmolality. Neurosurgical input in extreme cases for ventricular drainage can be considered.

Further Reading

Zepeda-Orozco D, Quigley R (2012). Dialysis disequilibrium syndrome. *Paediatric Nephrology* 227(12): 2205–2211.

200. D) New pericardial effusion

The diagnosis in this case is scleroderma renal crisis. Whilst the development of ACE inhibitors has greatly improved the management of scleroderma renal crisis, the severity of the condition necessitates that those at increased risk of crisis are closely monitored.

Those at increased risk are those with:

- Diffuse cutaneous involvement
- Positive anti-polymerase antibodies
- Early disease course (scleroderma <4 years)
- Rapid progression of skin disease
- Recent anaemia
- Acute or subacute congestive cardiac failure or pericardial effusion
- Use of high dose corticosteroids

The following are not risk factors:

- Previous renal impairment
- Pre-existing hypertension
- Scl-70 or anti-centromere antibodies
- Abnormal urinalysis

Tutorial

Accelerated hypertension or rapidly progressive oliguric renal failure in a patient with systemic sclerosis is a renal crisis and is seen in 10% of patients with diffuse systemic sclerosis, but only 1% of those with limited systemic sclerosis.

Symptoms, if present, are non-specific and include severe headache, blurred vision, and shortness of breath. Seizures may occur. Damage to the endothelium with narrowed arterioles and ischaemia of the juxtaglomerular apparatus leads to increased renin secretion and the production of large amounts of angiotensin II potentiating hypertension and further renal ischaemia. Fibrinoid necrosis and fibrin thrombi are seen within vessels (thrombotic microangiopathy) with 'onion-skin' intimal thickening. Collapsed and ischaemic glomeruli and acute tubular necrosis is often seen.

A rapidly rising creatinine, which often continues to increase days after blood pressure has been controlled, is seen with a bland urine dipstick. Plasma renin values are often 30–40 times normal before treatment. Congestive cardiac failure and arrhythmias are often seen, which may be potentiated by a microangiopathic haemolytic anaemia with thrombocytopaenia.

Before ACE inhibitors less than 10% of patients survived scleroderma renal crisis and bilateral nephrectomies were attempted as a salvage therapy. Now survival at eight years is 85%, but roughly half of these require long-term dialysis due to irreversible renal damage.

Renal function usually initially worsens following the introduction of antihypertensive therapy due to impaired autoregulation of blood flow. However, this is made much worse if blood pressure is lowered too rapidly. A BP reduction of 10–15 mmHg/day is the target. Calcium channel blockers may be used in addition to ACE inhibition, but beta blockers should not be used. Angiotensin receptor blockers should be used with caution as they may worsen renal failure. Normotensive scleroderma renal crisis is also sometimes seen, and ACE inhibitors also improve outcome in these patients.

Further Reading

Mouthon L, Bussone G, Berezné A, Noël L-H, Guilevin L (2014). Scleroderma renal crisis. *Journal of Rheumatology* 41(6): 1040–1048.

201. D) MRI of her spine should be performed

The radiograph shows significant cystic disease in liver and kidneys. With the finding of impaired renal function, haematuria, and mild proteinuria, the most likely diagnosis is autosomal dominant polycystic kidney disease (ADPKD).

Flank pain in such a patient may be due to chronic cyst pain or, if acute, renal colic, or infection or haemorrhage within a cyst. The pain described in this case is more consistent with sciatica. Patients with ADPKD have increased abdominal girth: this is particularly likely in this patient due to the size of her liver and kidneys. This leads to an increase in lumbar lordosis, predisposing such patients to intervertebral disc disease. This possibility should therefore be investigated further in this patient. Eighty-five per cent of ADPKD patients have a mutation of the PKD1 gene on chromosome 16. Discussion about screening for berry aneurysms should be considered if there is a positive family history of ruptured intracerebral aneurysm or stroke before the age of 50.

Tutorial

The prevalence of ADPKD ranges from 1 in 400 to 1 in 800. It is characterized by the development of multiple renal cysts leading to end-stage renal failure and is associated with a number of extrarenal abnormalities. It is inherited in an autosomal dominant manner from mutations in the genes PKD-1 (chromosome 16) and PKD-2 (chromosome 4). PKD-1 is found in 85% and is associated with more aggressive disease, whereas PKD-2 often does not lead to end-stage renal disease. Non-visible haematuria and/or proteinuria (usually <1 g/day) can occur. Loin pain can occur due to mass effect from enlarged kidneys, bleeding into cysts (which can also cause visible haematuria), cyst infection, or renal calculi. PKD1 patients develop renal failure earlier than PKD2 patients. Patients may of course be asymptomatic.

Hypertension is more prevalent in PKD1 than PKD2. Intracerebral berry aneurysms around the Circle of Willis are found around five times more commonly in ADPKD patients compared to the general population. BP control is important for decreasing the rate of rupture of berry aneurysms and prevention of other cardiovascular complications in ADPKD. Since the majority of berry aneurysms never rupture and prophylactic surgical or radiological intervention carries significant risk, screening for aneurysms in asymptomatic ADPKD patients is not routinely performed. When it is considered, the potential risks and benefits should be discussed carefully with the patient in a specialist clinic. Factors favouring screening with a view to intervention include symptoms suggestive of an aneurysm (e.g. headaches or cranial nerve lesions), or patients with a positive family history (ruptured intracerebral aneurysm or stroke before the age of 50). The prevalence of mitral valve prolapse is increased in ADPKD patients and can lead to mitral regurgitation.

Liver cysts normally develop later than renal cysts in ADPKD. They are often asymptomatic. An increase in GGT or ALP may be seen, but AST and bilirubin are rarely elevated. Pancreatic, intracranial arachnoid, seminal vesicle, ovarian, and splenic cysts can occur but are usually asymptomatic. Renal cell carcinoma is not more common in ADPKD but is more often bilateral, multicentric, and sarcomatous. The differential diagnosis of von Hippel-Lindau disease (in which there is an increased risk of renal cell carcinoma) as a cause of polycystic kidneys should not be forgotten.

Ultrasound remains the investigation of choice in reaching a diagnosis. In an adult with a positive family history and/or cysts in the liver, an ultrasound showing bilaterally enlarged kidneys with multiple cysts of various sizes in the cortex and medulla is diagnostic of ADPKD. However, diagnosis in an adult with renal cysts but no family history, or pre-symptomatic diagnosis in a young individual with a positive family history is less straightforward. Currently the Ravine criteria are used, as summarized in Table 10.2.

Table 10.2 Ravine criteria for diagnosing ADPKD

Age	Positive family history	Negative family history
<30 years	2 cysts in either kidney	5 cysts in either kidney
30–60 years	4 cysts in either kidney	5 cysts in either kidney
>60 years	8 cysts in either kidney	8 cysts in either kidney

Reprinted from *The Lancet*, 343, Ravine D, et al., Evaluation of ultrasonographic diagnostic criteria for autosomal dominant polycystic kidney disease 1, pp. 824–827, Copyright 1994, with permission from Elsevier.

Detection of a mutation in both PKD genes is now available in PKD1 and PKD2 but may be difficult to interpret due to the size of the genes and number of potential mutations. Genetic testing and counselling is therefore not carried out at present outside specialist centres.

Tolvaptan is a competitive vasopressin receptor 2 antagonist which is used in PKD to antagonize the effects of vasopressin in the collecting ducts, leading to aquaresis (and hence loss of excess fluid in PKD patients) and improvement in sodium levels. Additionally it reduces the rate of kidney cyst proliferation in PKD. Side effects can include elevated liver enzymes, volume depletion, and hypernatraemia.

Further Reading

Pei Y, Obaji J, Dupuis A, et al. (2009). Unified criteria for ultrasonographic diagnosis of ADPKD. *Journal of American Society of Nephrology* 20(1): 205–212.

Simms R (2016). Autosomal dominant polycystic kidney disease. *British Medical Journal* 352.

202. E) TINU syndrome

The findings of the renal biopsy are consistent with a tubulointerstitial nephritis but the visual impairment from uveitis further characterizes this as part of TINU syndrome.

Sarcoidosis can also lead to uveitis and tubulointerstitial nephritis, but non-caseating granulomas are also often seen in the biopsy. The light microscopy findings are non-specific in Alport's syndrome and diagnosis is made when electron microscopy shows a thinning of the glomerular basement membrane with a characteristic basket-weave appearance (splitting of the lamina densa into several irregular layers which branch and rejoin). Segmental or diffuse mesangial hypercellularity with an increase in mesangial matrix (which may lead to segmental sclerosis) is seen on light microscopy in IgA nephropathy.

Tutorial

The definition of ATIN is a clinic-pathological one consisting of acute kidney injury with a predominantly interstitial infiltrate of lymphocytes, monocytes with or without eosinophils in the interstitium. *The glomeruli are normal.* A worse prognosis is seen in those with fibrosis of the interstitium which indicates a chronic tubulointerstitial nephritis. It is often associated with interstitial oedema and some degree of tubular damage, meaning it can be difficult to differentiate from acute tubular necrosis if the inflammatory infiltrate is mild. The term ATIN is preferred to the older term of acute interstitial nephritis (AIN) to emphasize that tubular and interstitial changes are present.

Table 10.3 lists the causes of ATIN, for which 70–90% of cases are caused by drugs.

Table 10.3 Causes of ATIN

Causes	Examples
Drugs (over 120 drugs have been implicated)	NSAIDS, penicillins, cephalosporins, rifampicin, sulphonamides, diuretics, allopurinol, PPIs, antiretrovirals, anticonvulsants
Systemic infections	*Streptococcus*, tuberculosis, legionella, *Corynebacterium diphtheriae*
Renal parenchymal infection	Bacterial, fungal, parasitic or viral
Immunological	Cryoglobulinaemia, IgA nephropathy, SLE, Sjögrens, renal transplant rejection, Wegener's granulomatosis
Metabolic	Hyperoxaluria, hyperuricosuria
Neoplastic	Melanoma, lymphoma
Idiopathic	Without or with uveitis (TINU)

These patients present acutely with acute kidney injury and oliguria in 40% of cases 3–21 days after the provoking insult, but it may be several months after. Systemic symptoms of fever, arthralgia, and maculopapular rash may occur. Flank pain may occur due to distension of the renal capsule. Eosinophilia is seen in up to 40%. Urinalysis may show haematuria, sterile pyuria, and WBC casts. Proteinuria is generally mild (<1 g/24hrs).

Aside from identifying and stopping the offending agent or treating the underlying disease causing the ATIN, treatment is supportive. Although clear evidence is lacking, corticosteroids are widely used to treat ATIN and may hasten the recovery of renal function. Outcome is generally good with the majority, including dialysis dependent ATIN, regaining independent renal function.

TINU is the term given to patients presenting with ATIN and visual impairment from anterior uveitis (often bilateral). It is classically seen in young women who may also have weight loss, anaemia, raised ESR, and deranged liver function tests. Corticosteroid therapy is given to achieve remission but disease recurrence means longer term immunosuppression is often required. An urgent ophthalmology opinion is required on presentation.

Further Reading

Ragahaven R, Eknoyan G (2014). Acute interstitial nephritis—a reappraisal and update. *Clinical Nephrology* 82(3): 149–162.

Rossert J (2001). Drug induced acute interstitial nephritis. *Kidney International* 60(2): 804–817.

203. A) 0.9% NaCl 1 ml/kg/hr for 12 hours pre- and 12 hours post-procedure

This is a common clinical problem, yet there is little agreement as to which interventions are definitely beneficial. The only preventative measure shown to be of clear benefit is answer B. Many reports have been written about the other agents, with conflicting answers, leading many candidates to be nervous about the above question not having one clear answer.

Tutorial

RCN is defined as an otherwise unexplained acute deterioration of renal function after intravascular administration of contrast media. Ten per cent of inpatient acute kidney injury is due at least in part to RCN and may lead to irreversible decline in renal function, especially in those with pre-existing renal impairment.

Whilst contrast is directly toxic to proximal tubular cells it also leads to a prolonged decrease in renal blood flow (after a transient increase). The end result is acute tubular necrosis (ATN). This is compounded by a post contrast diuresis. Higher risk is seen with the older high osmolar ionic contrast mediums and larger volumes of contrast. Other risk factors for RCN are: (1)

volume depletion and hypotension; (2) concurrent use of nephrotoxic drugs; (3) chronic kidney disease; (4) diabetic nephropathy; (5) congestive cardiac failure.

The decrease in GFR may not be reflected in a creatinine increase until 24–48 hours and usually starts to decline within 3–7 days. Strict fluid balance measurement after contrast is essential as oliguria is often the earliest sign. The fractional excretion of Na+ is <1% in RCN.

Proposed prophylactic strategies prevent RCN are best divided into:

1) Hydration
2) N-acetylcysteine
3) Other

IV fluids reverse volume depletion and increase renal blood flow as well as minimizing the pre-renal effects of a post contrast diuresis. The following are three typical regimes that are a guide. However, it is essential to assess the patient's individual fluid balance first; if the patient is dehydrated then larger volumes of fluid are required and you may need to delay the procedure until hydration is achieved. The opposite situation may be the case if the patient is volume overloaded:

- 0.9% NaCl 1 ml/kg/hr for 12 hours pre and 12 hours post procedure
- 0.45% NaCl 1 ml/kg/hr for 12 hours pre and 12 hours post procedure
- 1.26% NaHCO$_3$ 3 ml/kg/hr for 1 hour pre and 1 ml/kg/hr for 6 hours during and post procedure

The antioxidant properties of NAC have been studied for the prevention of RCN. There are large numbers of published studies, but many randomized control trials and meta-analyses show no clear benefit. Also, NAC may decrease creatinine independently of GFR by interference with tubular handling (cf trimethoprim tubular effects) leading to a false positive result. However, it remains a strategy in many hospital protocols *always used in conjunction with IV hydration* as it is inexpensive and has few side effects.

A wide range of other strategies have been looked at in small studies but are yet to show clear benefit. These include endothelin receptor antagonism, adenosine A1 receptor antagonists, prostaglandin E1, theophylline and 1-Arginine administration. Haemofiltration or haemodialysis to remove contrast has also yet to show clear benefit.

It should always be remembered that a key differential of RCN is renal atheroembolic disease as most of the patients undergoing vascular studies have diffuse atherosclerotic disease.

Further Reading

Luk L, Steinman J, Newhouse J (2017). Intravenous contrast-induced nephropathy—the rise and fall of a threatening idea. *Advances in Chronic Kidney Disease* 24(3): 169–175.

Subramaniam R, Suarez-Cuervo C, Wilson R, et al. (2016). Effectiveness of prevention strategies for contrast-induced nephropathy: a systematic review and meta-analysis. *Annals of Internal Medicine* 164(6):406–416.

204. E) Thin membrane disease

Thin basement membrane disease (TMD) is a relatively common disorder where the only abnormal finding on renal biopsy is diffuse thinning of the glomerular basement membranes (GBM) on electron microscopy.

The normal renal ultrasound is against a diagnosis of autosomal recessive polycystic kidney disease, as is the age of presentation. C1q nephropathy would involve heavy deposition in the mesangium and elsewhere, often with secondary focal segmental glomerulosclerosis. A degree of renal impairment would be expected with acute tubular necrosis, and flattened tubular cells and mitotic figures would be seen on biopsy. The light microscopy and immunofluorescence are normal in both Alport's syndrome and thin membrane disease but the GBM has a characteristic basket-weave appearance (splitting of the lamina densa into several irregular layers which branch and rejoin) in Alport's syndrome and is simply thinner (<200 nm) in thin membrane disease.

Tutorial

Microscopic haematuria, minimal proteinuria with a GBM of less than 200 nm thick (normal ~350 nm) is seen in TMD which may also be termed benign familial haematuria. A family history of haematuria is found in 30–50% of cases. It must be distinguished from the other common glomerular causes of isolated haematuria: IgA nephropathy and Alport's syndrome. TMD has an excellent long-term prognosis but some authors suggest follow-up yearly with urine dipstick, blood pressure, and creatinine levels. Interestingly, some TMD patients are heterozygous for mutations on COL4A3 and COL4A4, suggesting that TMD is the heterozygous state of autosomal recessive Alport's syndrome. TMD can be difficult to distinguish from Alport's syndrome. Alport's syndrome is an inherited disorder that results in the production of defective type IV collagen. The worldwide incidence is ~1:10,000.

Type IV collagen is a triple helix of alpha chains, and an abnormality in any of these will result in defective collagen. Of the six collagen alpha chains: COL4A3, COL4A4, and COL4A5 are seen in the glomerular basement membrane. In 80% of cases, Alport's syndrome is caused by an X-linked mutation in COL4A5. The rest of the inheritance is autosomal recessive, with mutations in COL4A3 and COL4A4 which are located on chromosome 2.

Males have persistent or intermittent microscopic haematuria, with episodes of gross haematuria often brought on by exercise or respiratory infections. A mild proteinuria progresses to nephrotic range in 30% of patients. In males the majority progress to ESRF by the fourth decade. High frequency sensorineural hearing loss is present in 30–50%. Heterozygous females generally have mild disease and have microscopic haematuria. Patients can also have signs in the eye visible on fundoscopy. 'Oil droplet in water' is the term given to the dark disc at the centre of the papillary region in the anterior lenticonus which is seen in 15–30% of Alport's syndrome patients. This is due to abnormal type IV collagen.

The diagnosis of TMD is confirmed on renal biopsy. Whilst light microscopy findings are non-specific and immunofluorescence staining is usually negative, electron microscopy is key and shows a thinning of the GBM (less than 250 nm) with a characteristic basket-weave appearance (splitting of the lamina densa into several irregular layers). In practice, due to the risks of a renal biopsy, patients with isolated haematuria, with no hypertension, proteinuria, or deranged renal function are usually not biopsied and observed with a presumptive diagnosis of TMD, and a biopsy only then performed if the clinical features change to suggest an alternate diagnosis (i.e. hypertension, renal impairment, or proteinuria).

As no specific treatment for Alport's syndrome exists, good control of blood pressure and use of ACE inhibitors are the mainstay of treatment. Family members should be screened for haematuria and hypertension. Alport's is not a contraindication to transplantation but patients can develop anti-GBM antibodies after renal transplantation (donor α5 type collagen is recognized as non-self). In this situation the risk of anti-GBM glomerulonephritis is <5%.

Further Reading

Savige J, Gregory M, Gross O, Kashtan C, Ding J, Flinter F (2013). Expert guidelines for the management of Alport syndrome and thin basement membrane nephropathy. *Journal of American Society of Nephrology* 24(3): 364–375.

205. E) Urinary sodium excretion will decrease during admission whilst on intravenous rehydration

This patient is clinically hypotensive and has hyponatremia, hypokalemia, hypocalcaemia, and a hypochloraemic metabolic alkalosis. The biochemical picture fits with a diagnosis of Bartter's syndrome which is due to loss of function of the NKCC2 transporter in the thick ascending limb of the loop of Henle. This is the same transporter upon which furosemide and other loop diuretics act on. Whilst this patient has a short stature that is often associated with Bartter's syndrome, she also suffers from anorexia and has a low BMI. Taking the whole clinical picture into account and the fact that Bartter's syndrome is first, very uncommon and second, often presents in early childhood, loop diuretic abuse should be suspected in this case. She may have obtained these from her parents who suffer from hypertension. As such, whilst admitted to hospital the patient will no longer be able take this medication and her kidneys will then be able to appropriately retain sodium and her urinary sodium excretion will decrease.

The patient is on tenofovir which is known to cause Fanconi's syndrome by interfering with various proximal tubule transporters. Classically this causes hypophosphataemia due to hyperphosphaturia. The patient's low phosphate may be due to her anorexia, or it may indeed be due to proximal tubule dysfunction. Fanconi's syndrome can cause hyponatraemia and hypokalaemia, but with a renal tubular acidosis, rather than an alkalosis as is seen here. To differentiate between whether the patient's hypophosphataemia is due to anorexia or proximal tubule dysfunction, urinary phosphate excretion would need to be assessed to determine if there is indeed a degree of proximal tubule dysfunction. Fractional excretion of phosphate of over 2% for any serum phosphate, and over 1% if the serum phosphate is less than 0.8 suggests proximal tubule dysfunction.

As the patient's condition is likely due to medication abuse, rather than a genetic condition her family members will not be affected. Similarly, high salt and high potassium diet is not necessary, nor is use of a potassium sparing diuretic as sometimes used in potassium wasting tubulopathies such as Bartter's, Gitelman's, or Liddle's syndromes.

Tutorial

For a detailed discussion on congenital tubulopathies, their presentations and characteristics, please read the tutorial for question 65. For a detailed discussion on Fanconi's syndrome, please read the tutorial for question 178.

206. C) Liver

The patient presents with nephrotic syndrome. The long history of joint pains and hand examination findings suggest a long history of rheumatoid arthritis. Clinically therefore amyloid secondary to rheumatoid arthritis is a likely cause of nephrotic syndrome in this case.

The renal biopsy confirms amyloid with Congo red positivity of amyloid fibrils. Immunofluorescence is negative for light chains in AA amyloid (as in this case) and usually positive in AL amyloid. Serum amyloid A protein is an acute phase protein produced by the liver. It can accumulate during chronic inflammation of any cause, with classic examples including inflammatory arthropathies, hepatitis C infection, chronic skin ulcers, and chronic osteomyelitis. Although some cases of AL amyloid will be negative for immunofluorescence of light chains at renal biopsy, B cells or bone marrow are not listed in the stems of the MCQ.

Tutorial

Amyloidosis is characterized by extracellular tissue deposition of proteins which undergo a misfolding event that makes them prone to self-aggregation and as fibrils in β-pleated sheets. They are classified by the precursor protein that forms the fibrils and the major types are shown in Table 10.4.

Within the kidney, deposition occurs throughout the mesangium, tubules, interstitium, capillary walls, and glomeruli, with the degree of glomeruli involvement dictating the degree of proteinuria, which can range from mild proteinuria to nephrotic syndrome. Amyloid is a cause of enlarged kidneys on ultrasound but in most patients they are of normal size. Symptoms and signs associated with other organ involvement may also be seen.

Diagnosis requires the demonstration of amyloid deposits histologically. The fibrils bind Congo red leading to apple green birefringence under polarized light. Electron microscopy confirms fibrils, but this may be patchy in distribution. Immunostaining using antibodies against the known amyloid proteins is used to distinguish the type of amyloid. Severe amyloid mesangial deposition in the kidney can resemble the appearance of nodular lesions in diabetic nephropathy but amyloid protein will only weakly stain periodic acid-Schiff stain compared to the nodules seen in diabetic nephropathy.

If AL amyloid is suspected protein electrophoresis, serum free light chain quantification, and bone marrow aspirate and trephine may be carried out. Half of patients will have slightly increased plasma cell numbers in the bone marrow and about 15% will overtly have myeloma (with significantly raised plasma cells). Lambda light chains are more often seen than kappa light chains in AL amyloid, whereas kappa chains are seen more often than lambda in myeloma. Mass spectrometry of amyloid proteins and DNA sequencing can be used to diagnose rarer forms of amyloidosis.

Dialysis (haemodialysis and peritoneal dialysis) associated amyloidosis occurs when serum levels of β-2 microglobulin, which is normally cleared by glomerular filtration and tubular catabolism, increase in renal failure leading to amyloid deposition. Accumulation is seen in synovial membranes and osteoarticular sites leading to carpal tunnel syndrome and tenosynovitis as well as subchondral cysts and fractures. Visceral and cardiovascular involvement is rare. There is no curative treatment. High-flux dialysis, which is now the current standard across the UK, results in an enhanced β-2 microglobulin and so this form of amyloid is now rare.

Table 10.4 Types of amyloidosis

Disease	Precursor protein	Amyloid protein	Comments
Primary AL amyloid	Monoclonal Ig light chain	AL	Usually lambda light chain or fragments produced by a plasma cell dyscrasia
Reactive AA amyloid	Serum amyloid A (SAA)	AA	Seen in patients with underlying inflammatory conditions (see explanation)
AH Amyloidosis	Monoclonal Ig heavy chain	AH	Very rare and involving kidneys predominantly
Hereditary/familial amyloid	Transthyretin	ATTR	
	Fibrinogen Aα chain	AFib	
	Apolipoprotein AI	AApoAI	
	Apolipoprotein AII	AApoAII	
	Lysozyme	ALys	
	Gelsolin	AGel	Cranial nerves predominantly
	Cystatin C	ACys	Cerebral amyloid angiopathy of cerebral vessels
Dialysis related amyloidosis	β2-microglobulin	Aβ2M	Mainly musculoskeletal deposition
Senile systemic amyloidosis	Wild type transthyretin	ATTR	

Treatment of amyloidosis is mainly supportive of organ impairment, such as dialysis in the case of renal failure, or diuretics and beta blockers for cardiac amyloid. Treating the underlying case of the amyloid protein, for example treatment of plasma cell dyscrasia or underlying rheumatoid arthritis, helps prevent progression of disease and to an extent also gradually clears the deposited amyloid, but recovery of organ function is variable as damage can often be permanent. New drugs are in development which include RNA inhibitors, fibril formation stabilizers and inhibitors, and immunotherapeutic targeting of amyloid deposits, all of which hold promise for the future.

Further Reading

Wechalekar A, Gillmore J, Hawkins P (2016). Systemic amyloidosis. *Lancet* 387: 2641–2654.

207. B) Cryoglobulins precipitating after five days

The patient is known to be hepatitis C positive and now presents with a vasculitic rash, arthralgia, signs of neuropathy, renal impairment, and haematuria/proteinuria. The renal biopsy confirms a mesangiocapillary glomerulonephritis. In association with hepatitis C infection this is most likely secondary to cryoglobulin deposition in the medium and small vessels in the skin, joints, and glomerulus fixing complement and causing local inflammation. This is a type II mixed essential cryoglobulinaemia. Detection of serum cryoglobulins is undertaken on a blood sample taken at 37°C without anticoagulants. Serum is then removed after it has clotted and incubated at 4°C. Type I cryoglobulins precipitate in the first 24 hours, whereas type II and III take up to seven days. Spectrometry and immunologic assays can then determine concentration and type. The rash is a leukocytoclastic vasculitis which is ANCA negative. Serum complement measurement shows decreased C4 and normal C3 in most cases. Rheumatoid factor is positive in type II cryoglobulinaemia (hepatitis C-infected B cells secrete auto-antibody which is a rheumatoid factor).

Tutorial

Cryoglobulinaemia is characterized by the presence in the serum of immunoglobulins which undergo reversible precipitation at temperatures <37°C and are known as cryoglobulins. They are grouped by the Brouet classification into three types:

- Type I cryoglobulinaemia (simple cryoglobulinaemia) is the result of a monoclonal Ig. This is usually IgM but may also occur with IgG, IgA, or free light chains. It is associated with lymphoproliferative disease such as myeloma, CLL, Waldenstrom's macroglobulinaemia and lymphoma. It presents with features of hyperviscosity syndrome and thrombosis: retinal haemorrhage, Raynaud's phenomenon, digital ulceration, purpura, acrocyanosis, livedo reticularis, and arterial thrombosis.

- Type II cryoglobulinaemia (mixed essential cryoglobulinaemia) consists of a monoclonal IgM with polyclonal IgG. It is associated with hepatitis C or autoimmune disease (e.g. SLE, Sjögrens syndrome). The IgM is a rheumatoid factor.

- Type III cryoglobulinaemia consists of a polyclonal IgM that also has a rheumatoid factor activity. It is seen at low level and is associated with viral infection and autoimmune disease and may become type II with time.

Type II and III cryoglobulinaemia present most typically with musculoskeletal involvement (including arthralgia and myalgia), cutaneous vasculitis, and peripheral neuropathy with renal involvement due to immune complex deposition. Renal involvement may also be seen in type I cryoglobulinaemia due to thrombosis.

In secondary cryoglobulinaemia, diagnosis and treatment of the underlying condition is required; this then often leads to suppression of the cryoglobulinaemia. Cases in which there is no associated underlying disorder are termed essential or idiopathic cryoglobulinaemia. These are treated with immunosuppressive agents such as glucocorticoids with either rituximab or cyclophosphamide and, in some patients, plasmapheresis.

Further Reading

Retamozo S, Brito-Zerón P, Bosch X, Stone J, Ramos-Casals M (2013). Cryoglobulinemic disease. *Oncology (Williston Park)*. 27(11): 1098–1105.

208. C) She has class III lupus nephritis

The patient has more than four features that meet the American College of Rheumatology criteria for lupus (see discussion below). She has malar rash, oral ulcers, proteinuria, positive ANA, and positive anti ds-DNA. The renal biopsy confirms class III lupus nephritis (Table 10.5). A guide to disease activity can also be assessed by measurement of antibodies to double stranded DNA (dsDNA), complement (C3 and C4), erythrocyte sedimentation rate (ESR), and C-reactive protein (CRP). Elevated ESR and dsDNA and decreased C3 and C4 are associated with active nephritis. CRP is not elevated in patients with SLE unless infection or significant arthritis are present. ANAs appear early in SLE and are highly sensitive and specific. Anti-C1q antibodies are also associated with lupus nephritis being more specific but less sensitive than anti-dsDNA antibodies.

Tutorial

SLE is a multisystem disease resulting from production of auto-antibodies directed against nuclear elements along with impaired immune complex clearance. The diagnosis of SLE is based on symptoms, signs, and blood tests. The American College of Rheumatology diagnostic criteria for SLE requires 4 out of 11 features in its 1997 update (Table 10.6) but in 2012 the Systemic Lupus International Collaborating Clinics (SLICC) Group expanded the number of criteria from 11 to 17 by adding further acute and chronic rashes, alopecia, further neurological manifestations, hypocomplementaemia, and direct Coombs test positivity. The SLICC group classified a person as having SLE if 4 of the 17 diagnostic criteria were present (at least 1 clinical and 1 immunologic) or the presence of biopsy proven lupus with ANA or anti-dsDNA antibodies.

Identifying the class of renal involvement through biopsy is important as early detection and treatment can significantly improve renal outcome. The histology seen can be varied but has important therapeutic and prognostic implications and the International Society of Nephrology (ISN)/Renal Pathology Society (RPS) classification is used (Table 10.6).

The aim of treatment of lupus nephritis is to induce and maintain renal remission whilst minimizing drug toxicity. Class I lupus nephritis rarely requires treatment unless there is involvement of other organs. Class II nephritis may require treatment if proteinuria is high (>1 g/24 hours). Class III or IV nephritis is initially treated with high dose oral steroids and mycophenolate. For non-responders to initial therapy, cyclophosphamide or rituximab is considered. Management of class V nephritis is not clear: spontaneous remission may occur and if proteinuria is low and renal function normal no immunosuppression may be needed. If significant proteinuria occurs then treatment similar to class III and IV is considered. Hydroxychloroquine is used if disease is mainly limited to skin and joints. In all cases of lupus nephritis general measures include BP control to <130/80 mmHg and commencement of ACE inhibitors or angiotensin receptor blockers if significant proteinuria is present (>1 g/day).

Table 10.5 International Society of Nephrology (ISN)/Renal pathology Society (RPS) 2003 classification of lupus nephritis.

Class	Light microscopy	Immunofluorescence and electron microscopy	Usual associated clinical manifestations
I *Minimal mesangial lupus nephritis*	Normal	Mesangial immune deposits	Mild proteinuria
II *Mesangial proliferative lupus nephritis*	Mesangial hypercellularity or mesangial matrix expansion with mesangial immune deposits	Mesangial immune deposits; few subepithelial and subendothelial deposits possible	Asymptomatic haematuria or proteinuria
III *Focal lupus nephritis* *A-active and/or* *C-chronic*	Active or inactive focal, segmental, or global glomerulonephritis involving <50% of all glomeruli	Subendothelial and mesangial immune deposits	Generalized active SLE. Mild-moderate haematuria and proteinuria. Worsening renal function in minority.
IV *Diffuse lupus nephritis* *S-Segmental or* *G-Global* *A-Active and/or* *C-Chronic*	Active or inactive diffuse, segmental or global glomerulonephritis	Subendothelial immune deposits	Hypertension, oedema, active urinary sediment, worsening renal function, and nephrotic range proteinuria in most cases. Active extrarenal SLE in most cases.
V *Membranous lupus nephritis*	Thickening of glomerular basement membrane without inflammatory infiltrate. Subepithelial deposits and spikes. May show advanced sclerosis. May occur in combination with class II or IV.	Subepithelial and intramembranous immune deposits. Subendothelial deposits when associated with proliferative component.	Usually nephritic syndrome
VI *Advanced sclerosis lupus nephritis*	Advanced glomerular sclerosis, interstitial fibrosis and tubular atrophy		Significant renal impairment or end-stage renal disease unlikely to reverse with medical therapy

Reprinted from *Kidney International*, 65(2), Weening J, D'Agati V, Schwartz M, et al. The classification of glomerulonephritis in systemic lupus erythematosus revisited, pp. 521–530. Copyright 2004, with permission from Elsevier and the International Society of Nephrology.

Table 10.6 American College of Rheumatology Criteria For SLE, based upon 1997 update of the 1982 revised criteria for the classification of systemic lupus erythematosus

Four or more of the following meets the criteria for SLE. Those with 2–3 features often go on to develop SLE

Malar rash	Butterfly fixed erythematous rash
Discoid rash	Raised patches that scar
Photosensitivity	
Oral ulcers	Usually painless
Arthritis	Two or more peripheral joints
Serositis	Pleuritis or pericarditis

Table 10.6 Continued

Renal disease	Persistent proteinuria or cellular casts
Neurological disorder	Psychosis or seizures
Haematological disorder	Haemolytic anaemia, leukopaenia, or lymphopaenia on two or more occasions, thrombocytopaenia
Immunological disorder	Positive anticardiolipin, anti-dsDNA, or anti-Sm antibodies or false positive syphilis serology
Positive anti-nuclear factor	In the absence of drugs known to cause positive ANA

Adapted with permission from Tan E, Cohen A, Fries J, et al. (1982). The 1982 revised criteria for the classification of systemic lupus erythematosus. *Arthritis and Rheumatology* 25(11): 1271–1277.

Data from Hochberg M (1997). Updating the American College of Rheumatology revised criteria for the classification of systemic lupus erythematosus *Arthritis and Rheumatolgy* 40(9): 1725.

Further Reading

Hochberg M (1997). Updating the American College of Rheumatology revised criteria for the classification of systemic lupus erythematosus. *Arthritis and Rheumatology* 40(9): 1725.

Tan E, Cohen A, Fries J, et al. (1982). The 1982 revised criteria for the classification of systemic lupus erythematosus. *Arthritis and Rheumatology* 25(11): 1271–1277.

Weening J, D'Agati V, Schwartz M, et al. (2004). The classification of glomerulonephritis in systemic lupus erythematosus revisited. *Kidney International* 65(2) 521–530.

209. C) ADAMTS13 activity 2% of normal is diagnostic

The history and laboratory features are consistent with thrombotic thrombocytopaenic purpura (TTP) with microangiopathic haemolytic anaemia (MAHA), thrombocytopaenia, neurological features, and purpura. Whilst haemolytic uraemic syndrome (HUS) is a possibility, the lack of renal involvement with hypertension, and predominance of neurological features is more in keeping with TTP. The absence of diarrhoea would suggest that if it were HUS it would be D-HUS which may be due to a mutation in factor H rather than an increase in factor H. Mutations in ADAMTS13 are seen in TTP as discussed below. A decreased von Willebrand factor (vWF) is seen in von Willebrand's disease, and haemophilia A and B involve decreases in factor VIII and IX respectively. The normal D-dimer and normal fibrinogen are against a diagnosis of disseminated intravascular coagulation.

Tutorial

The combination of MAHA, thrombocytopaenia, and tissue ischaemia (due to occlusion by platelet aggregates and thrombus) characterizes thrombotic microangiopathies (TMA). All TMAs may involve the kidneys, leading to thrombi in the glomerular capillaries and ischaemia. The main causes of TMAs are as follows:

- TTP
- HUS
- HELLP syndrome (haemolysis (H), elevated liver enzymes (EL) and low platelet count (LP)) and pre-eclampsia
- Disseminated intravascular coagulopathy (DIC)
- Malignant hypertension
- SLE, systemic sclerosis, rheumatoid arthritis, vasculitis
- Antiphospholipid syndrome
- Paroxysmal nocturnal haemoglobinuria

- Metastatic disease
- HIV
- Drugs

TTP involves impairment of the proteinase ADAMTS13 which normally cleaves the large vWF multimers released from endothelial cells. Inherited mutations in ADAMTS13 or auto-antibodies directed against it result in the larger vWF multimers activating platelets, leading to the microangiopathy seen in TTP. TTP secondary to drugs (e.g. clopidogrel and ticlopidine) involves IgG auto-antibodies to ADAMTS13. Features of TTP include fever, MAHA, thrombocytopaenia, purpura, central nervous system involvement (confusion, fits, or any other neurological abnormality), and renal involvement. Red cell fragments are seen on film, along with thrombocytopaenia, raised LDH, and decreased haptoglobins. These parameters can be used to monitor disease activity. Low ADAMTS13 activity (<5% normal) is diagnostic of TTP in the setting of appropriate clinical findings. Normal or mildly elevated D-dimer and normal or high fibrinogen differentiates TTP from DIC in which raised D-dimers and decreased fibrinogen are seen. Management of TTP aims to recover ability to cleave vWF. Daily plasma exchange with fresh frozen plasma removes vWF cleaving protein inhibitor and allows plasma infusion in large volume (providing ADAMTS13 replacement). It should be continued until platelet count and LDH have normalized (usually 1–2 weeks). If plasma exchange is not available, platelet-depleted fresh frozen plasma or cryosupernatant infusion can be used. Platelet infusion should be avoided unless there is severe life-threatening bleeding as it precipitates further thrombosis which causes further tissue ischaemia and organ damage. Response to treatment is good if instituted promptly but resistant disease may require plasma exchange twice daily or the addition of steroids, intravenous immunoglobulin, or rituximab. Aspirin and anticoagulants have no clear benefit in TTP.

HUS is defined by the concurrent characteristic triad of microangiopathic haemolytic anaemia, thrombocytopaenia, and AKI. The most common cause of HUS is Shiga toxin-producing *Escherichia coli* (STEC), causing D+ (diarrhoea-positive) HUS. D+ HUS is associated with *E. coli* O157:H7, *Shigella dysenteriae* serotype 1, *Salmonella*, *Campolobacter*, and *Yersinia*. The Shiga-like exotoxin translocates the bowel wall and binds to intrarenal vasculature and platelets with release of large vWF multimers and prothrombogenic factors from endothelial cells.

Complement-mediated HUS accounts for most of the D-HUS (otherwise known as atypical HUS). The proposed pathogenesis of complement-mediated HUS is that a trigger (e.g. infection) causes uninhibited continuous activation of the alternate complement pathway in a susceptible individual with either gene mutations or antibodies to complement proteins (e.g. Factor H deficiency). This results in renal endothelial damage leading to thrombotic microangiopathy. Quinine, tacrolimus, cyclosporine, ciprofloxacin, OCP, heparin, and rapamycin have been associated with drug-induced D-HUS. *Pneumoniae*, *Neisseria meningitidis*, *Mycoplasma*, *Legionella*, and *Rickettsia* are potential infective causes. Multi-organ failure may ensue. Pregnancy-associated HUS may occur in the setting of pre-eclampsia and may progress to a full-blown HELLP syndrome. The same laboratory features are seen in HUS as in TTP although no reduction in ADAMTS13 is seen. Renal involvement is more common and more severe than in TTP, though platelets are not as severely reduced, and hypertension with fluid overload is more common. In clinical practice, the platelet count can often help distinguish between TTP vs aHUS. The platelet count is seldom above 30×10^9/L (and usually less than 20×10^9/L) with TTP, and so a higher count should point the clinician away from this diagnosis. However, it should be noted that the reverse is not necessarily true. A platelet count of less than 30×10^9/L does not confirm a diagnosis of TTP or refute an alternate differential diagnosis.

Management of HUS is supportive, including dialysis as required. Antibiotics are not given in D+ HUS as they may increase toxin release. Plasma exchange does not improve outcome in D+ HUS and there is no role for anticoagulation. Platelet transfusions may increase thrombotic risk.

Treatment of atypical HUS includes supportive care and either plasma exchange or eculizumab as soon as the diagnosis is made. Eculizumab is a humanized monoclonal antibody which acts as a terminal complement pathway (C5) inhibitor. It is an effective therapy, but is extremely expensive and its usage is approved only on a case-by-case basis.

Further Reading

George J, Nester C (2014). Syndromes of thrombotic microangiopathy. *New England Journal of Medicine* 371: 654–666.

Jokiranta T (2017). HUS and atypical HUS. *Blood* 129(21): 2847–2856.

Page E, Kremer Hovinga J, Terrell D, Vesely S, George J (2017). Thrombotic thrombocytopenic purpura: diagnostic criteria, clinical features, and long-term outcomes from 1995 through 2015. *Blood Advances* 1: 590.

210. E) Rasburicase 200 mg/kg/day IV

The patient is at high risk of tumour lysis syndrome when undergoing treatment for his AML, and has developed this complication within the first three days of treatment as evidenced by hyperuricaemia, acute on chronic renal failure, hyperphosphataemia, and hypocalcaemia. He is dehydrated but not yet oligoanuric and should therefore be given aggressive IV rehydration with close monitoring of his fluid balance, electrolytes, and calcium. A complication of hyperuricaemia is urate stones, which can cause an obstruction, and hydronephrosis and this should also be ruled out with ultrasound investigation.

Alkalinization of urine to pH 7.0 was in the past recommended as it promotes urine solubility; however, both xanthine and hypoxanthine, the precursors of uric acid (see Figure 10.1) precipitate under alkaline conditions. More importantly, the patient has G6PD deficiency and so rasburicase is contraindicated as it may cause haemolytic anaemia and methaemoglobinaemia. Allopurinol needs dose reduction in renal impairment. Allopurinol inhibits the conversion of xanthines to uric acid, reducing the effectiveness of rasburicase and so the two should not be given together.

Tutorial

Tumour lysis syndrome is a constellation of life-threatening metabolic complications that can occur after the initiation of cytotoxic treatment of a cancer, particularly bulky/large treatment-responsive tumours. It is due to the rapid necrosis of large numbers of neoplastic cells releasing cellular products acutely into the circulation. It can occur immediately or up to three days after the initiation of treatment. Hyperkalaemia (often rapid and to dangerous levels) and hyperphosphataemia result due to cellular release. Nucleic acid purines that are released are converted to uric acid by hepatic xanthine oxidase, leading to hyperuricaemia. Uric acid is freely filtered and forms crystal casts in excess which obstruct tubules leading to AKI (compounded when patients are volume depleted). Hyperphosphataemia leads to phosphate-calcium binding (with concurrent hypocalcaemia) and deposition in the vasculature and kidneys (further compounding renal failure). Magnesium levels also fall. Symptoms may be variable but include cardiac dysrhythmias, tetany, seizures, cramp, and nausea and vomiting.

Hydration is key in managing tumour lysis syndrome. Aggressive hydration and enhanced urinary flow promote the excretion of uric acid and phosphate. The use of diuretics to increase urinary flow should not be used in patients with hypovolaemia or obstructive uropathy. Additionally, due to the possible complications (metabolic acidosis and calcium/phosphate precipitation) along with no clear evidence of benefit, alkalinization of urine is not routinely recommended in the treatment of tumour lysis syndrome. Allopurinol is a xanthine oxidase inhibitor used to reduce hypoxanthine to uric acid. It may be given orally or intravenously. A side effect can be the precipitation of xanthine crystals in the renal tubules. Care also has to be taken given its interaction with azathioprine and

6-mercaptopurine, both of which are commonly used in chemotherapy. Rasburicase is recombinant urate oxidase. Urate oxidase is not normally expressed in humans. It catalyses highly insoluble uric acid to soluble allantoin. It acts rapidly, usually decreasing uric acid levels to undetectable levels within six hours. Haemodialysis may be required in the interim if indications are met (hyperkalaemia and/or volume overload, oliguria, and/or acidosis, and/or uraemia).

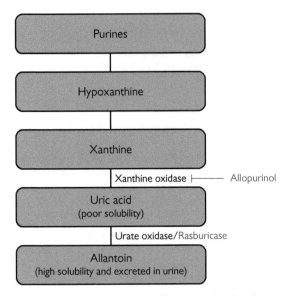

Figure 10.1 Purine catabolism and sites of action of allopurinol and rasburicase.

Further Reading

Jones G, Will A, Jackson G, Webb N, Rule S (2015). Guidelines for the management of tumour lysis syndrome in adults and children with haematological malignancies on behalf of the British Committee for Standards in Haematology. *British Journal of Haematology* 169 (5): 661–671.

211. B) McArdle's disease

The patient presents with rhabdomyolysis after a period of exercise with a history of previous myalgic episodes including during childhood. There is no history of traumatic, drug/toxin, or infective causes of rhabdomyolysis. The history is therefore suggestive of an underlying myopathy. Glycogen storage disease is the result of defects in enzymes that convert glycogen compounds to glucose. Of the 14 glycogen storage diseases, four cause clinically significant muscle weakness: Pompe disease (GSD type II, acid maltase deficiency), Cori disease (GSD type II, debranching enzyme deficiency), McArdle's disease (GSD type V, myophosphorylase deficiency) and Tarui disease (GSD type VII, phosphofructokinase deficiency). The muscle biopsy in this case confirms McArdle's disease as the enzyme histochemistry reveals absence of myophosphorylase. A history of exercise-induced myalgia and rhabdomyolysis in the absence of other causes of rhabdomyolysis should raise suspicion of an underlying myopathy.

Tutorial

Rhabdomyolysis means breakdown of skeletal muscle. It is the name given to a clinical syndrome caused by leakage of muscle cell contents (including myoglobin, K+, phosphate, creatine kinase, and LDH) into the circulation. Table 10.7 lists the causes of rhabdomyolysis.

Renal failure as a result of rhabdomyolysis is caused by:

1) Volume depletion due to fluid sequestering in inflamed muscle tissue.

2) Further injury from renal vasoconstriction due to activation of the renin-angiotensin system in response to hypovolaemia, but also the release of vasoconstrictors and decrease in vasodilators due to myoglobin oxidative injury. This can lead to tubular ischaemia.

3) Direct oxidative tubular injury from myoglobin (when in excess the ferric form (Fe^{3+}) of myoglobin is freely filtered, when in excess and tubular degradation in acidic conditions leads to toxic ferryl-myoglobin (Fe^{4+}) and tubular damage).

4) Tubular obstruction from both Tamm-Horsfall protein-myoglobin complex, and also cellular casts from sloughed tubular cells.

5) Uric acid stones.

The symptoms, if present, include myalgia, weakness, dark urine, or oliguria. Recurrent rhabdomyolysis after exertion or infections should raise the suspicion of an underlying myopathy. Urine dipstick testing is unable to distinguish between myoglobin and haemoglobin.

Biochemical features include raised creatine kinase, AKI (with low urea:creatinine ratio), hyperkalaemia, hyperphosphataemia/hypocalcaemia (phosphate binding calcium with deposition of calcium-phosphate complexes in soft tissues: hypercalcaemia occurs on recovery as this deposited calcium is mobilized), high anion gap metabolic acidosis, hypermagnesaemia, and hyperuricaemia.

It is essential to investigate for and treat any underlying cause, whilst instituting supportive care. Hyperkalaemia should be managed appropriately and dialysis instituted if indicated. Strict fluid assessment is vital and in the early phase aggressive fluid resuscitation may prevent complications. As much as 12 L of fluid a day may be needed to achieve an adequate urine output.

The role of urinary alkalinization remains controversial. Possible benefits include: (1) solubilization of Tamm-Horsfall protein-myoglobin complex; (2) inhibition of direct tubular oxidative injury; (3) reduced metmyoglobin vasoconstriction due to alkalinized urine. A potential disadvantage is potentiating hypocalcaemia by reducing the free plasma calcium concentration. Not all clinical studies have shown clear benefits. Use of diuretics is equally controversial, with three potential benefits: (1) increasing urinary flow and flushing of nephrotoxins; (2) creating an osmotic gradient extracting fluid from injured muscle and therefore helping hypovolaemia; (3) free radical scavenging. Mannitol is preferred but its use is not supported by any randomized control trial.

Table 10.7 Causes of rhabdomyolysis

Trauma/direct injury	Crush syndrome
	Immobilization (compression)
	Compartment syndrome
	Electrical shock
Excessive muscle activity	Strenuous exercise
	Seizures
	Alcohol withdrawal syndrome
Hereditary enzyme defects/myopathies	McArdle's disease
	Cori disease
	Pompe disease
	Tarui disease
	Poly/dermatomyositis
Other medical causes	
Drugs and toxins	Statins, fibrates, antimalarials, alcohol, amphetamines, heroin, zidovudine, snake and insect venoms

Table 10.7 Continued

Muscle hypoxia	Sickle cell disease, muscle vessel occlusion
Temperature alterations	Neuroleptic malignant syndrome/malignant hyperthermia Heat stroke
Metabolic(non-hereditary)/ endocrine	↓K+ ↓Ca+ ↓Po4 ↓↑Na+ Hypothyroidism Hyperglycaemic emergencies
Infections	Influenza Legionella EBV Coxsackie Primary HIV Tetanus Salmonella Malaria Gas gangrene (*Clostridium*, *Strep. pyogenes*, *Staph. aureus*)

Further Reading

Allison R, Bedsole D (2003). The other medical causes of rhabdomyolysis. *American Journal of Medical Science* 326(2): 79–88.

Bosch X, Poch E, Grau J (2009). Rhabdomyolysis and acute kidney injury. *New England Journal of Medicine* 361: 62–72.

van Adel B, Tarnopolsky M (2009). Metabolic myopathies: Update 2009. *Journal of Clinical Neuromuscular Disease* 10: 97–121.

212. C) If the patient does not recover renal function, renal transplantation is possible in the long term

The patient presents with a pulmonary renal syndrome. The diagnosis is anti-GBM disease as evidenced by the renal biopsy and anti-GBM positive titre. Around a third of patients will also be ANCA positive and these patients usually have a better outcome. The patient has no ENT symptoms of granulomatosis with polyangiitis and the biopsy is not pauci-immune and does not show granulomata. Therefore, the patient does not, at least at this moment in time, have clinical evidence of granulomatosis with polyangiitis. However, it is very possible that unlike patients who are only seropositive for anti-GBM, those who are 'double hit positive' will go on to get a disease relapse as they appear to truly have a hybrid disease phenotype.

Treatment involves steroids and cyclophosphamide +/− plasma exchange. Pulsed methyl-prednisolone 0.5–1 g daily for three days then prednisolone 1 mg/kg/day is given with cyclophosphamide 1–2 mg/kg/day (max 150 mg) orally, or pulsed intravenously.

Prednisolone and cyclophosphamide are then continued for 3–6 months. The benefits of treatment have to be weighed up against side effects and patient co-morbidity. A creatinine >500 μmol/L, dialysis dependent renal failure, or oliguria <200 ml/day implies severe glomerular damage and most of these patients do not show a response to plasma exchange. Those with less renal damage may have renal benefit from plasma exchange. Pulmonary haemorrhage has a good response to plasma exchange and should be treated even if severe renal damage is present. Plasma exchange is instituted early and 8–10 treatments in over 10–14 days are given initially and then continued if required.

Anti-GBM titre is used to measure response and guide treatment. Patients must be discouraged from smoking. Those who have end-stage renal disease secondary to anti-GBM disease can be treated with renal transplantation; however, anti-GBM disease can recur in the graft. Patients are therefore not considered for transplantation until they have a negative ant-GBM titre for six months. Don't forget anti-GBM disease can arise *de novo* in renal transplants in Alport's syndrome (see question 204).

Tutorial

Anti-GBM disease (Goodpasture's disease) involves serum antibodies (usually IgG1+4 but also IgA) directed against two epitopes (E_a and E_b) of the α3 chain of type 4 collagen (found in the basement membranes of the glomerulus and alveolus). These epitopes are inaccessible to antibody unless the α3.α4α3-NC1 hexamer in which they reside is dissociated. Environmental factors are believed to act as triggers. Cigarette smoke, gasoline, oxygen toxicity, and other irritants have been implicated as aggravating or initiating factors, possibly playing a role in revealing the α3 chain epitope.

Commonly in men in their late 20s or women over 60 years of age, the presentation may be gradual over months to years or more acute and dramatic. Manifestations are renal, pulmonary, and systemic/other with patients presenting with some or all of these symptoms:

- Renal
  - Visible haematuria, then dysmorphic red cells and red cell casts in later disease.
  - Loin pain.
  - Renal failure (acute or chronic) degree correlates well to anti-GBM titre.
  - Proteinuria (<3 g/24hours).
- Pulmonary
  - Cough, dyspnoea.
  - Pulmonary haemorrhage (about 50% of patients) with or without haemoptysis. Anti-GBM titre correlates poorly with degree of haemorrhage.
- Systemic/other
  - Loss of weight.
  - Fever.
  - Ocular abnormalities such as retinal detachment.

Demonstration of anti-GBM antibodies in the circulation or fixed to the kidney confirms the diagnosis. The renal biopsy shows segmental and mesangial matrix expansion and hypercellularity with focal and proliferative glomerulonephritis and total necrosis and crescent formation with increasing severity. Linear staining for anti-GBM (IgG) is seen on immunostaining (IgA, C3, or IgM can also be seen in a third of cases). Lung tissue is less useful as it can have a large amount of autofluorescence. Increased KCO is seen on pulmonary function tests if alveolar blood is present.

Further Reading

Hudson B, Tryggvason K, Sundaramoorthy M, Neilson E (2003). Alport's syndrome, Goodpasture's syndrome, and type IV collagen. *New England Journal of Medicine* 348: 2543–2556.

McAdoo S, Tanna A, Hrušková Z, et al. (2017). Patients double-seropositive for ANCA and anti-GBM antibodies have varied renal survival, frequency of relapse, and outcomes compared to single-seropositive patients. *Kidney International* 92(3): 693–702.

213. B) An M type phospholipase A2 receptor antibody can be identified in 70% of cases of primary idiopathic MGN

The patient presents with a membranous nephropathy. Primary MGN has recently been associated with IgG4 antibodies to the M type phospholipase A2 receptor (PLA2R) (expressed on podocytes) in up to 70% of cases. It can now be assayed on serum samples in the UK with high specificity for primary membranous nephropathy. Its level correlates with disease activity and the titre is useful in monitoring response to therapy as its decrease precedes the decline in proteinuria. Membranous nephropathy may be idiopathic (in 85% of cases) or secondary (described in Table 10.8). Focal segmental glomerular sclerosis (FSGS) is more common in patients of Afro-Caribbean origin, not MGN. Serum complement levels are unaffected in MGN and only a third of patients will undergo spontaneous remission if untreated.

Tutorial

Presentation is typically with nephrotic syndrome or nephrotic range/significant proteinuria. Haematuria and hypertension occur variably. Renal impairment may or may not be a feature and may also be secondary to volume changes secondary to hypoalbuminaemia. Essential investigations include FBC, clotting screen, Alb, LFTs, adjusted Ca^{2+}, Chol/LDL, immunoglobulins, viral hepatitis screen, and urine protein quantification. However, features of an underlying secondary cause may also be present and should be sought in the history, examination, and investigations.

A renal biopsy is required unless contraindicated. Typically thickening and 'spikes' of GBM extending around subepithelial deposits are seen (best seen on silver stain). Loss of podocyte foot processes occurs. There are granular IgG +/− C3 deposits on immunostaining. Note: early in the disease, light microscopy may be normal and changes only seen on electron microscopy and immunofluorescence.

In secondary membranous nephropathy, treatment of the underlying cause usually leads to resolution of the nephrotic syndrome. Supportive measures as described above may also be needed. With regard to idiopathic membranous nephropathy, as a global rule the natural history of membranous nephropathy follows *'the rule of thirds'*: one third progress to end-stage renal disease, one third achieve remission, and one third have persistent proteinuria and reduced but stable renal function or a relapsing remitting course.

Patients can, however, be risk-stratified into low-risk, medium-risk, and high-risk groups.

- **Low-risk group**
  - Normal renal function, age <50 and <4 g/day proteinuria.
  - Low risk for progression and therefore should not be given aggressive immunotherapy and treated conservatively.
    - (1) Reduce proteinuria with an ACEi and/or ARB
    - (2) Reduce blood pressure to ≤125/75 mmHg) and monitor
- **Medium risk group**
  - Normal renal function and persistent proteinuria 4–8 g/day.
  - This group has a higher risk of a poor outcome than the rule of thirds suggests. Therefore, treatment of cycling cytotoxic drugs and steroids may be considered (particularly if proteinuria is showing no evidence of decline with ACE-I/ARB).
- **High risk group**
  - Worsening renal function, age >50 and proteinuria >8 g/day over a six-month period.
  - These patients should receive aggressive therapy with the possibility of newer protocols and be advised that dialysis is a very real eventual possibility.

Treatment of the secondary effects of nephrotic syndrome must also be addressed: (1) lipid abnormalities (commonly raised total cholesterol, VLDL, IDL, and LDL with normal or low HDL) should be treated with dietary changes and statins; (2) hypercoagulability, prophylactic treatment with anticoagulants is based on a risk/benefit analysis, including serum albumin level and previous history of thrombosis; (3) oedema is treated with loop diuretics +/− a distally acting diuretic with strict fluid balance assessments to avoid depletion of circulating volume. Intravenous albumin only provides a temporary effect but may improve the efficacy of diuretics. Salt restriction to <2 g/day; (4) infections should be treated promptly with a particularly low threshold for covering capsulated organisms (such as *Pneumococcus* and *Meningococcus*) due to low IgG levels.

Table 10.8 Secondary causes of membranous nephropathy

Neoplastic	Solid tumours (lung, colon, breast, kidney, gastric)
	Lymphoma (Non-Hodgkin's lymphoma, Hodgkin's disease)
Multisystemic/autoimmune disease	SLE
	Autoimmune thyroiditis
	Sarcoidosis
	Dermatitis herpetiformis
	Rheumatoid arthritis
	Antiphospholipid syndrome
	Sjögren's syndrome
	Autoimmune hepatitis
Medication	Captopril
	Gold
	D-penicillamine
	NSAIDs
Infection	Hepatitis B+C
	Malaria
	Streptococcal infection
	Syphilis/leprosy
	Schistosomiasis
Other	Diabetes
	Renal allograft, de novo disease
	Mercury
	Sickle cell disease

Further Reading

Bomback A, Fervenza F (2018). Membranous nephropathy: approaches to treatment. *American Journal of Nephrology* 47: 30–42.

Couser W (2017). Primary membranous nephropathy. *Clinical Journal of American Society of Nephrology* 12(6): 983–997.

214. B) The patient has focal and segmental sclerosis and the glomerular tip lesion indicates a better prognosis

The patient presents with nephrotic syndrome and the biopsy shows changes consistent with FSGS and not minimal change disease (see Tutorial below). A finding of thickening and 'spikes' of GBM extending around subepithelial deposits with loss of podocyte foot processes would be expected with membranous nephropathy. The glomerular tip lesion suggests a better prognosis in FSGS, whereas the collapsing variant implies a worse prognosis. Recurrence of FSGS is seen in about 30–40% of adults who undergo renal transplantation.

Tutorial

Minimal change disease and FSGS both lead to nephrotic syndrome. It is undecided as to whether they represent two diseases or two parts of the same disease process. It is important to remember that both pathologies can occur in children and adults, but minimal change disease is the most common cause of nephrotic syndrome in children and is less common in adults. The majority of cases are idiopathic for both FSGS and minimal change disease. Secondary causes of minimal change include: (1) drugs (NSAIDS, rifampicin, penicillin/ampicillin, lithium); (2) infection (infectious mononucleosis, HIV); and (3) neoplastic (lymphoma, post bone marrow transplant). Secondary causes of FSGS include reflux nephropathy, renal dysplasia, renovascular disease, obesity, diabetic nephropathy, HIV associated nephropathy, pre-eclampsia, membranous nephropathy, sickle cell disease, Alport's syndrome, and bisphosphonates. Any glomerulonephritis with scarring can also cause FSGS.

Adults present with oedema although it is often less rapid in onset when compared to the presentation in children. Hypertension is often present in adults. Impaired renal function is more commonly seen in adults with FSGS than children with minimal change disease. It should be remembered that in both cases acute kidney injury may be seen due to hypovolaemia and diuresis.

Due to the fact that the majority will respond completely to a course of steroids (and response to this treatment is highly supportive for a diagnosis of minimal change disease) a renal biopsy is not indicated in children with *typical* symptoms. In adults a steroid responsive disease is less likely and wider differential of causes of nephrotic syndrome exists, therefore a biopsy is performed unless there are any contraindications.

Histology of minimal change disease as its name suggests is minimal. Light microscopy and immunostaining are normal. Changes of podocyte foot process effacement may be seen on electron microscopy. For FSGS focal (only some glomeruli), segmental (only part of glomerular tuft) sclerosis, hyalinosis, and mesangial matrix expansion is seen with effacement of foot processes and podocyte degeneration. Immunostaining may show IgM and C3. Of the five FSGS histological variants, two are of note for MRCP: tip lesion (sclerosis affecting the outer tip of the glomerulus near the proximal tubule) implies a better prognosis and collapsing lesion a worse prognosis (glomerular collapse and severe rapid progressive nephrotic syndrome and renal failure is usually seen). It should be noted that a small sample biopsy may miss a sclerotic area as disease is focal, hence may be misdiagnosed as minimal change disease.

For adult minimal change disease 80–90% will be in remission by 12 weeks but can take as long as six months. The general recommendation is to give 1 mg/kg of prednisolone (maximum 80 mg) until remission is achieved and taper prednisolone fortnightly with not less than 12 weeks treatment. This obviously has to be weighed up against steroid side effects as per individual patients. Relapse should be treated, if possible, with another course of steroids but tapering as soon as remission is achieved. Recurrent relapses may occur. At this point a repeat biopsy is considered to verify that the diagnosis is not FSGS. Treatment options at that stage include tacrolimus, ciclosporin, cyclophosphamide, or mycophenolate.

Chance of progression to end-stage renal disease in FSGS is dependent on: (1) degree of proteinuria (especially >14 g/24 hours); (2) response to steroids; (3) collapsing variant (worse)/ glomerular tip lesion (better); and (4) progressive CKD. FSGS responds less frequently and more slowly to steroids than minimal change disease. Prednisolone 1 mg/kg/day should be given for 16–24 weeks if tolerated. If remission of nephrotic syndrome occurs (seen in a third of cases), steroids are tapered for another 12 weeks. Those that relapse during tapering are 'steroid dependent' and those that do not respond at all are 'steroid resistant'. Alternative treatments then include tacrolimus, ciclosporin, or cyclophosphamide.

Further Reading

Rosenberg A, Kopp J (2017). Focal segmental glomerulosclerosis. *Clinical Journal of American Society of Nephrology* 12(3): 502–517.

215. **C)** Hepatitis C

This patient has presented with a membranoproliferative glomerulonephritis (MPGN). Immune complex-mediated MPGN can be seen with many conditions: infectious, autoimmune, and even malignancy. The main underlying cause is a chronic antigenaemia driving immune-complex formation. It is unclear, why some infections are more prone to cause MPGN than others, or why some individuals develop this complication whilst others don't. Intravenous drug use is associated with numerous infective risk factors for kidney disease including bacterial endocarditis, hepatitis C, hepatitis B, HIV, and infected leg ulcers. Of these, hepatitis C is the most strongly associated with MPGN, and therefore is the correct answer. It is worth noting though, that all the aforementioned infections cause various different histological lesions in the kidney, and also cause varying clinical syndromes from nephrotic syndrome, to nephritic syndrome, or proteinuric progressive kidney disease.

Tutorial

MPGN is a pattern of glomerular injury which is characterized on renal biopsy which encompasses: (1) glomerular hypercellularity (proliferation of mesangial cells); (2) expansion of the mesangial matrix; and (3) thickening of capillary walls (giving rise to the classic double-contouring or 'tram-track appearance'). Historically, it was divided up into three types based on electron microscopy appearance corresponding to the location of deposits within the glomerulus. However, this classification system was subjective, often resulting in 'overlap' conditions, and perhaps, most importantly, did not help in identifying underlying causes or provide insights into underlying pathophysiology of the disease.

The updated classification of MPGN depends on what is seen on immunofluorescence staining of the glomerulus. The division hinges on whether immunoglobulins (along with but not necessarily complement) can be detected by immunofluorescence, or whether there is only predominant complement staining. This division helps to identify underlying causes of the MPGN, but also reflects the underling pathophysiological pathways that cause the diseases: immune complex-mediated MPGN which is mediated via the classic complement pathway vs complement-mediated MPGN which is mediated by the alternate complement pathway.

Figure 10.2 demonstrates the updated classification of MPGN and Table 10.9 lists the common causes of immune-complexed mediated MPGN. Identifying causes of C3 glomerulopathy (the term used to describe complement mediated MPGN) is a rapidly developing field, whilst there are two histological variants, depending on the presence of pathognomonic 'dense deposits': dense deposit disease (DDD) vs C3 glomerulonephritis (C3GN). Both conditions share many clinical features, but appear to represent two distinct pathophysiological entities, and have some distinct characteristics in that DDD more commonly presents in younger patients, is associated with lower C3, and is more commonly associated with a crescentic glomerulonephritis, but the prognosis for both conditions in terms of progression to end-stage kidney diseases is similar. Most cases of C3 glomerulopathy (i.e. both DDD and C3GN) are thought to be due to genetic mutations in complement regulatory proteins, with new culprit mutations constantly being identified. Some are *de novo*, whilst others such as CFHR5 nephropathy, which is due to a mutations in complement factor H-related 5 (CFHR5) identified in Cypriot families, is hereditary. In other cases, a causal antibody: C3 nephritic factor (an antibody to C3 convertase which stabilizes the enzyme, resulting in excessive activation of C3 into C3a and C3b) has been identified as causing C3 glomerulopathy.

The mainstay of treatment for immune-complex mediated MPGN is to treat the underlying cause, for example the plasma cell dyscrasia, infection, or auto-immune condition, if it is truly idiopathic; then immunosuppressive regimes can be tried, but have varying response. Treatment for C3 glomerulopathies is an evolving field based mainly on case reports and small centre series. Plasma-exchange, mycophenolate, and even eculizumab are appropriate (an antibody which prevents activation of C5, which is the terminal step in both the classical and alternate complement pathway, resulting in the formation of the 'membrane attack complex'). Treatment results and recurrence of disease often occurs after renal transplantation, and this is most likely because the C3 glomerulopathies are a result of a heterogenous group of genetic or acquired deficiencies in complement regulation,

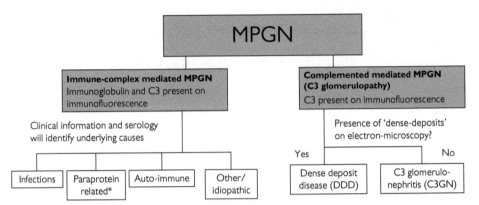

Figure 10.2 Algorithm for differentiating immune-complex mediated MPGN vs complement mediated MPGN (C3 glomerulopathy).

* Paraprotein related MPGN, usually due to plasma cell dyscrasias, is due to a pathological monoclonal antibody being produced which forms immune-complex deposits in the glomerulus, resulting in disease.

Table 10.9 Causes of immune-complex mediated MPGN

Infection	• Hepatitis B • Hepatitis C • Infective endocarditis • Abscesses • HIV Less commonly (though possible under diagnosed/reported): • Protozoa, for example malaria • Helminths, for example schistosomiasis • Mycoplasma
Auto-immune	• SLE • Cryoglobulinemia • Sjögren's syndrome • Sarcoidosis • Systemic sclerosis
Monoclonal gammopathies/ paraproteinaemias	• Myeloma • Lymphomas • CLL • MGUS (more correctly MGRS: mono-clonal gammopathy of RENAL significance)
Idiopathic/other	• Idiopathic • Drugs

Further Reading

Cook H, Pickering M (2015). Histopathology of MPGN and C3 glomerulopathies. *Nature Reviews Nephrology* 11(1): 14–22.

Sethi S, Nester C, Smith R (2012). Membranoproliferative glomerulonephritis and C3 glomerulopathy: resolving the confusion. *Kidney International* 81(5): 434–441.

216. E) *Staphylococcus epidermidis*

PD peritonitis is the most common and potentially serious complication of PD. Although less than 5% of peritonitis episodes result in death, peritonitis is the direct or major contributing cause of death in around 16% of PD patients. In addition, up to 50% of technique failures can be attributed to PD peritonitis. The most common organism is the skin commensal *Staphylococcus epidermidis*.

Tutorial

PD peritonitis can be diagnosed when at least two of the following are present:

(1) Clinical features consistent with peritonitis, that is, abdominal pain and/or cloudy dialysis effluent.
(2) Dialysis effluent white cell count > 100/μL or >0.1 × 10⁹/L (after a dwell time of at least two hours), with >50% polymorphonuclear cells.
(3) Positive dialysis effluent culture.

Clinical assessment should include examination of the exit site and tunnel for infection and the abdomen for signs of intra-abdominal pathology. An abdominal X-ray is not always indicated. At least 20 ml of freshly drained dialysate should be sent for culture.

Abdominal pain and pyrexia are key symptoms but very variable, and in some patients are not a feature until the bags have been cloudy for some days. On starting peritoneal dialysis, patients should be trained to report a cloudy bag as soon as they see one regardless of whether they have any other symptoms. If there is delay in diagnosis, or failure to respond to treatment, the fluid becomes increasingly turbid and eventually looks like 'pea soup'. Drainage can then become poor as the catheter becomes blocked. Even in milder cases, fibrin can form and block the catheter. Loss of ultrafiltration is also a feature of peritonitis, and may persist even after the episode has cleared.

Empirical antibiotic treatment, which should be given intra-peritoneally as first line, should cover for both Gram positive and negative organisms and should be commenced immediately whilst awaiting specific sensitivities. Most units will opt for a triple therapy regimen: a third generation cephalosporin (e.g. ceftazidime), an aminoglycoside (e.g. gentamicin), and a glycopeptide (e.g. vancomycin). A mixed bacterial growth, especially if associated with anaerobes should dictate early surgical assessment, catheter removal, and laparotomy. Catheter removal is likely if there is an associated tunnel infection or a failure to respond to antibiotics over the next few days.

The severity of an episode of peritonitis depends on the causative organism. The need for hospitalization depends on the severity and on the ability of the patient to carry out the treatment regimen. In general, patients with minimal pain could be treated on an outpatient basis with intraperitoneal (IP) antibiotic therapy if this can be arranged. No organisms are grown from about 20% episodes (usually mild). *S. epidermidis* peritonitis is often clinically mild. Episodes due to *S. aureus* or Gram-negative infections are much more severe and have a worse prognosis.

Patients with cloudy effluent may benefit from the addition of heparin 500 units/L IP to prevent occlusion of the catheter by fibrin. Depending on the severity of symptoms, some patients would require analgesics for pain control.

Most cases are mild and respond quickly to antibiotics. Complications occur when the diagnosis is delayed, or there is a poor response to treatment. They include:

- Failure to respond to antibiotics, necessitating catheter removal and transfer to haemodialysis.
- Loss of ultrafiltration (fluid removal).
- Loss of appetite and increased catabolism resulting in malnutrition.
- Fungal peritonitis after repeated courses of intraperitoneal antibiotics.
- Persistent intra-abdominal sepsis requiring laparotomy and drainage.
- Formation of adhesions and later catheter malfunction.
- Ileus (in severe infections).
- Death (rare).

Further Reading

Li P, Szeto C, Piraino B, et al. (2016). ISPD peritonitis recommendations: 2016 update on prevention and treatment. *Peritoneal Dialysis International* 36(5): 481–508.

217. E) Renal artery stenosis

In this scenario, the blood test results indicate a secondary hyperaldosteronism, which could be secondary to renal artery stenosis. In renal artery stenosis, the reduced blood supply across the juxtaglomerular apparatus stimulates the production of renin and subsequently aldosterone.

Tutorial

Secondary hypertension accounts for around 5% of all patients with arterial hypertension. The work up for causes is costly and should be reserved for those with a true clinical suspicion. It should be suspected in patients with severe or resistant hypertension (i.e. those with hypertension despite concurrent use of adequate doses of three antihypertensive agents from different classes, including a diuretic), aged less than 30, not obese, not black, and have no family history of hypertension, and patients with malignant or accelerated hypertension.

In adults, renal artery stenosis is more commonly due to atherosclerotic lesions, particularly in the older population, males, smokers, and those with evidence of atherosclerosis elsewhere. A cause of renal artery stenosis that particularly affects young women is fibromuscular dysplasia.

Examination findings can include an abdominal bruit. Clinical suspicion should be raised when there is a rise in serum creatinine of at least 30% after administration of ACE inhibitor or angiotensin II receptor blocker (ARB), recurrent episodes of flash pulmonary oedema, diffuse atherosclerotic disease, and worsening hypertension in arteriopaths. Screening imaging can be performed using duplex ultrasound, CT, or MRI. However, the diagnosis is made by angiography to detect a significant trans-lesional gradient. The pathophysiology and imaging of renal artery stenosis is discussed further in the tutorial to question 28.

Other causes of secondary hypertension are discussed in Table 10.10

Table 10.10 Overview of the most common causes of secondary hypertension

Cause	Prevalence in hypertensive patients	Clinical symptoms and findings	Investigations
Primary hyperaldosteronism	1.4–10%	Fatigue, polyuria, polydipsia, muscle weakness.	Hypokalaemia, hypernatraemia, metabolic alkalosis, increased urinary sodium excretion. Elevated renin aldosterone ratio. Confirmatory tests with sodium loading or captopril suppression can be performed.
Cushing's syndrome	0.5%	High BMI with centripetal obesity, striae, ecchymoses, and proximal muscle weakness.	Increased 24-hour urinary cortisol, hyperglycaemia, hyperlipidaemia, hypokalaemia
Phaeochromo-cytoma	0.2–0.5%	Paroxysmal elevations in blood pressure (which may be superimposed upon stable chronic hypertension). Headache, palpitations, and sweating.	24-hour urine catecholamines and metanephrine or plasma fractionated metanephrine. If positive proceed to imaging with CT or MRI.

Table 10.10 Continued

Cause	Prevalence in hypertensive patients	Clinical symptoms and findings	Investigations
Hypo/ hyperthyroidism	1–2%	Hypothyroidism: weight gain, fatigue constipation, bradycardia, myxoedema. Hyperthyroidism: weight loss, palpitations, anxiety. AF, tachycardia, exopthalamos.	Hypothyroidism: high TSH, low T4, high cholesterol. Hyperthyroidism: high TSH, low T4.
Coarctation of the aorta	<1%	Hypertension in the upper extremities (>20/10 mmHg difference between upper and lower limbs), diminished or delayed femoral pulses ('brachial-femoral delay')	Echocardiography is the screening method of choice. CT or MRI may also be performed.
Obstructive sleep apnoea	>5–15%	Daytime somnolence, snoring, and irritability. Assessed sleepiness using Epworth Sleepiness scale. Severity of OSA is classified based on the apnoea-hypopnoea index.	Overnight pulse oximetry.

Adapted from: Rimoldi S, Scherrer U, Messerli F (2014). Secondary arterial hypertension: when, who, and how to screen? *European Heart Journal* 35(19): 1245–1254. By permission of the European Society of Cardiology.

Further Reading

Rimoldi S, Scherrer U, Messerli F (2014). Secondary arterial hypertension: when, who, and how to screen? *European Heart Journal* 35(19): 1245–1254.

218. C) Membranous nephropathy

Patient with membranous nephropathy are more prone to renal vein thrombosis. A study conducted by Barbour et al. demonstrated that the incidence of venous thromboembolic events was much higher in membranous nephropathy (7.9%) and focal segmental glomerulosclerosis (3.0%) than in IgA nephropathy (0.4%) in a cohort of 1313 patients with idiopathic glomerular disease due to membranous nephropathy, focal segmental glomerulosclerosis, or IgA nephropathy. The histologic diagnosis remained a predictive factor for thrombosis after adjustment for the degree of proteinuria (which was much higher at presentation in membranous nephropathy and focal segmental glomerulosclerosis (median 5.6 and 3.7 g/day versus 1.6 g/day in IgA nephropathy)) and the serum albumin concentration.

Tutorial

Patients with nephrotic syndrome are in a hypercoagulable state, making them prone to both arterial and venous thromboses. The absolute risk of venous thrombosis has previously been reported as 1.0% per year, which is eight times higher than the age- and sex-matched annual incidence. The overall prevalence is unknown, however, and is likely to be underdiagnosed.

The reasons for the hypercoagulable state are not fully understood. Various mechanisms have been described, including excessive urinary protein loss associated with decreased antithrombin III, protein S, and plasminogen, and a relative excess of fibrinogen, leading to a propensity to clot. Platelet aggregation is also stimulated by hypoalbuminaemia. The mechanism is believed to be due to increased availability of normally albumin-bound arachidonic acid, leading to increased formation of thromboxane A2 in platelets. In addition, elevated levels of LDL cholesterol is thought to stimulate platelet aggregation. As well as these factors, intravascular volume depletion that typically occurs in patients with nephrotic syndrome due to the use of diuretics further predisposes patients to venous thromboembolism. The degree of thrombosis appears to be greater in patients with an albumin of less than 20 g/L, and for this reason many centres will empirically anticoagulate patients with nephrotic syndrome who have an albumin lower than this.

Presentation of renal vein thrombosis can be variable and the majority of patients are asymptomatic. There has been no proven benefit for screening for RVT in patients with nephrotic syndrome. It is also not useful to evaluate for RVT in a patient who experiences an overt embolic event such as PE as the management would not be altered.

The diagnostic method of choice at present is imaging with CT as this has a higher specificity and sensitivity as compared with Doppler ultrasonography.

As well as nephrotic syndrome, other risk factors for renal vein thrombosis include:

- Renal cell carcinoma
- Renal allograft
- Antiphospholipid syndrome
- Behçets disease
- Other hypercoagulable states

Management of renal vein thrombosis mainly involves anticoagulation and attempts to reduce urinary protein loss. If renal vein thrombosis is associated with pulmonary emboli, anticoagulation should be continued for as long as nephrotic syndrome persists. Streptokinase may also be used to lyse acute thrombosis, although the number of patients in which this has been attempted remains small.

Further Reading

Barbour S, Greenwald A, Djurdjev O, et al. (2012). Disease-specific risk of venous thromboembolic events is increased in idiopathic glomerulonephritis. *Kidney International* 81(2): 190.

Wysokinski W, Gosk-Bierska I, Greene E, Grille D, Wiste H, McBane R (2008). Clinical characteristics and long-term follow-up of patients with renal vein thrombosis. *American Journal of Kidney Disease* 51: 224–232.

219. B) A lateral abdominal radiograph can be used to detect the presence or absence of vascular calcification

This patient has chronic kidney disease—mineral bone disorder (CKD-MBD) which has likely arisen due to poor compliance with calcium supplementation and phosphate binders. The patient has a high bone turnover as indicated by the elevated alkaline phosphatase and hypocalcaemia. The clinical challenge is to maintain bone mineral density by optimizing serum calcium levels, whilst reducing the complication of 'over-calcification' and systemic vascular calcification. Current 2017 KDIGO (Kidney Disease: Improving Global Outcomes) guidelines state that a 'lateral abdominal radiograph can be used to detect the presence or absence of vascular calcification as a reasonable alternative to computed tomography-based imaging and an echocardiogram can be used to detect the presence or absence of valvular calcification, as reasonable alternatives to computed tomography-based imaging.'

Reprinted from *Kidney International Supplements*, 7, 1, Kidney Disease: Improving Global Outcomes (KDIGO) CKD-MBD Update Work Group, 2017. *KDIGO 2017 Clinical Practice Guideline Update for the Diagnosis, Evaluation, Prevention, and Treatment of Chronic Kidney Disease–Mineral and Bone Disorder (CKD-MBD)*, pp. 1–59. Copyright 2017, with permission from Elsevier and the International Society of Nephrology.

Hypercalcaemia should be avoided and serum calcium levels should be maintained in the normal range.

Tutorial

CKD-MBD is an important cause of morbidity and mortality in patients with renal insufficiency. As renal function declines, the kidney's ability to excrete phosphate decreases, leading to hyperphosphataemia and hyperparathyroidism. The renal hydroxylation of 25-hydroxycholecalciferol to the active form of vitamin D: 1,25-hydroxycholecalciferol is also diminished, causing a reduction in calcium absorption in the gut and thereby again contributing to hyperparathyroidism.

Another protein that is implicated in CKD-MBD is fibroblast growth factor 23 (FGF 23). This is a protein which is secreted by osteoclasts in response to elevated 1,25(OH2)D and also phosphate levels. Its physiological role is to promote renal excretion of phosphate by decreasing the expression of the proximal tubule NPT2, a sodium-phosphate cotransporter, which results in phosphaturia. FGF 23 also raises PTH levels and reduces renal vitamin D hydroxylation as a negative feedback mechanism. In CKD, as phosphate levels progressively rise due to nephron loss, FGF 23 levels begin to rise, and with it PTH levels also rise and vitamin D levels fall. As there is already impaired renal excretion of phosphate due to diminished nephron number, the expected increased phosphaturia as a result of FGF 23 (and PTH itself) acting on the remaining nephrons does not offset the raised serum phosphate.

These changes affect both bone modelling in growth and bone remodelling throughout adulthood. Complications of MBD include renal osteoporosis and osteodystrophy, pathologic fractures, and the development of Brown tumours. In addition, there have been concerns regarding extra-skeletal calcification, that is, arterial calcification leading to both cardiovascular and peripheral vascular disease, thus contributing to the morbidity and mortality of these patients.

Management of CKD-MBD focuses on maintaining calcium and phosphate within normal ranges, and PTH to a supra-normal level (2–10 times normal, depending on severity of CKD). This is because supressing PTH to normal levels through phosphate binders and vitamin D supplementation actually causes low bone turnover which is known as adynamic bone disease which also results in bones becoming more prone to fracture. There are various reasons for this but in summary uraemia confers downstream resistance to PTH in the bone, so a 'normal' level in a patient with ESKD is actually sub-physiological.

KDIGO guidelines recommend that in CKD stage 5, serum calcium and phosphorus should be checked every 1–3 months and PTH every 3–6 months. No other markers need to be measured. In this patient, although the calcium and phosphate levels are not hugely abnormal (partly because blood tests are often taken after dialysis at which point electrolytes will be temporarily 'corrected'), the extent of the MBD can be seen by the extremely elevated PTH and alkaline phosphatase indicating an extremely high bone turnover.

Treating CKD-MBD requires a multidisciplinary team. Dietician input is essential for patients in advising on low phosphate diets and providing alternate food sources of nutrients. Vitamin D and calcium supplements are prescribed in addition to phosphate binders. In severe cases, cinacalcet can also be used. This drug increases the sensitivity to calcium of the calcium sensing receptor of the parathyroid gland thus reducing PTH secretion. When patients have suffered from secondary hyperparathyroidism for a long time, changes occur in the parathyroid gland resulting in secretion of PTH in a manner autonomous to serum calcium levels. This is known as tertiary hyper-parathyroidism. The result is normal or even high calcium levels with an inappropriately raised PTH level, resulting in aggressive bone lytic lesions. In this case, cinacalcet can be used but the definitive treatment is surgical parathyroidectomy of some or all of the hyperactive glands.

Further Reading

Jüppner H (2011). Phosphate and FGF-23. *Kidney International* (Suppl.) 79(121): S24–27.

Kidney Disease: Improving Global Outcomes (KDIGO) CKD-MBD Update Work Group (2017). KDIGO 2017 Clinical practice guideline update for the diagnosis, evaluation, prevention, and treatment of chronic kidney disease–mineral and bone disorder (CKD-MBD). *Kidney International* (Suppl.) 7(1): 1–59.

220. **C)** Medullary sponge kidney

This patient has medullary sponge kidney (MSK), a diagnosis which relies on the typical radiological appearances as described in the case. It is associated with chronic renal impairment, distal renal tubular acidosis, haematuria, and urinary tract infections.

Tutorial

MSK is a benign congenital disorder (also known as Cacchi-Ricci disease) characterized by malformation of the terminal collecting ducts in the pericalyceal region of the renal pyramids. This collecting duct dilatation is associated with the formation of both microscopic and large medullary cysts that are often diffuse but do not involve the cortex.

The exact prevalence of MSK is unknown, although the frequency in the general population has been estimated to be 1 case per 5000 population. Women are affected by MSK more frequently than men.

Some patients with MSK have mutations in the gene for REarranged during Transfection (RET) proto-oncogene and glial cell-derived neurotrophic factor (GDNF), which play a role in renal development. Most patients with MSK have no family history of the condition, although a rare, familial, autosomal dominant form of the disease has been described. The genetic mutation in these patients has yet to be identified.

Patients with MSK are usually asymptomatic but can present with renal calculi, haematuria, recurrent urinary tract infections, and distal renal tubular acidosis. Symptoms typically occur in adulthood and rarely can cause renal insufficiency. Management revolves around symptom control. Infections should be treated promptly and aggressively. In order to prevent renal stone formation, patients are advised to drink plenty of fluid and have a low purine diet. A 24-hour urine collection should be performed to rule out risk factors for stone disease. In patients in whom a distal renal tubular acidosis is suspected, potassium citrate supplementation should be commenced to increase the urinary pH to a maximum of 7.0–7.2. The prognosis for patients is good, with less than 10% developing renal insufficiency. Morbidity commonly results from recurrent infections or stone formation.

Further Reading

Gambaro G, Danza F, Fabris A (2013). Medullary sponge kidney. *Current Opinion in Nephrology and Hypertension* 22: 421–424.

221. **B)** Black ethnicity

Patients who are identified as 'high risk' may require more aggressive immunosuppressive regimens. The 2009 KDIGO clinical practice guidelines identified the following factors as 'high risk' for acute rejection:

- One or more human leukocyte antigen (HLA) mismatches
- Younger recipient and older donor age
- African-American ethnicity (in the USA)
- Panel reactive antibody (PRA) greater than 0%
- Presence of a donor-specific antibody (DSA)
- Blood group incompatibility

- Delayed onset of graft function
- Cold ischaemia time greater than 24 hours

Tutorial

Acute rejection following transplantation is a major cause of morbidity and mortality. Risk benefit approach should be used to ascertain the adequate level of immunosuppression which is required to dampen the immune response to the allograft with the overall risk of infection and malignancy.

The induction therapy immunosuppression regimens used for kidney transplant patients may vary according to the 'risk' status of the patient and protocols vary across centres. Following induction therapy, maintenance immunosuppressive therapy is administered to all renal transplant recipients to help prevent acute rejection and the loss of the renal allograft. Most centres used a combination of triple therapy in this setting, consisting of:

- Calcineurin inhibitors (CNIs)—tacrolimus or ciclosporin
- Antimetabolite—mycofenalate mofetil or azathioprine
- Prednisolone—weaning regimen used, which often varies between centres

Alternatives to CNIs include mTOR inhibitors (e.g. sirolimus) or belatacept (CTLA4 agonist), for example for patients who cannot continue CNIs due to toxicity, or who develop a new cancer after transplantation.

Further Reading

Kidney Disease: Improving Global Outcomes (KDIGO) Transplant Work Group (2009). KDIGO clinical practice guideline for the care of kidney transplant recipients. *American Journal of Transplantation* (Suppl.)9: S1–S155.

222. C) Levetiracetam

Levetiracetam is an anti-epileptic medication. Although it has a low level of protein binding (<10%), it has a large volume of distribution similar to total body water, which makes it poorly dialysable (see tutorial). Carbamazepine also has a relatively large volume of distribution and is highly protein bound, yet the molecular weight is relatively small, so high flux haemodialysis can be used in this setting.

A commonly used mnemonic for recalling which drugs are dialyzable is BLAST: barbituates, lithium, alcohol (methanol/ethanol), salicylate, theophylline.

Tutorial

Haemodialysis comes in standard as well as high-efficiency or high-flux modalities, both of which use clearance by diffusion. The major difference is the pore size of the membrane, the type of membrane, and the amount of dialysate flow that occurs. Typically, with flux or high-efficiency HD, membranes with a larger pore size (as large as 20 kDa) are available for the clearance of intoxications.

Factors influencing dialysis

- Molecular weight—smaller molecular weight substances will pass through the dialysis membrane more easily than larger molecular weights.
- Protein binding—drugs with a high degree of protein binding will have a small plasma concentration of unbound drug available for dialysis, making them poorly dialysable or requiring multiple sessions, for example digoxin.

- Volume of distribution—drugs with large volumes of distribution, usually due to lipid solubility and low plasma protein binding, are poorly dialysable.
- Plasma clearance—although plasma clearance may be beneficial, increasing plasma clearance will decrease dialysis clearance.
- Dialysis flow rates—greater degrees of dialysis can be achieved with faster dialysate flow rates if the dialysate drug concentrations is low. As the concentration of drug is increased in the dialysate, the flow rate needs to be lowered.

The introduction of high flux haemodialysis has resulted in the clearance of more drugs, including those which are highly protein bound, but often not to a degree that would allow clinical significance. Other forms of clearance include the use of continuous renal replacement therapy in the intensive care setting or peritoneal dialysis. In the acute accident and emergency setting, the handbook of dialysable drugs can be consulted to ascertain which form of clearance would be best suited.

For further reading regarding dialysis and dialysis complications please see the tutorial for question 199.

Further Reading

Bunchman T, Ferris M (2011). Management of toxic ingestions with the use of renal replacement therapy. *Pediatric Nephrology* 26(4): 535–541.

223. B) Kimmelstiel-Wilson glomerulosclerosis

This patient is suffering from diabetic nephropathy, which is the single most common cause of end-stage renal disease worldwide. The clinical features fit with the diagnosis. However, on histology the findings in type II diabetes can be diverse and difficult to distinguish from other conditions. Therefore, in order to accurately ascertain the diagnosis, the history, clinical picture, laboratory investigations, and (if a renal biopsy is warranted) histological findings, must all be considered.

Patients with diabetes can be affected by multiple glomerulonephropathies which must be differentiated from diabetic nephropathy. Clinical features include increasing proteinuria accompanied by hypertension and impairment of glomerular filtration. Histologically, diabetic nephropathy is characterized by diffuse or nodular glomerulosclerosis (i.e. Kimmelstiel-Wilson nodules), tubulointerstitial fibrosis, and atrophy, with variable degrees of hyaline arteriolosclerosis and arterial sclerosis.

Although a renal biopsy is the gold standard for diagnosis, the majority of diabetic patients with renal involvement are not biopsied. There is a significant bleeding risk from renal biopsies, which should be carefully weighed up against the proposed benefits. Typically, a histological diagnosis will not change the management of a patient with diabetic nephropathy—tight blood pressure and glycaemic control (this is discussed in further detail in the tutorial to question 224). Many nephrologists would only proceed with a renal biopsy should an immunological or viral screen be suggestive of an alternate pathology, or the degree of renal impairment was not in keeping with the patient's diabetic burden. For example, the absence of diabetic eye disease is often used as a rough clinical guide to prompt referral for a kidney biopsy.

Tutorial

Diabetic nephropathy can occur as a complication of both type I and type II diabetes mellitus and most commonly leads to diffuse scarring of the glomeruli, eventually leading to chronic kidney disease.

Various mechanisms have been identified for the process of injury in diabetic nephropathy. It is thought that reactive oxygen species cause glomerular damage causing proteinuria. The protein accumulation in Bowman's space causes distinct periodic-acid Schiff nodules to form, that is,

Kimmelstiel-Wilson nodules. Other mechanisms for injury include glomerular hyperfiltration, mesangial expansion due to hyperglycaemia, increased circulating ACE, and activation of cytokines, profibrotic elements, inflammation, and vascular growth factors (vascular endothelial growth factor, VEGF).

Four classes of glomerular lesions in diabetes have been defined by the Renal Pathology Society and are as follows:

- Class I: isolated glomerular basement membrane thickening. There is no evidence of mesangial expansion, increased mesangial matrix, or global glomerulosclerosis involving >50% of glomeruli.
- Class II: mild (class IIa) or severe (class IIb) mesangial expansion. Severe areas are those with expansion larger than the mean area of a capillary lumen, present in >25% of the total mesangium.
- Class III: at least one Kimmelstiel-Wilson lesion (nodular intercapillary glomerulosclerosis) is observed on biopsy and there is <50% global glomerulosclerosis.
- Class IV: advanced diabetic sclerosis. There is >50% global glomerulosclerosis that is attributable to diabetic nephropathy.

The mainstay of treatment involves optimization of glycaemic control, diabetic control, and angiotensin inhibition with ACE inhibitors and ARB. Recently, it has also been found that the use of sodium-glucose cotransporter 2 (SGLT-2) inhibitors (e.g. dapafiglozin) can reduce progression of kidney disease, although the mechanism remains unclear at present. Secondary prevention measures such as weight loss, a low salt diet, blood pressure control, and reduction of hyperlipidaemia, also play an important role.

Further Reading

Tervaert T, Mooyaart A, Amann K, et al. (2010). Pathologic classification of diabetic nephropathy. *Journal of American Society of Nephrology* 21: 556–563.

224. A) CKD G3a A1

CKD is a condition that affects >10% of the population. It describes an abnormality of the kidney structure or renal function for more than three months. CKD is classified based on eGFR and albuminuria.

Proteinuria should be measured in an early morning urine sample and a urine albumin to creatinine ratio is the preferred measurement. Rapid progression is defined as a sustained decline in eGFR of more than 5 ml/min/1.73 m2/yr. The stages of CKD are summarized in Table 10.11, the higher the stage, the worse the GFR. Whilst the specific prognosis of each stage varies on the underlying cause of the kidney disease, the presence of proteinuria regardless of underlying cause confers a more rapid progression to end-stage kidney failure.

Table 10.11 Stages of CKD by eGFR

Stage of CKD	eGFR (ml/min//1.73m²)
1	≥90
2	60–89
3a	45–59
3b	30–44
4	15–29
5	<15

Tutorial

Management of CKD involves the following:

Blood pressure

Adults with CKD in whom BP is consistently >140 mmHg systolic or >90 mmHg diastolic should be treated with antihypertensive medication to maintain a BP that is consistently around 140 mmHg systolic and 90 mmHg diastolic. Adults with urine albumin excretion of 3 mg/mmol whose BP is consistently >130 mmHg systolic or >80 mmHg diastolic should be treated with antihypertensive medication to maintain a BP that is consistently kept below 130 mmHg systolic and 80 mmHg diastolic. An ARB or ACE-I can be used in both diabetic and non-diabetic adults with CKD and urine albumin excretion >30 mg/mmol.

Anaemia

Anaemia in adults with CKD is diagnosed when the Hb concentration is less than 13.0 g/dl in males and 12.0 g/dl in females. Anaemia in CKD occurs for two reasons—first, due to impaired iron absorption from the gut as a result of increased circulating levels of hepcidin (a protein which is renally cleared), which results in decreased absorption of iron by enterocytes. Second, as CKD progresses, there is decreased erythropoietin production by the kidney. Target Hb for patients with CKD is 10–11.5 g/dl, as studies have shown that aiming to normalize haemoglobin levels using synthetic erythropoietin results in a significant rise in cardiovascular and other adverse events. It is important to stress, however, that patients with mild CKD do not typically become anaemic, especially not profoundly so, and therefore should still be investigated for iron deficiency anaemia and potential GI tract malignancy.

Metabolic bone disease

Measure serum levels of calcium, phosphate, PTH, and alkaline phosphatase activity at least once in adults with GFR <45 ml/min/1.73 m. The management of bone disease in CKD patients is discussed in more detail in the tutorial to question 219.

Acidosis

CKD with serum bicarbonate concentrations of <22 mmol/l should be treated with oral bicarbonate supplementation to maintain serum bicarbonate within the normal range.

Diet

Individuals with CKD should receive expert dietary advice, tailored to the severity of CKD, advising on the need to moderate salt, phosphate, potassium, and protein intake where indicated.

Glycaemic control

A target haemoglobin A1c (HbA1c) of 53 mmol/mol should be maintained to prevent or delay progression of the microvascular complications of diabetes, including diabetic nephropathy. However, as patients' GFR decreases, a more relaxed target HbA1c of 60 mmol/mol is recommended due to the risk of hypoglycaemia as a result of impaired insulin clearance. It may become necessary to further relax the HbA1c target for patients who become established on dialysis, if they are experiencing peri-dialysis hypoglycaemias.

Further Reading

Anders H, Huber T, Isermann B, Schiffer M (2018). CKD in diabetes: diabetic kidney disease versus nondiabetic kidney disease. *Nature Reviews Nephrology* 14(6): 361–377.

Drawz P, Rahman M (2015). Chronic kidney disease. *Annals of Internal Medicine* 162(11): ITC1–16.

225. **D)** Metolazone

Initial management of fluid overload in patients with CKD consists of fluid restriction and encouraging a low salt diet. In this situation, adding a thiazide diuretic would be the most efficacious way to enhance this patient's diuresis. The patient is already on furosemide, which is a potent loop diuretic commonly used to treat fluid overload, hypertension, and occasionally hypercalcaemia.

Metolazone is a thiazide diuretic which would have a synergistic effect (see mechanism of action below). The effect of additional metolazone can be potent, and close monitoring of the patient, including daily weights and monitoring of electrolytes, would be recommended. Spironolactone and amiloride are potassium sparing diuretics and in this context would not be appropriate due to the risk of hyperkalaemia, particularly as the patient is also on an ACE inhibitor. Mannitol is an osmotic diuretic which results in a weak diuresis and would not be appropriate given the degree of symptoms.

Tutorial

Diuretics are often used in patients with chronic kidney disease for symptom control and their mechanisms of action are summarized below according to classes:

Loop diuretics: for example furosemide, bumetanide. These compete for the Cl site on the Na-K-2Cl carrier in the thick ascending limb of the loop of Henle, thus reducing net reabsoprtion. They can lead to the excretion of up to 25% of filtered sodium at maximal dose. In addition, passive paracellular reabsorption of both magnesium and calcium, which normally occurs due to the positive electrochemical gradient created by back leak of K^+ as opposed to absorbed Na^+ and Cl^-, is diminished. This leads to an increased calcium excretion. Potential adverse effects include nephrocalcinosis and renal stone formation.

Thiazide diuretics: for example bendroflumethiazide, metolazone. These inhibit NaCl reabsorption primarily in the distal convoluted tubule. Thiazide diuretics alone have a smaller natriuretic effect than loop diuretics, as the fractional reabsorption of sodium in this segment of the nephron is usually quite small. However, when used in conjunction with loop diuretics (which impair sodium reabsorption in the loop of Henle), a greater fraction of sodium reaches the distal convoluted tubule and thus in this circumstance, thiazide diuretics have a more potent effect.

As thizaide diuretics inhibit the reabsorption of sodium in the distal tubule, this gives a positive transluminal charge resulting in increased reabsorption of calcium. The resulting hypocalciuria is the reason why thiazide diuretics are sometimes used in the treatment of renal calculi.

Potassium sparing diuretics: for example spironolactone, eplerenone, amiloride. These are competitive antagonists that compete with either aldosterone (thereby reducing ENaC and Na^+/K^+ anti-porter expression) or directly block sodium channels. They result in the inhibition of sodium reabsorption in the principal cells of the collecting duct. Whilst this does have a natriuretic effect, there is also impaired secretion of potassium and hydrogen ions, and thus this class of diuretics can cause or worsen both metabolic acidosis and hyperkalaemia. The naturesis achieved by potassium-sparing diuretics alone is small, with the maximal excretion of sodium of only 1–2% under normal physiological circumstances. So they are often used in combination with other diuretics which increase the percentage of filtered sodium reaching this part of the nephron.

These drugs are also, as their name suggests, potassium sparing agents. This is due to their effect of increasing distal potassium reabsorption, and can be useful to counter the profound hypokalaemia that can occur as a result of loop diuretic use. However, this problem is less common in patients with chronic kidney disease.

Carbonic anhydrase inhibitors: for example acetazolamide. Carbonic anhydrase is important for proximal bicarbonate, sodium, and chloride reabsorption. In clinical practice, however, they have a very weak diuretic effect and so are not used for this indication.

Osmotic diuretics: for example mannitol—a non-reabsorbable sugar alcohol. These act on the proximal tubule and loop of Henle, by reducing the osmotic gradient against which water is absorbed from the tubules. However, their initial effect can be to induce volume expansion, due to osmotic effects in the intracellular space, and therefore osmotic diuretics are not used clinically for oedematous patients. Mannitol is used in some neurosurgical emergencies because of its effects in reducing CSF pressure.

Further Reading

Jentzer J, DeWald T, Hernandez A (2010). Combination of loop diuretics with thiazide-type diuretics in heart failure. *Journal of the American College of Cardiology* 56:(19): 1527–1534.

226. **A 24-year-old man presented with a sudden onset of breathlessness and right-sided pleuritic chest pain. He had no significant past medical history but smoked ten cigarettes per day. On examination he was dyspnoeic at rest, with a respiratory rate of 24 breaths per minute. His pulse rate was 105 beats per minute and blood pressure was 134/85 mmHg. Oxygen saturations were 94% on room air. There was reduced chest expansion and air entry on the right.**

    A chest radiograph revealed a right-sided pneumothorax with a 3.5 cm rim of air. The patient was given high-flow oxygen and 600 mL of air was aspirated from the chest. The patient's breathlessness improved, but he still complained of chest pain on deep inspiration. Repeat oxygen saturations were 96% on room air. A repeat chest CXR showed 2.5 cm rim of air.

    What should be the next step in managing this patient?

    A. Continue high-flow oxygen and insert intercostal drain

    B. Continue high-flow oxygen and repeat aspiration of pneumothorax

    C. Prescribe analgesia, allow home with a repeat CXR in seven days

    D. Prescribe analgesia, continue high-flow oxygen, and admit and observe for 24 hours, followed by a repeat CXR

    E. Prescribe analgesia, continue high-flow oxygen for three hours and repeat CXR

227. **A 68-year-old male presented with a four-month history of intermittent pleuritic, left-sided chest discomfort. Over the preceding two weeks he had noticed progressive breathlessness on exertion. There was no history of cough, sputum production, or haemoptysis. He reported a loss of appetite with weight loss of 8 kg over the previous two months. His past medical history included hypertension and rheumatoid arthritis. He had smoked 20 cigarettes per day for nearly 40 years.**

   On examination he was afebrile, respiratory rate was 20 breaths per minute, pulse was 84 beats per minute, and BP was 154/90 mmHg. He had no clubbing and there were no palpable lymph nodes. Jugular venous pressure was not elevated. Auscultation of the lung fields revealed reduced air entry at the left base, and fine inspiratory crackles at the right base. There was bilateral lower limb oedema.

```
Investigations:
    Hb                      122 g/L
    WCC                     12 × 10⁹/L
    Sodium                  138 mmol/L
    Potassium               3.9 mmol/L
    Urea                    11 mmol/L
    Creatinine              142 μmol/L
    AST                     25 iU/L
    ALT                     35 iU/L
    ALP                     90 iU/L
    Bilirubin               13 μmol/L
    Albumin                 24 g/L
    Protein                 50 g/l
    LDH                     300 iU/L
    Glucose                 5.4 mmol/L
    Urinalysis              protein 2+
    ECG                     sinus rhythm, left ventricular
                            hypertrophy
    CXR                     moderate left pleural effusion
Pleural aspirate:
    Protein                 26 g/L
    LDH                     240 iU/L
    Glucose                 3.2 mmol/L
```

   What is the next best investigation?

   A. A 24-hour urine collection for protein
   B. Bronchoscopy
   C. Contrast-enhanced CT scan
   D. Echocardiogram
   E. Serum rheumatoid factor

228. **A 64-year-old man with COPD presented with sudden onset of left-sided pleuritic infrascapular pain. On examination, his respiratory rate was 22 breaths per minute, pulse rate was 110 beats per minute, blood pressure was 145/90 mmHg, and oxygen saturations were 94% on air. Auscultation of the chest revealed no wheeze, but reduced air entry on the left. A CXR confirmed the suspicion of a left pneumothorax with a 2 cm rim of air between the edge of the lung and the ribs.**

What is the best management?

A. Aspiration of the pneumothorax

B. Insertion of intercostal drain

C. Insertion of intercostal drain with suction

D. Prescribe analgesia and allow home with a repeat CXR in seven days

E. Prescribe analgesia and supplemental oxygen and admit for observation

229. **A 68-year-old man presented with a six-month history of worsening breathlessness on exertion. He reported a non-productive cough, general malaise, lethargy, loss of appetite, and a 5 kg weight loss. He had been given multiple courses of antibiotics for both upper and lower respiratory tract infections by his GP to varied response. His past medical history included ischaemic heart disease with percutaneous coronary intervention five years previously, and late onset asthma diagnosed a year previously. He had no smoking history and had previously worked as a shipbuilder for over 20 years.**

On examination he had a temperature of 37.4°C, a respiratory rate of 22 breaths per minute, oxygen saturations of 95% on room air, a pulse of 84 beats per minute, and blood pressure of 150/90 mmHg. Heart sounds were normal and JVP was seen at 5 cm. Auscultation of the chest revealed a diffuse expiratory wheeze. There was also mild pitting oedema to the lower shins.

```
Investigations:
   Hb                       130 g/L
   WCC                      12 × 10⁹/L
   Neutrophils              7.1 × 10⁹/L
   Lymphocytes              2.3 × 10⁹/L
   Eosinophils              1.6 × 10⁹/L
   Sodium                   134 mmol/L
   Potassium                4.2 mmol/L
   Urea                     6.1 mmol/L
   Creatinine               96 µmol/L
   Urinalysis               no blood, nitrites, protein, glucose,
                            or ketones
   ECG                      sinus rhythm, inferior Q waves
   CXR                      normal heart size, pleural plaques,
                            clear lung fields
   FEV₁                     2.2 L (2.5–3.1 L)
   FVC                      4.1 L (3.4–4.3 L)
Partial improvement with beta-agonist challenge.
```

What is the most likely diagnosis?

A. Carcinoma of the lung

B. COPD

C. Congestive cardiac failure

D. Eosinophilic granulomatosis with polyangiitis (EGPA, formerly Churg-Strauss syndrome)

E. Interstitial lung disease

230. **A 82-year-old female was admitted with a three-day history of left-sided chest pain, breathlessness, and a non-productive cough. Her previous medical history included hypertension, hypercholesterolaemia, and osteoarthritis for which she had undergone a right total hip replacement one week previously. She smoked 10–15 cigarettes per day.**

Physical examination revealed a large body habitus, a temperature of 37.1°C, pulse rate of 112 beats per minute, respiratory rate of 30, oxygen saturations of 91% on room air, and blood pressure of 145/ 80 mmHg. Heart sounds were soft but audible with no murmurs. The venous pressure was not elevated. Auscultation of the chest revealed normal breath sounds. There was bilateral pitting ankle oedema. The calves were soft and non-tender.

```
Investigations:
  Hb                  130 g/L
  WCC                 10.2 × 10⁹/L
  Platelets           440 × 10⁹/L
  CRP                 26 mg/L
  Sodium              134 mmol/L
  Potassium           4.2 mmol/L
  Urea                6.1 mmol/L
  Creatinine          143 µmol/L
  Troponin            0.6 µmol/L (<0.14)
  ECG                 sinus tachycardia, LBBB, ST depression,
                      and T-wave changes V1-V4.
  CXR                 cardiomegaly, unfolded aorta, left basal
                      consolidation
  ABG (air)           pH 7.48
  pO2                 8.1 kPa (11.3-12.6)
  pCO2                3.2 kPa (4.7-6.0)
  HCO3-               26 kPa (22-28)
```

What is the most likely diagnosis?

A. Acute cardiac failure

B. Acute coronary syndrome

C. Pericardial effusion

D. Pneumonia

E. Pulmonary embolism

231. **A 42-year-old female was admitted with severe breathlessness following a two-day history of a non-productive cough and breathlessness. She had recently returned from a holiday in Thailand and was a smoker.**

On examination she had a temperature of 37.7°C, pulse rate of 145 beats per minute, respiratory rate of 36 breaths per minute, oxygen saturations of 87% on room air, and blood pressure of 71/44 mmHg. She was drowsy but opened her eyes to voice. The venous pressure was elevated. Heart sounds were normal. The chest was clear to auscultation. She was resuscitated with oxygen and fluids but her blood pressure remained low at 76/48 mmHg.

```
Investigations:
    Hb                      142 g/l
    WCC                     11 × 10⁹/L
    Platelets               440 × 10⁹/L
    CRP                     44 mg/L
    PT                      13 seconds
    APTT                    36 seconds
    ECG                     sinus tachycardia
    CXR                     clear lung fields
    ABG (air)               pH 7.51
    pO2                     7.1
    pCO2                    3.1
    HCO3-                   24
    Echocardiogram          small non-dilated LV with good LV
                            systolic function
Dilated RV with hypokinesis of RV free wall
No thrombus visible in the main pulmonary artery
No pericardial effusion
```

What are the next most important steps in this patient's management?

A. CT pulmonary angiography and then heparin if indicated

B. Escalation to intensive care and administration of noradrenaline

C. Heparin and then urgent CT pulmonary angiography

D. Immediate thrombolysis and then heparin

E. Start ACS protocol and 'blue light' patient for primary percutaneous intervention

232. **A 49-year-old banker presented with breathlessness and increasing confusion. Over the preceding week he had complained of a non-productive cough, fevers, headaches, and profound lethargy. He had returned from a business trip to Italy two weeks previously but was well during his trip. He did not smoke, and had no significant medical history.**

On examination the temperature was 39.1°C, pulse rate was 120 beats per minute, respiratory rate was 36 per minute, oxygen saturations were 89% on room air, and blood pressure was 112/80 mmHg. There were no palpable lymph nodes. Auscultation of the lung fields revealed coarse crepitations in the right axilla. He was disorientated in time and place. Examination of the nervous system revealed mild neck stiffness and with no focal signs.

```
Investigations:
  Hb                      126 g/L
  WCC                     13.4 × 10⁹/L
  Neutrophils             10.7 × 10⁹/L
  Lymphocytes             1.4 × 10⁹/L
  Platelets               240 × 10⁹/L
  CRP                     175 mg/L
  Sodium                  122 mmol/L
  Potassium               4.9 mmol/L
  Urea                    11.4 mmol/L
  Creatinine              162 µmol/L
  ALT                     80 iU/L
  AST                     85 iU/L
  ALP                     110 iU/L
  Bilirubin               27 µmol/L
  Albumin                 25 g/L
  Protein                 48 g/l
  Gamma GT                105 iU/L
  Corrected calcium       1.7 mmol/L
  Phosphate               0.7 mmol/L
  ECG                     sinus tachycardia
  CXR                     right lower lobe consolidation
  ABG (air)               pH 7.41
  pO₂                     8.1
  pCO₂                    3.8
  HCO₃⁻                   20
```

What is the likely diagnosis?

A. Carcinoma of the lung with adrenal metastases

B. Klebsiella pneumonia

C. Legionella pneumonia

D. Mycoplasma pneumonia

E. Streptococcal pneumonia

233. **A 48-year-old Afro-Caribbean male presented with worsening breathlessness on exertion and ongoing productive cough. He was a heavy smoker but had no significant medical history.**

On examination his fingers appeared clubbed, his pulse rate was 80 beats per minute, oxygen saturations were 96% on room air, and blood pressure was 136/72 mmHg. Auscultation of the lung fields revealed coarse crepitations at the left base and diffuse expiratory wheeze.

```
Investigations:
  Hb                      166 g/L
  WCC                     9.5 × 10⁹/L
  Platelets               380 × 10⁹/L
  CRP                     25 mg/L
  Sodium                  132 mmol/L
  Potassium               4.1 mmol/L
  Urea                    6.4 mmol/L
  Creatinine              102 µmol/L
  CXR                     increased bronchovascular markings
  ABG (air)               pH 7.42
  pO₂                     9.8
  pCO₂                    3.8
  HCO₃⁻                   23
  Flow-volume loop:       Figure 11.1
```

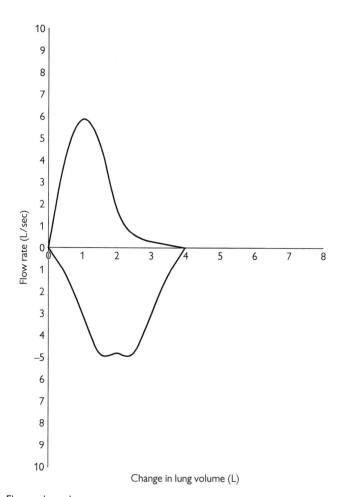

Figure 11.1 Flow-volume loop.

What is the most likely diagnosis?

A. Asthma
B. Bronchiectasis
C. Carcinoma of the lung
D. COPD
E. Interstitial lung disease

234. **A 44-year-old female presented with a productive cough and breathlessness. She had a history of type I diabetes and was under investigation for a lump in her neck. She smoked 5–10 cigarettes per day and had a number of pets, including a budgerigar and a parrot. She was admitted to hospital and after responding well to treatment, was discharged home.**

```
Investigations:
    Hb                          136 g/L
    WCC                         11.5 × 10⁹/L
    Platelets                   380 × 10⁹/L
    CRP                         65 mg/L
    Glucose                     5.8 mmol/L
    TSH                         2.8 mU/L
    CXR                         normal
    Urinlaysis                  protein +
    ABG (air)                   pH 7.42
    pO2                         9.8
    pCO2                        3.8
    HCO3-                       23
Flow-volume loop on admission: Figure 11.2
```

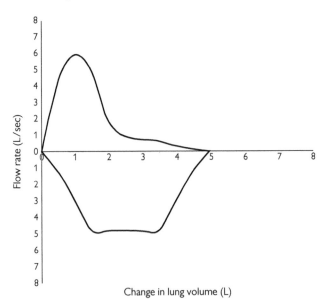

Figure 11.2 Flow-volume loop on admission.

She was seen in the respiratory clinic four months later still complaining of mild breathlessness. In addition, she complained of persistent diplopia. She was otherwise active and reported no other neurological symptoms. On examination her pulse rate was 72 beats per minute, oxygen saturations were 98% on room air, and blood pressure was 119/70 mmHg. She was noted to have a diffuse thyroid swelling with

no associated lymphadenopathy. **The chest was clear to auscultation. There was no dysphonia or dysarthria. There was obvious strabismus with diplopia in all directions of gaze. The remainder of the neurological examination was unremarkable. Repeat spirometry was performed.**

Flow-volume loop in clinic: Figure 11.3

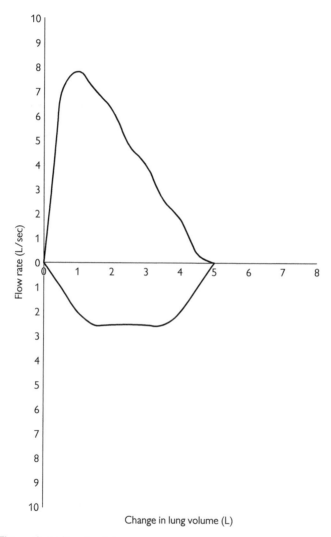

Figure 11.3 Flow-volume loop in clinic.

What was the most likely diagnosis at her initial presentation?

A. Carcinoma of the lung

B. Exacerbation of asthma

C. Exacerbation of COPD

D. Extrinsic allergic alveolitis

E. Interstitial lung disease

What is the cause of her shortness of breath in clinic?

A. Botulism
B. Carcinoma of the lung
C. Graves' disease
D. Multiple endocrine neoplasia type II
E. Myasthenia gravis

235. **A 67-year-old female presented with fever, cough, and breathlessness. She had no significant past medical history. On examination her temperature was 38.1°C, pulse rate was 90 beats per minute, respiratory rate was 24 per minute, oxygen saturations were 96% on room air, and blood pressure was 132/80 mmHg. She was able to speak in full sentences. There were no palpable lymph nodes. Auscultation of the lung fields revealed coarse crepitations at the right base.**

```
Investigations:
   Hb                        126 g/L
   WCC                       14.5 × 10⁹/L
   Neutrophils               10.7 × 10⁹/L
   Platelets                 440 × 10⁹/L
   CRP                       105 mg/L
   Sodium                    132 mmol/L
   Potassium                 4.1 mmol/L
   Urea                      6.4 mmol/L
   Creatinine                112 µmol/L
   ALT                       31 iU/L
   AST                       26 iU/L
   ALP                       72 iU/L
   Bilirubin                 8 µmol/L
   Albumin                   25 g/L
   Protein                   46 g/l
   ECG                       sinus rhythm
   CXR                       left basal consolidation
```

What is the best management?

A. Inpatient treatment intravenous co-amoxiclav
B. Inpatient treatment intravenous amoxicillin and oral clarithromycin
C. Outpatient patient treatment with oral amoxicillin
D. Outpatient treatment with oral amoxicillin and oral clarithromycin
E. Outpatient treatment with oral co-amoxiclav

236. **A 62-year-old farmer presented with progressive breathlessness over the preceding six months accompanied with 5 kg weight loss. He also reported a cough preceding this by many years, typically worse in the evenings and occasional fevers and flu-like symptoms. He denied chest pain. His past medical history included a myocardial infarction five years previously, resulting in coronary artery bypass surgery, and a subsequent admission to hospital two years later with left ventricular failure requiring percutaneous coronary revascularization and optimization of diuretics therapy. He had a 40 pack-year smoking history.**

Physical examination revealed a temperature of 37.1°C, pulse rate of 120 beats per minute, respiratory rate of 28 breaths per minute, oxygen saturations of 88% on room air and blood pressure of 162/80 mmHg. Jugular venous pressure was elevated. Heart sounds revealed no murmurs, but a prominent second heart sound was noted. Inspiratory crackles were heard bilaterally. There was mild peripheral oedema.

```
Investigations:
   Hb                  110 g/L
   WCC                 7 × 10⁹/L
   CRP                 35 mg/L
   ESR                 47 mm/h
   ECG                 sinus tachycardia; anterior Q waves
   CXR                 cardiomegaly; reticulonodular shadowing
                       in mid-zones
   ABG (air)           pH 7.47
   pO2                 7.1
   pCO2                3.2
   HCO3-               23
   Spirometry          FEV1 2.0
   FVC                 2.1
   TLC                 3.2
   KCO                 60%
```

What is the diagnosis?

A. Decompensated congestive cardiac failure

B. Exacerbation of chronic obstructive pulmonary disease

C. Hypersensitivity pneumonitis

D. Organic dust toxic syndrome

E. Pneumoconiosis

237. A 41-year-old taxi driver presented with a five-day history of headaches, fever, sore throat, cough, and breathlessness. He smoked, and drank 20–30 units of alcohol per week. There was no other significant medical history.

On examination he had a temperature of 38.9°C, pulse rate of 124 beats per minute, respiratory rate of 28 breaths per minute, oxygen saturations of 92% on room air, and a blood pressure was 132/82 mmHg. There were no palpable lymph nodes. Examination of the ears, nose, and throat revealed oropharyngeal inflammation without exudates and erythematous tympanic membranes. Maculopapular lesions resembling rings were noted on the arms. Heart sounds were normal with a pericardial rub. The venous pressure was not elevated. Auscultation of the lung fields revealed coarse crepitations in the right axilla. Abdominal examination was unremarkable. Examination of the nervous system revealed mild neck stiffness with no focal signs.

```
Investigations:
  Hb                        98 g/L
  WCC                       10.1 × 10⁹/L
  Platelets                 140 × 10⁹/L
  CRP                       123 mg/L
  Blood film                red cell agglutination and
                            thrombocytopenia
  Sodium                    130 mmol/L
  Potassium                 4.2 mmol/L
  Urea                      6.4 mmol/L
  Creatinine                112 µmol/L
  ALT                       91 iU/L
  AST                       65 iU/L
  ALP                       101 iU/L
  Bilirubin                 21 µmol/L
  Albumin                   23 g/L
  Protein                   44 g/l
  Troponin                  <0.3
  ECG                       sinus tachycardia; anterolateral
                            T wave inversion
  CXR                       right middle lobe consolidation
  Echocardiogram            good biventricular function
Normal valves
Small rim of pericardial fluid (<0.5 cm)
```

What is the best treatment?

A. Amoxicillin

B. Clarithromycin

C. Co-amoxiclav

D. Doxycycline

E. Erythromycin

238. A 30-year-old female presented with progressive shortness of breath and fatigue. She reported struggling to walk even 150 m on the flat and had not been able to work or visit the gym over the previous four months. She had been diagnosed with asthma and used salbutamol and beclomethasone inhalers to some benefit. She also had a diagnosis of bulimia. She smoked occasionally but did not drink alcohol. She kept a budgerigar as a pet.

Examination revealed a pulse rate of 104 beats per minute, respiratory rate of 22 breaths per minute, oxygen saturations of 94% on room air, and BP of 102/74 mmHg. Auscultation of the heart sounds were normal. The JVP was 3 cm above the sternal notch with a double waveform. Chest expansion was symmetrical but reduced, with a resonant percussion note throughout. On auscultation there was reduced air entry throughout, with a mild expiratory wheeze. Abdominal examination revealed a palpable liver edge 3 cm below the costal margin. There was no splenomegaly and no clinical evidence of ascites. There was pitting oedema up to her shins.

```
Investigations:
   Hb                        170 g/L
   WCC                       10 × 10⁹/L
   Platelets                 140 × 10⁹/L
   Sodium                    134 mmol/L
   Potassium                 3.5 mmol/L
   Urea                      2.8 mmol/L
   Creatinine                60 µmol/L
   AST                       55 iU/L
   ALT                       85 iU/L
   ALP                       530 iU/L
   Bilirubin                 36 µmol/L
   Albumin                   24 g/L
   Protein                   52 g/l
   Urinalysis                protein +
   ECG                       sinus tachcyadia
   CXR                       normal heart size; hyperlucent and
                             oligaemic lung fields
   FEV₁                      1.9 L (predicted 3.9 L)
   FVC                       3.8 L (predicted 5.1 L)
   TLC                       6.9 L (predicted 5.2 L)
   KCO                       0.6 mmol/L/kPa (predicted
                             1.4 mmol/L/kPa)
   ABG (air)                 pH 7.39
   pO₂                       9.1
   pCO₂                      5.7
   HCO₃⁻                     29
```

Which test will confirm the diagnosis?

A. A 24-hour urine collection for protein

B. Avian precipitins

C. Liver biopsy

D. Right and left heart catheter

E. Serum α-1 antitrypsin

239. **A 42-year-old male was referred to the respiratory outpatient clinic. He had a six-month history of progressive breathlessness on exertion. He had a past medical history of hereditary haemorrhagic telangiectasia, complicated by recurrent epistaxis treated successfully by nasal cauterization four years previously. He took no regular medications but smoked 5–10 cigarettes per day and drank 20–30 units of alcohol a week.**

On examination there were multiple telangiectasia visible around the mouth, tongue, and buccal mucosa. The pulse rate was 74 beats per minute, respiratory rate was 18 breaths per minute, oxygen saturations were 99% on room air, and BP was 112/80 mmHg. The venous pressure was normal. Auscultation of chest revealed reduced air entry at the right base, but was otherwise clear to auscultation. The following results are available.

```
Investigations:
   CXR                  normal heart size; clear lung fields
   ECG                  sinus rhythm
   ABG (air)            pH 7.39
   pO2                  14.1
   pCO2                 4.1
   HCO3-                23
   Spirometry           FEV₁ 4.1 L (predicted 4.5 L)
   FVC                  5.1 L (predicted 5.8 L)
   TLC                  4.9 L (predicted 5.2 L)
   KCO                  0.9 mmol/L/kPa (predicted 1.4 mmol/L/kPa)
```

Which is the next best investigation?

A. Contrast-enhanced CT chest

B. Echocardiogram

C. Full blood count

D. Liver function tests

E. Serum α-1 antitrypsin levels

240. A 35-year-old Caucasian male was admitted to hospital with lethargy, dry cough, and breathlessness. He denied chest pain or haemoptysis but had lost 6 kg in weight over four months. Eight months previously he had been admitted to hospital with fevers, joint aches, headaches, painful rash on his shins, and a cough following return from a caving expedition in Greece. He was diagnosed with pneumonia and treated with antibiotics. He reported still being troubled by a dry cough and intermittent fevers for which he had tried further courses of antibiotics. He worked as a labourer at a large plastics factory making polyurethane foam and rubber. He had a 15 pack-year smoking history but did not drink alcohol.

On examination his temperature was 37.6°C, the pulse rate was 84 beats per minute, respiratory rate was 18 breaths per minute, and oxygen saturations were 99% on room air, with a blood pressure of 132/84 mmHg. The venous pressure was normal. Auscultation of chest revealed reduced air entry at the left base. Abdominal examination revealed a palpable liver edge 2 cm below the costal margin.

```
Investigations:
   Hb                        90 g/L
   WCC                       3.5 × 10⁹/L
   Platelets                 140 × 10⁹/L
   CRP                       85 mg/L
   Sodium                    132 mmol/L
   Potassium                 4.5 mmol/L
   Urea                      9.4 mmol/L
   Creatinine                102 µmol/L
   AST                       35 iU/L
   ALT                       25 iU/L
   ALP                       135 iU/L
   Bilirubin                 11 µmol/L
   Albumin                   32 g/L
   Protein                   68 g/l
   PT                        13 s
   APTT                      30 s
   Corrected calcium         2.7 mmol/L
   Phosphate                 1.1 mmoml/L
   Serum ACE                 60 U/L (normal range 0–20 U/L)
   ECG                       sinus rhythm
   CXR                       prominent left hilar lymph nodes;
                             well circumscribed 2 cm non-calcified
                             nodule in left lower lobe
```

```
ABG (air)              pH 7.36
pO₂                    10.1
pCO₂                   4.1
HCO₃⁻                  23
Spirometry
FEV₁                   4.2 L (predicted 4.4 L)
FVC                    5.3 L (predicted 6.0 L)
TLC                    5.9 L (predicted 6.2 L)
KCO                    1.2 mmol/L/kPa (predicted 1.4 mmol/
                       L/kPa)

Blood cultures         negative
Tuberculin test        negative
```

Which is the diagnosis?

A. Carcinoma of the lung
B. Chemical worker's lung
C. Coccidioidomycosis
D. Histoplasmosis
E. Sarcoidosis

241. A 32-year-old female smoker presented with a persistent non-productive cough, joint pains, and breathlessness over the preceding year. Over the previous six months she complained of weight loss and increasing thirst and urinary frequency. Whilst on holiday in the Pyrenees three months before, she had been admitted to hospital with sudden onset sharp right-sided chest pain. She was diagnosed with a pneumothorax and required intercostal drain insertion. She worked at a local garage as a spray-painter and was on the combined oral contraceptive pill.

On examination her temperature was 37.6°C, the pulse rate was 84 beats per minute, respiratory rate was 20 breaths per minute, oxygen saturations were 97% on room air, and blood pressure was 112/70 mmHg. Auscultation of chest revealed normal breath sounds.

```
Investigations:
  Hb                     110 g/L
  WCC                    6 × 10⁹/L
  Platelets              180 × 10⁹/L
  Sodium                 132 mmol/L
  Potassium              4.1 mmol/L
  Urea                   6.4 mmol/L
  Creatinine             112 µmol/L
  AST                    35 iU/L
  ALT                    25 iU/L
  ALP                    165 iU/L
  Bilirubin              11 µmol/L
  Albumin                31 g/L
  Corrected calcium      2.7 mmol/L
  Glucose                5.7 mmol/L
  Serum ACE              50 U/L (normal range 0–20U/L)
  CXR                    no hilar lymphadenopathy; bilateral
                         reticulonodular infiltrates in the
                         upper and midzones
  Spirometry             FEV₁ 2.4 L (predicted 4.4 L)
  FVC                    4.2L (predicted 5.8 L)
  TLC                    5.0 L (predicted 6.5 L)
  KCO                    1.8 mmol/L/kPa (predicted
3.2 mmol/L/kPa)
```

What is the most likely diagnosis?

A. Histiocytosis X
B. Hypersensitivity pneumonitis
C. Lymphangioleiomyomatosis
D. Occupational asthma
E. Sarcoidosis

242. **A 58-year-old smoker presented with a productive cough, wheeze, and breathlessness. He had recently been diagnosed with type II diabetes and initiated on metformin 500 mg tds. Given his smoking history and hype-inflated lungs on CXR, an underlying diagnosis of COPD was suspected and he was treated for an exacerbation.**

He responded well to titrated oxygen, nebulizer therapy, oral corticosteroids, and oral antibiotics. After 48 hours he was off oxygen supplementation and switched to inhalers and felt near his baseline. A repeat arterial blood gas was performed prior to discharge.

```
Investigations:
Repeat arterial blood gas
    pH                      7.2
    pO2                     9.6
    pCO2                    5.4
    HCO3-                   27
    BE                      -1.5
    Sodium                  135
    Potassium               4.1
    Urea                    8.1
    Creatinine              112
    Chloride                102
    Glucose                 13.1 mmol/L
```

Which is the next step?

A. Increase steroid dose
B. Initiate non-invasive ventilation
C. Repeat arterial blood gas
D. Re-instate nebulizers
E. Stop metformin

243. **A 72-year-old male with COPD presented with a productive cough, breathlessness, and wheeze having already started on oral amoxicillin and oral steroids three days earlier. Despite using inhalers regularly, his breathing had progressively deteriorated and he had become confused. He was brought to A&E by paramedics having been found hypoxic and being stabilized with nebulizers and high-flow oxygen.**

On examination he was confused (GCS = 13, E3V4M6), his temperature was 37.9°C, pulse rate was 122 beats per minute, respiratory rate was 24 per minute and oxygen saturations were 96% on oxygen, and blood pressure was 155/70 mmHg. Auscultation of chest revealed poor air entry with diffuse expiratory wheeze. Neurological examination was otherwise normal, with no lateralizing signs.

```
Investigations:
  ABG (room air)        pH 7.26
  pO₂                   12.1
  pCO₂                  12.8
  HCO₃⁻                 30
  BE                    +5.1
```

What is the most appropriate management?

A. Commence non-invasive ventilation

B. Continue nebulizers and start intravenous aminophylline infusion

C. Replace oxygen with 24% venturi mask

D. Replace oxygen with 4 L Hudson mask

E. Urgent anaesthetic opinion and intubation

244. **A 62-year-old female was seen in the respiratory outpatient clinic. She reported a two-year history of progressive breathlessness and frequent daily productive cough with white sputum. Her exercise tolerance had reduced from being unrestricted to 200 metres whilst walking on the flat. She reported no weight loss or haemoptysis. She had recently been started on a salbutamol inhaler with some therapeutic effect. She had a 40 pack-year smoking history but had given up six months previously.**

On examination her pulse rate was 92 beats per minute, respiratory rate was 18 per minute, oxygen saturations were 94% on room air, and blood pressure was 125/70 mmHg. The JVP was not elevated. Auscultation of the chest revealed poor air entry with expiratory wheeze.

```
Investigations:
   CXR                        hyperinflated lung fields
Spirometry
   FEV1                       1.5 L (48% predicted)
   FVC                        2.9 L (80% predicted)
ABG (room air) pH 7.41
   pO₂                        9.1
   pCO₂                       4.1
   HCO₃⁻                      25
```

What is the most appropriate management?

A. A long-acting β_2-agonist inhaler

B. A long-acting β_2-agonist inhaler and a long-acting muscarinic antagonist inhaler

C. A long-acting muscarinic antagonist inhaler

D. A long-acting muscarinic antagonist inhaler and inhaled corticosteroid

E. An inhaled corticosteroid

245. **A 58-year-old male presented with a swollen right calf. There was no history of chest pain or breathlessness. His past medical history included chronic myeloid leukaemia, for which he was on hydroxyurea and imatinib mesylate. He was a non-smoker.**

On examination he was a afebrile, his pulse rate was 72 beats per minute, respiratory rate was 16 breaths per minute, oxygen saturations were 99% on room air, and blood pressure was 135/75 mmHg. Auscultation of heart and chest was normal. The right calf was swollen and tender.

```
Investigations:
  Hb                      100 g/L
  WCC                     107 × 10⁹/L
  Platelets               840 × 10⁹/L
  CRP                     35 mg/L
  Sodium                  135
  Potassium               4.1
  Urea                    8.1
  Creatinine              112
  CXR                     normal heart size; clear lung fields
  ECG                     sinus rhythm; RBBB; normal axis
  ABG (room air)          pH 7.39
  pO₂                     7.1
  pCO₂                    4.8
  HCO₃⁻                   24
  BE                      -0.5
  Doppler USS             right calf DVT
  VQ scan                 low probability for PE
```

What is the most likely cause of the low pO_2?

A. Atrial septal defect
B. Methaemoglobinaemia
C. Pulmonary embolism
D. Pulmonary leucostasis
E. Spurious hypoxaemia

246. **A 74-year-old male presented with a productive cough, breathlessness, and confusion. He had a 60 pack-year smoking history and been given a salbutamol inhaler by his GP many years previously. Over the preceding week he had become progressively breathless despite using his inhaler and a short course of steroids and antibiotics.**

On examination his temperature was 38.1°C, GCS was 11(E3V3M5), pulse rate was 124 beats per minute, respiratory rate was 24 per minute, oxygen saturations were 84% on room air, and blood pressure was 91/50 mmHg. He was peripherally cyanosed. The JVP was not elevated. Auscultation of the chest revealed poor air entry and diffuse marked expiratory wheeze.

```
Investigations:
   Hb                          166 g/L
   WCC                         13.5 × 10⁹/L
   Platelets                   480 × 10⁹/L
   CRP                         225 mg/L
   Sodium                      133 mmol/L
   Potassium                   4.1 mmol/L
   Urea                        9.4 mmol/L
   Creatinine                  132 µmol/L
   ECG                         sinus tachycardia; RBBB
   CXR                         hyperinflated lung fields
ABG (room air) pH 7.22
   pO₂                         5.1
   pCO₂                        12.1
   HCO₃⁻                       32
   BE                          +6
```

What is the most appropriate management?

A. 24% oxygen (venturi mask); nebulizers; and steroids

B. 24% oxygen (venturi mask); nebulizers; intravenous aminophylline; and steroids

C. High-flow oxygen; nebulizers; intravenous co-amoxiclav; and steroids

D. Nebulizers; steroids; and non-invasive ventilation

E. Urgent anaesthetic review and ventilation

247. **A 55-year-old cattle and sheep farmer present with fever, headache, dry cough, and breathlessness. He had started to notice these symptoms intermittently over the previous six months. On a typical day, his symptoms would begin in the late afternoon as he would finish his work, and persist until late in the evening. However, over the last month he had started to note that these symptoms had become persistent. He was fond of pets and he kept three dogs and two budgerigars. He did not smoke.**

On examination his temperature was 38.1°C, pulse rate was 104 beats per minute, respiratory rate was 24 per minute, oxygen saturations were 89% on room air, and blood pressure was 121/80 mmHg. Auscultation of chest revealed poor air entry and bronchial breathing at the left base. Cardiovascular and abdominal examination was unremarkable.

```
Investigations:
    Hb                        156 g/L
    WCC                       13.5 × 10⁹/L
    Platelets                 450 × 10⁹/L
    CRP                       115 mg/L
    Sodium                    137 mmol/L
    Potassium                 3.9 mmol/L
    Urea                      8.4 mmol/L
    Creatinine                122 µmol/L
    AST                       55 iU/L
    ALT                       60 iU/L
    ALP                       132 iU/L
    Bilirubin                 13 µmol/L
    Albumin                   22 g/L
    Protein                   48 g/l
    ECG                       sinus tachycardia
    CXR                       indistinct left hemidiaphragm;
                              normal heart size
ABG (room air) pH 7.46
    pO₂                       8.8
    pCO₂                      3.2
    HCO₃⁻                     24
    BE                        -0.5
    Avian precipitins         positive
    Micopolyspora faenia precipitins positive
```

What is the most likely cause for this presentation?

A. Avian influenza
B. Bird fancier's lung
C. Farmer's lung
D. Psittacosis
E. Q fever

248. **A 46-year-old male presented with a week-long history of a productive cough, fever, and breathlessness. This had been preceded by two weeks of fevers, myalgias, sore throat, and coryzal symptoms. He had no other significant medical history and had previously been fit and well. He worked as a journalist and travelled worldwide frequently. He lived alone, was an occasional smoker, and drank 10–15 units of alcohol per week. He denied any loss of appetite or weight loss.**

On examination his temperature was 38.3°C, pulse rate was 102 beats per minute, respiratory rate was 24 breaths per minute, oxygen saturations were 97% on room air, and blood pressure was 103/80 mmHg. There were no palpable lymph nodes. Examination of the chest revealed bronchial breathing in the left lower zone.

```
Investigations:
  Hb                     136 g/L
  WCC                    18.5 × 10⁹/L
  Neutrophils            14.7 × 10⁹/L
  Lymphocytes            0.7 × 10⁹/L
  Platelets              110 × 10⁹/L
  CRP                    221 mg/L
  ECG                    sinus tachycardia
  CXR                    left-sided lower zone cavitating
                         lung lesion
```

What is the most likely cause of his lung pathology?

A. Aspergilloma

B. *Klebsiella pneumoniae*

C. Lobar adenocarcinoma

D. *Mycobacterium tuberculosis*

E. *Staphylococcus aureus*

249. **A 71-year-old female with a long-standing history of rheumatoid arthritis was admitted to hospital with a fractured neck of femur. She was a non-smoker. Two days following her right hip replacement she became acutely breathless and confused. There was no cough, sputum, or haemoptysis.**

On examination she was confused (GCS = 13, E3V4M6), her temperature was 38.1°C, pulse rate was 122 beats per minute, respiratory rate was 24 breaths per minute, oxygen saturations were 92% on room air, and her blood pressure was 111/80 mmHg. The venous pressure was not elevated. Auscultation of the chest revealed decreased air entry bibasally. A petechial rash was noted over her arms and trunk.

```
Investigations:
  Hb                         96 g/L
  WCC                        9.5 × 10⁹/L
  Platelets                  90 × 10⁹/L
  CRP                        105 mg/L
  Sodium                     132 mmol/L
  Potassium                  4.9 mmol/L
  Urea                       9.4 mmol/L
  Creatinine                 142 µmol/L
  PT                         15 s
  APTT                       33 s
  Fibrinogen                 1.1 g/L
  ECG                        sinus tachycardia
  CXR                        bilateral diffuse perihilar
                             infiltrates

ABG (room air) pH 7.45
  pO₂                        8.9
  pCO₂                       3.5
  HCO₃⁻                      22
```

What is the most likely diagnosis?

A. Disseminated intravascular coagulation

B. Fat embolism

C. Post-operative pneumonia

D. Pulmonary embolism

E. Thrombotic thrombocytopenic purpura

250. **A 71-year-old male with a long-standing history of COPD was reviewed in the respiratory clinic. Over the preceding year he reported progressive breathlessness with a significant reduction in exercise tolerance. He also had had three hospitals admissions for infective exacerbations. He reported a chronic cough and progressive ankle swelling but no increased sputum production, chest pain, or orthopnoea. He had stopped smoking five years previously.**

His medications include Ventolin, Seretide and serevent inhalers, uniphyllin and furosemide. On examination he was apyrexial, pulse rate 94 beats per minute, respiratory rate 18 per minute, oxygen saturations 91% on room air, and blood pressure 151/80 mmHg. He was peripherally and centrally cyanosed. The JVP was elevated and he had a loud second heart sound. Auscultation of chest revealed poor air entry and mild expiratory wheeze. A smooth liver edge was palpable 1 cm below the costal margin with pitting ankle oedema up to the shins.

```
Investigations:
    Hb                      186 g/L
    WCC                     5.5 × 10⁹/L
    Platelets               480 × 10⁹/L
    CRP                     5 mg/L
    Sodium                  137 mmol/L
    Potassium               3.9 mmol/L
    Urea                    8.4 mmol/L
    Creatinine              132 µmol/L
    ECG                     sinus rhythm; RBBB
    CXR                     hyperinflated and hyperlucent
                            lung fields; increased pulmonary
                            vasculature at the hilar; normal
                            heart size

ABG (room air) pH 7.47
    pO₂                     7.8
    pCO₂                    6.7
    HCO₃⁻                   29
    BE                      +6
    Spirometry
    FEV1                    1.3 (30% predicted)
    FVC                     2.4 (70% predicted)
```

What is the most appropriate management?

A. Initiate carbocisteine

B. Initiate inhaled corticosteroid therapy

C. Initiate long-term oxygen therapy

D. Initiate low dose corticosteroid therapy

E. Initiate spironolactone

251. **A 68-year-old male of Pakistani origin presented with a six-month history of productive cough, haemoptysis, weight loss, and ankle swelling. He had no other past medical history. He was a poultry farmer and had a 40 pack-year smoking.**

On examination, the pulse rate was 84 beats per minute, respiratory rate 22 breaths per minute, oxygen saturations 95% on room air, and blood pressure 141/90 mmHg. His fingers were clubbed. Auscultation of chest revealed coarse crepitations in the left upper zone with mild expiratory wheeze. Abdominal examination was unremarkable. There was pitting oedema of the lower limbs extending up to knees.

```
Investigations:
    Hb                      126 g/L
    WCC                     5.5 × 10⁹/L
    Platelets               390 × 10⁹/L
    CRP                     15 mg/L
    Sodium                  137 mmol/L
    Potassium               3.9 mmol/L
    Urea                    8.4 mmol/L
    Creatinine              132 µmol/L
    AST                     45 iU/L
    ALT                     40 iU/L
    ALP                     82 iU/L
    Bilirubin               13 µmol/L
    Albumin                 21 g/L
    Protein                 38 g/l
    Corrected calcium       2.5 mmol/L
    Phosphate               0.8 mmol/L
    Urinalysis              protein 3+
    Mantoux test            positive
```

What is the most likely diagnosis?

A. Bronchiectasis

B. Extrinsic allergic alveolitis

C. Interstitial lung disease

D. Lung malignancy

E. Pulmonary tuberculosis

252. **A 35-year-old female presented with worsening cough, breathlessness, and wheeze. She had long-standing asthma with Ventolin and Becotide inhalers. Her symptoms had begun a few days prior, and she had been trialled on a course of antibiotics and oral steroids for an infective exacerbation of asthma. She was a non-smoker. On examination she was afebrile, her pulse rate was 130 per min, her respiratory rate was 28 breaths per minutes, oxygen saturations were 85% on room air, and her blood pressure was 110/65 mmHg. Auscultation of the lung fields reveals diffuse expiratory wheeze.**

    She was treated with high-flow oxygen (15 L) via a re-breather bag, salbutamol, and Atrovent® nebulizers, and intravenous hydrocortisone. CXR demonstrated clear lung fields with no evidence of pneumothorax.

    ```
    An arterial blood gas analysis:
       pH                    7.31
       pO₂                   13.9
       pCO₂                  6.8
       HCO₃⁻                 23
    ```

    What is the most appropriate management?

    A. Intravenous aminophylline
    B. Intravenous magnesium sulphate
    C. Intubation and ventilation
    D. Non-invasive ventilation
    E. Reduce oxygen to 24% via venture mask and repeat arterial blood gas

253. **A 45-year-old male presented with a two-day history of fever, frank haemoptysis, and breathlessness, preceded by a two-week history of fatigue, dry cough, and headaches. His only past medical history was of longstanding rhinitis. He worked as a zookeeper at a wildlife park which required handling of birds and had recently returned from a three-week visit to a large wildlife park in Croatia. He was a non-smoker.**

On examination he was afebrile, his pulse rate was 110 beats per min, respiratory rate was 24 breaths per minute, oxygen saturations were 90% on room air, and blood pressure was 120/65 mmHg. There was no clubbing or lymphadenopathy. The venous pressures was decreased and seen at 2 cm. Heart sounds were normal. Auscultation of the lung fields revealed diffuse bilateral crepitations. Abdominal examination was unremarkable.

```
Investigations:
  Hb                    77 g/L
  WCC                   14 × 10⁹/L
  Platelets             240 × 10⁹/L
  CRP                   285 mg/L
  Sodium                133 mmol/L
  Potassium             5.5 mmol/L
  Urea                  18.4 mmol/L
  Creatinine            322 µmol/L
  Urinalysis            blood +++ protein++
  ECG                   sinus tachycardia
  ABG (air)             pH 7.35
  pO2                   8.1
  pCO2                  3.1
  HCO3-                 18
  BE                    -6.7
  CXR                   Figure 11.4
```

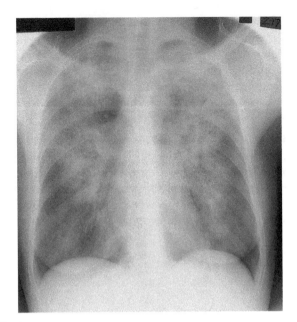

Figure 11.4 CXR of patient.

Reproduced with permission from, *Oxford Textbook of Medicine*, Fifth Edition, edited by Warrell D, Cox T, Firth J, Fig. 18.14.1.1, p. 3426, Oxford University Press, Oxford, UK, Copyright © 2010.

What is the most likely diagnosis?

A. Acute histoplasmosis

B. Acute hypersensitivity pneumonitis

C. Goodpasture's syndrome

D. Granulomatosis with polyangiitis (GPA, formerly Wegner's granulomatosis)

E. Legionella pneumonia

254. **A 58-year-old Indian male presented with a two-month history of fever, cough, weight loss, and dizziness. He had a previous history of tuberculosis (TB), diagnosed four years previously and received treatment for six months. He had a long-standing history of renal stones and asthma. He had worked in the shipbuilding industry his entire life. He was a smoker and drank ten units of alcohol per week.**

On examination he was apyrexial, pulse rate was 100 per minute, oxygen saturations were 95% on oxygen, respiratory rate was 20, and blood pressure was 105/85 mmHg but dropped to 88/71 mmHg on standing. There was no evidence of finger clubbing. Auscultation of the lung fields reveals reduced air entry and crackles at the left apex.

```
Investigations:
   Hb                          110 g/L
   WCC                         10 × 10⁹/L
   Neutrophils                 7.2 × 10⁹/L
   Eosinophils                 0.7 × 10⁹/L
   Lymphocytes                 2.0 × 10⁹/L
   Platelets                   240 × 10⁹/L
   CRP                         115 mg/L
   Sodium                      128 mmol/L
   Potassium                   5.1 mmol/L
   Urea                        6.4 mmol/L
   Creatinine                  112 µmol/L
   CXR                         cavitating lesion at the left
                               upper zone
   Urinalysis                  blood ++ protein +
Precipitins for A. fumigatus positive
```

What is the most likely diagnosis?

A. Aspergilloma

B. Granulomatosis polyangiitis (GPA, formerly Churg-Strauss syndrome)

C. Lung malignancy

D. Re-activation of tuberculosis

E. *Staphylococcus aureus* pneumonia

255. **A 27-year-old female with a past medical history of asthma was seen in the respiratory clinic. Her mediation included a PRN salbutamol inhaler, low-dose inhaled steroid inhaler twice daily, and a recently started regular salmeterol inhaler. Over the preceding three months she had required her salbutamol inhaler every 2–4 hours. She reported an ongoing dry cough and a reduction in exercise tolerance affecting her work as a shop floor assistant. She was a non-smoker and had kept a pet dog for the preceding five years.**

On examination she was afebrile, her pulse rate was 80 breaths per min, oxygen saturations were 97% on room air, respiratory rate was 22 breaths per minute, and blood pressure was 120/65 mmHg. Auscultation of the lung fields revealed mild diffuse expiratory wheeze.

```
Arterial blood gas:
   pH                      7.41
   pO₂                     11.9
   pCO₂                    4.8
   HCO₃⁻                   25
```

What is the most appropriate management?

A. Add leukotriene receptor antagonist
B. Replace low-dose with high-dose inhaled steroid therapy
C. Stop salmeterol and add aminophylline
D. Stop salmeterol and add leukotriene receptor antagonist
E. Stop salmeterol and replace low-dose with high-dose inhaled steroid therapy

226. A) Continue high-flow oxygen and insert intercostal drain

This man, with no significant cardiorespiratory history, presents with a spontaneous primary pneumothorax, and has failed aspiration. This question tests the candidate's knowledge of the current British Thoracic Society (BTS) guidelines on the management of spontaneous primary pneumothoraces. If a patient has a pneumothorax with >2 cm of air, or has symptoms (pain and dyspnoea on minimal exertion), then aspiration is recommended. If this is successful, then the patient can be discharged with a repeat CXR in one week. If this is unsuccessful, insertion of an intercostal drain is recommended.

In the 2003 BTS guidelines, a repeat aspiration was recommended but this suggestion has been changed in the 2010 guidelines. A repeat aspiration should only be attempted if there is technical difficulty during the first attempt. Although analgesia and high-flow oxygen are important in the management of pneumothoraces, they are not the most appropriate next step without intercostal drainage.

Tutorial

Primary pneumothoraces occur in the absence of underlying respiratory disease. The reported incidence is 18–28/100,000 per year for males and 1.2–6/100,000 per year in females. They result from rupture of apical pleural blebs under the visceral pleura. They are typically observed in tall young individuals (often males) without underlying respiratory disease and 90% of patients are smokers. Smoking increases the risk of first spontaneous pneumothorax by 20-fold in men and 10-fold in women. The increased risk of pneumothorax and recurrence is approximately proportional to the number of cigarettes smoked. Recurrence of pneumothorax is common (15–40%) and up to 15% of recurrences can be on the contralateral side.

The BTS (2010) provide comprehensive guidance on management of primary pneumothoraces. If the patient is asymptomatic and the rim of air <2 cm, then the patients may be allowed home with a repeat CXR in 7–10 days. They should be given clear verbal and written advice to return if they develop breathlessness. The rate of resolution/reabsorption of a spontaneous primary pneumothorax is by slow absorption of air from the pleural cavity, and the rate of absorption is 1.22–1.8% of the volume of hemithorax every 24 hours. Intercostal drains are only used if aspiration is unsuccessful. There is no evidence that large tubes (20–24 F) are better than small tubes (10–14 F) in the management of pneumothoraces and thus standard practice is insertion of the latter using a guidewire system (Seldinger technique). However, a smaller tube may need to be replaced with a larger one if there is suspicion of a persistent air leak. Chest drain suctioning should not be applied directly after intercostal tube insertion due to increased risk of re-expansion pulmonary oedema. It can be added after 48 hours for persistent air leak or failure of a pneumothorax to expand. In the initial setting, high-volume and low-pressure systems are recommended (-10---20 cm H_2O). A suggested treatment algorithm can be found in Figure 11.5.

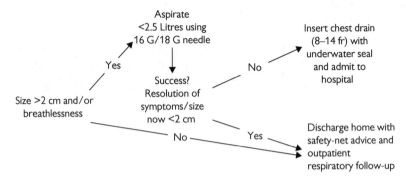

Figure 11.5 Suggested treatment algorithm for a primary pneumothorax.

NB: this is not applicable for secondary pneumothoraces, a suggested treatment algorithm for which can be found in Figure 11.6.

Further Reading

Macduff A, Arnold A, Harvey J (on behalf of BTS Pleural Disease Group) (2010). Management of spontaneous pneumothorax: British Thoracic Society pleural disease guideline 2010. *Thorax* 65 (2): ii18–ii31.

227. C) Contrast-enhanced CT scan

This patient with a heavy smoking history presents with weight loss, loss of appetite, and a left-sided pleural effusion. This history itself should lead one to suspect an underlying malignancy. There are many confounding factors in the history suggesting alternate diagnoses, besides malignancy, as causes for the pleural effusion. The presence of proteinuria, hypoalbuminaemia, and oedema may suggest nephrotic syndrome. A history of rheumatoid arthritis may suggest a diagnosis of a rheumatoid pleural effusion. The pleural fluid protein concentration is <30 g/L, suggesting a transudate, but it is important to interpret pleural fluid protein concentrations in the context of serum protein concentrations. Analysing the pleural aspirate results using the Light's criteria reveals an exudate, thus dismissing the diagnosis of nephrotic syndrome as the cause for the pleural effusion. The pleural fluid glucose concentration is low, which would be in keeping with a rheumatoid or malignant pleural effusion. Rheumatoid pleural effusions are often associated with very low pleural fluid glucose concentration (often <2 mmol/L). Moreover, malignancy is most in keeping with the other presenting symptoms. Therefore, the investigation of choice is a contrast-enhanced CT scan. Bronchoscopy is not helpful initially, as there are no specific features to suggest an underlying bronchial malignancy, such as haemoptysis.

An echocardiogram would be useful if congestive cardiac failure, which can present as unilateral pleural effusion, was suspected. Typically, this would be a transudate not an exudate; however, it is worth noting that in patients with long-standing effusions who are on furosemide, the effusion can become exudative. Serum rheumatoid factor is not indicated and is a non-specific test, although titres can be used to monitor progression of rheumatoid arthritis. The presence of lower limb oedema may be a side effect of amlodipine. The presence of proteinuria and hypoalbuminaemia does lead one to suspect nephrotic syndrome and can occur in the context of malignancy and rheumatoid arthritis. This would warrant further investigation with 24-hour urine collection, but this is not the next best investigation for the exudative pleural effusion.

Tutorial

Pleural effusions can be broadly classified into transudates and exudates. When interpreting pleural fluid results, it is important to interpret pleural fluid protein and LDH concentrations in the context of serum values. This becomes very important when protein concentrations are close to 30 g/L, a commonly used divider between transudates and exudates. Light's criteria, which more accurately define an exudate, have been summarized in Box 11.1. However, up to 25% of patients with transudates are mistakenly identified as having exudates using Light's criteria. Therefore, additional testing is needed if a patient is identified as having an exudate, with a clinical condition that would produce a transudate. In such cases, albumin levels in the blood and pleural fluid may be measured. If the difference between the albumin levels (serum-effusion) is greater than 12 g/L, it suggests a transudative pleural effusion.

A malignant pleural effusion is often bloodstained. Other causes giving similar appearances include pulmonary embolus, TB, and chest trauma. Thus, samples are often sent for cytology and microbiology. Malignancy is associated with a low pleural fluid glucose concentration and pH. The pleural fluid pH has a strong correlation with pleural fluid glucose concentration. If the pleural fluid pH <7.3, with a normal arterial blood pH, then the causes are the same as for low glucose concentration (Box 11.2). The presence of very low pleural fluid pH (<7.3) in the context of malignancy is significant as this is associated with more extensive pleural involvement, higher yield on cytology, decreased success rate of pleurodesis, and a shorter life expectancy. An elevated pleural amylase can also aid in diagnosis in selected cases (Box 11.3).

Box 11.1 Light's criteria for diagnosing an exudate

- Pleural fluid protein: serum protein >0.5
- Pleural fluid LDH: serum LDH >0.6
- Pleural fluid LDH >2/3 of the upper limit of normal serum value

Data from Light R, Macgregor M, Luchsinger P, Ball W (1972). Pleural effusions: the diagnostic separation of transudates and exudates. *Annals of Internal Medicine* 77 (4): 507–513. doi:10.7326/0003-4819-77-4-507. PMID 4642731.

Box 11.2 Causes of low glucose concentration and pH in pleural fluid

- Malignancy
- Empyema
- TB
- Oesophageal rupture
- Rheumatoid arthritis
- Systemic lupus erythematosus

Box 11.3 Causes of an elevated amylase in pleural fluid

- Pancreatitis
- Malignancy
- Bacterial pneumonia
- Oesophageal rupture

Further Reading

Hooper C, Lee Y, Maskell N (on behalf of BTS Pleural Disease Group) (2010). Investigation of a unilateral pleural effusion in adults: British Thoracic Society pleura pleural disease guideline 2010. *Thorax* 65(2): ii4–ii17.

228. B) Insertion of intercostal drain

This question tests the candidate's knowledge of the current BTS guidelines on the management of spontaneous secondary pneumothoraces. This 64-year-old man presents with a spontaneous secondary pneumothorax on the background of stable COPD. He is symptomatic and the rim of air is 2 cm. According to BTS guidelines, a rim of air ≥2 cm constitutes a large pneumothorax. Large secondary pneumothoraces, particularly in patients aged >50 years, should be considered a high risk of failure for simple aspiration and recurrence, and therefore intercostal drain insertion is recommended as the most appropriate initial treatment. Suction should not be applied immediately after tube insertion, but can be added after 48 hours.

Tutorial

There are many causes of a secondary pneumothorax (see Box 11.4). All patients with secondary pneumothoraces should be hospitalized for observation. Generally, all patients with secondary pneumothoraces require some degree of intervention and will therefore need admission to hospital. According to the BTS guidelines (2010) on secondary pneumothoraces, observation alone is only recommended with small pneumothoraces (<1 cm). If a patient has a pneumothorax of 1–2 cm an aspiration should be attempted. If this succeeds, the patient should be admitted for 24-hour observation. If this fails, a chest drain needs to be inserted. If the patient has pneumothorax ≥2 cm or is dyspnoeic, regardless of the size of the pneumothorax, they warrant a chest drain insertion. A suggested treatment algorithm can be found in Figure 11.6.

If a patient is hospitalized for observation, supplemental high-flow oxygen (10 L/min) should be given. Caution must be exercised in patients with COPD, where there is a risk of depressing the respiratory drive and hypercapnia. In such cases, the quantity of oxygen will need to be titrated accordingly. Inhalation of high-flow oxygen reduces the partial pressure of nitrogen and increases the pressure gradient between the pleural capillaries and the pleural cavity. This increases the absorption of nitrogen, the principal component of air, from the pleural cavity. The addition of high-flow oxygen has shown to result in a four-fold increase in rate of pneumothorax reabsorption during the periods of oxygen supplementation. Chest drain suctioning should not be applied directly after intercostal tube insertion. It can be added after 48 hours for persistent air leak or failure of a pneumothorax to expand. In this setting, high-volume and low-pressure systems are recommended (−10−−20 cm H_2O).

Box 11.4 The causes of secondary pneumothoraces

Respiratory disease

- COPD
- Asthma
- Cystic fibrosis
- Interstitial lung disease
- TB
- Malignancy
- Pneumonia
- Lung abscess
- Pneumoconiosis
- Sarcoidosis

Connective tissue disease

- Marfan syndrome
- Ehlers-Danlos syndrome
- Pseudoxanthoma elasticum

Lung cysts

- Lymphangioleiomyomatosis
- Langerhans cell histiocytosis X
- Tuberous sclerosis
- Neurofibromatosis

Iatrogenic

- Pleural aspiration
- Pleural biopsy
- Thoracentesis
- Central venous access (internal jugular or subclavian vein puncture)
- Pacemaker insertion
- Cardiopulmonary resuscitation

Trauma

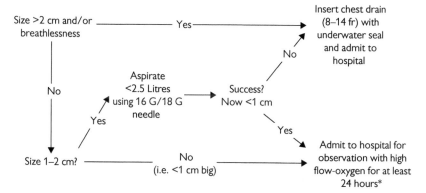

Figure 11.6 Suggested treatment algorithm for a secondary pneumothorax.

NB: this is not applicable for primary pneumothoraces, a suggested treatment algorithm for which can be found in Figure 11.5.

Further Reading

Macduff A, Arnold A, Harvey J (on behalf of BTS Pleural Disease Group) (2010). Management of spontaneous pneumothorax: British Thoracic Society pleural disease guideline 2010. *Thorax* 65(2): ii18–ii31.

229. D) Eosinophilic granulomatosis with polyangiitis (EGPA, formerly Churg-Strauss syndrome)

The key features in this question that constitute EGPA are a diagnosis of late-onset asthma and a marked eosinophilia >10%. It is likely he has also had sinusitis which has been treated with antibiotics by his GP. Given the obstructive deficit in lung function testing, COPD might seem like a good choice. However, given the absence of a smoking history this is less likely. In addition, COPD would not cause an eosinophilia. Given the history of ischaemic heart disease, evidence of old infarct on the ECG, and peripheral oedema, this may raise the suspicion of congestive cardiac failure. However, this is unlikely given clear lung fields, normal sized heart, and normal venous pressure. The mild peripheral oedema may reflect amlodipine therapy. A history of smoking, asbestos exposure (shipbuilding industry), and weight loss may raise the suspicion of lung malignancy or interstitial lung disease. Whilst the former, if causing a bronchial malignancy, could cause a wheeze, the latter would not and you would expect to hear crepitations on auscultation. Neither would account for the eosinophilia.

Constitutional symptoms such as malaise, fatigue, weight loss, and fever are common in EGPA, and whilst not specific for this diagnosis, in the context of a diagnosis of adult-onset asthma and eosinophilia make this the most likely diagnosis. Another consideration not mentioned here would be acute bronchopulmonary aspergillosis, which may present in a similar manner causing widespread wheeze and eosinophilia. When investigating this patient, total serum IgE and aspergillus precipitins (including IgE) would also be warranted. The lack of radiological changes on a chest radiograph should not go against this diagnosis of EGPA, as early changes may require high resolution CT.

Tutorial

EGPA is a small vessel vasculitis that affects the upper and lower respiratory tract, skin, kidneys, heart, gastrointestinal tract, and peripheral nerves, and is discussed in more detail in Table 11.1. The mean age at diagnosis is around 50 years. The diagnostic criteria for EGPA are shown in Box 11.5.

EGPA has three phases: (1) prodromal phase: asthma +/− allergic rhinitis; (2) eosinophilic phase: peripheral eosinophilia with eosinophilic tissue infiltration, such as eosinophilic pneumonia or eosinophilic gastroenteritis; and (3) vasculitic phase: systemic small-vessel vasculitis with granulomatous inflammation. The vasculitic phase often develops within three years of the onset of asthma, but this may be delayed for years.

Asthma symptoms are a central feature of EGPA, occurring in 97% of patients. They are usually persistent and therefore, patients are usually treated with steroids which may mask other features of the syndrome. Systemic eosinophilia (greater than 10% of the peripheral blood cell count) is also a hallmark of EGPA, and can be present even in the absence of systemic vasculitis. Antineutrophil cytoplasmic antibodies (ANCA) are present in approximately 35% of patients, with most of these being perinuclear-ANCA (or more specifically anti-myeloperoxidase (MPO) antibodies). Other findings include anaemia, elevated ESR, and CRP, increased serum IgE levels and hypergammaglobulinaemia; proteinuria, microscopic haematuria, and red blood cell casts in the urine. To note, normal renal function on blood testing does not preclude renal involvement.

The CXR can be normal in up to 25% of patients. Pulmonary opacities and infiltrates may be transient and can be found in up to 75% of cases. Localized parenchymal opacities usually are bilateral, peripheral, and patchy. Unlike granulomatosis with polyangiitis (Wegner's granulomatosis), lung cavitation is rare. Extensive air-space opacities with a drop in haemoglobin should raise the suspicion of a massive pulmonary haemorrhage. The characteristic pathologic changes in EGPA, found especially in the lung, include small necrotizing granulomas, as well as necrotizing vasculitis involving small arteries and venules. The granulomas are composed of a central eosinophilic core surrounded radially by macrophages and epithelioid giant cells.

Glucocorticoids alone are often effective for treatment of EGPA. Indications for the use of cyclophosphamide include renal insufficiency (serum creatinine >140 µmol/L), proteinuria, involvement of the gastrointestinal tract, involvement of the nervous system, or cardiomyopathy. Recent data has also implicated age >65 years as a poor prognostic marker.

Table 11.1 Clinical manifestations of EGPA

Organ system	Clinical manifestations
Constitutional symptoms	Malaise, fatigue, flu-like symptoms Weight loss (70%) Fever (60%) Myalgias (50%) Arthralgias (40%)
Respiratory	Asthma-like symptoms (97%) Allergic rhinitis, sinusitis, and/or nasal polyposis (60–80%) Pneumonitis Alveolar haemorrhage
Dermatological	Skin nodules Urticaria Necrotic bullae Leukocytoclastic angiitis with palpable purpura Livedo reticularis Digital ischaemia
Gastrointestinal	Eosinophilic gastritis Eosinophilic colitis Gastrointestinal bleeding Bowel ischaemia
Renal	Hypertension Renal impairment
Neurological	Mononeuritis multiplex (70%) Ischaemic stroke (5%)
Cardiac	Myocarditis Pericarditis Pericardial effusion Congestive cardiac failure

> **Box 11.5** American College of Rheumatology (ACR) 1990 diagnostic criteria for EPGA (at least four of the six criteria must be present)
>
> 1. Asthma
> 2. Eosinophilia >10%
> 3. Mono- or polyneuropathy
> 4. Migratory or transitory pulmonary infiltrates (not including fixed infiltrates)
> 5. Paranasal sinus abnormality
> 6. Extravascular eosinophils: biopsy including artery, arteriole or venule showing accumulations of eosinophils in extravascular areas.
>
> Reproduced with permission from Masi AT, et al., The American College of Rheumatology 1990 criteria for the classification of Churg-Strauss syndrome (allergic granulomatosis and angiitis), *Arthritis & Rheumatology* 33, 8, Copyright 2010, Wiley.

Further Reading

Jennette J, Falk R, Bacon P, et al. (2012). 2012 Revised international Chapel Hill consensus conference nomenclature of vasculitides. *Arthritis and Rheumatology* 54: 1–11.

Masi A, Hunder G, Lie G, et al. (1990). The American College of Rheumatology 1990 criteria for the classification of Churg-Strauss syndrome (allergic granulomatosis and angiitis). *Arthritis and Rheumatology* 33: 1094–1100.

Owen C, Clark S, Woolfson R (2015). A 77-year-old man with asthma and renal impairment—case review. *British Medical Journal* 350: h2021.

230. E) Pulmonary embolism

This elderly obese lady presents with chest pain and hypoxia, one week following a hip replacement. This raises the strong suspicion of pulmonary embolism (PE). The CXR demonstrates left basal consolidation that may represent infection, infarction, or malignancy. The WCC is normal, and CRP mildly raised in the context of a recent operation, both of which in the absence of a productive cough and fever make the diagnosis of pneumonia unlikely.

The presence of cardiomegaly on the CXR, LBBB on the ECG with a strong cardiovascular risk profile does raise the suspicion of underlying (chronic) heart failure, but clear lung fields and absence of suggestive features on CXR make acute decompensated cardiac failure unlikely.

Cardiomegaly on the CXR may also be consistent with pericardial effusion, but there are no pointers in the history for any specific aetiology. Furthermore, a symptomatic pericardial effusion would be associated with a raised JVP, muffled heart sounds, and hypotension (Beck's triad); and a pericardial effusion would not account for the hypoxia. The soft heart sounds in this case may merely reflect auscultation in an obese patient.

The history of chest pain in this patient with strong cardiovascular risk profile and LBBB on the ECG does raise the suspicion of an acute coronary syndrome. LBBB on the ECG may be due to myocardial infarction in the LAD territory, hypertension, or chronic heart failure. Additionally, T-wave inversion in the anterior leads may represent myocardial ischaemia, but are also seen with PE. A slightly elevated troponin may cause further confusion, but this can also be raised with a PE due to right ventricular strain or may just be raised due to the patient's renal impairment. It is also worth remembering that an acute coronary syndrome itself does not cause hypoxia, rather it is associated myocardial dysfunction with consequent pulmonary oedema which causes it. This patient's X-ray does not show that either.

Tutorial

PE is a common and potentially fatal condition that can occur in all age groups. The diagnosis should be confirmed or refuted if *any* suspicion of PE exists, as prompt diagnosis and treatment can dramatically reduce morbidity and mortality. The diagnosis is often missed, as it may present with only vague and non-specific symptoms. The initial suspicion should be prompted by a thorough history and enquiring about thromboembolic risk factors. These include recent surgery, malignancy, immobility, previous thromboembolism, oral contraceptive pill, pregnancy (and post-partum period), thrombophilic disorders (Factor V Leiden, protein S, protein C and antithrombin III deficiency).

The CXR is often normal, but radiographic features include: (1) Westermark sign (dilatation of the pulmonary vessels proximal to an embolism along with collapse of distal vessels (oligaemic lung fields); (2) atelectasis (with elevation of the hemidiaphragm); (3) pleural effusion; (4) consolidation; and (5) Hampton bump—a wedge-shaped or rounded pleural-based infiltrate with the apex pointed toward the hilum, often adjacent to the diaphragm (late sign). The most common ECG finding in pulmonary embolism is sinus tachycardia. Other ECG findings are summarized in Box 11.6. The d-dimer may be elevated in other causes such as infection or malignancy. However, a negative d-dimer reliably excludes PE if there is a low pre-test probability. A low d-dimer doesn't exclude PE if the pre-test probability is moderate or high. A V-Q scan should only be considered as a first-line investigation for PE, if the CXR is normal and there is no significant cardiopulmonary disease. A normal VQ scan in a patient with low pre-test probability reliably excludes a PE, but an intermediate scan should be followed up by CT pulmonary angiography, which remains the gold standard. A normal VQ scan in a patient with a high pre-test probability for PE should also be followed up by CT pulmonary angiography, as 4% of patients with PE can have a normal VQ scan. In pregnancy a Doppler ultrasound of the lower limbs is the first-line investigation, as if a DVT is identified treatment can begin without exposure to ionizing radiation.

The serum troponin has a critical role in the management of patients with ACS. However, troponin may also be elevated in patients with PE, indicating right ventricular strain and overload, and can significantly contribute to prognostic stratification. Elevated serum troponin is associated with adverse in-hospital outcomes in patients with PE and normal blood pressure.

Box 11.6 ECG findings in PE

- Sinus tachycardia (most common)
- Tall R wave in V_1
- Right ventricular strain
- Right bundle branch block (complete or incomplete)
- T wave inversion in V_1-V_3
- $S_1S_2S_3$ (classically described but rarely seen)
- $S_1Q_3T_3$ (classically described but rarely seen)
- Inferior ST elevation (rare, but has been described)
- Q waves in III and aVF (pseudo-infarction)
- New onset atrial arrhythmias

Further Reading

Becattini C, Vedovati M, Agnelli G (2007). Prognostic value of troponins in acute pulmonary embolism: a meta-analysis. *Circulation* 116(4): 427–433.

Bělohlávek J, Dytrych V, Linhart A (2013). Pulmonary embolism, part I: Epidemiology, risk factors and risk stratification, pathophysiology, clinical presentation, diagnosis and non-thrombotic pulmonary embolism. *Experimental and Clinical Cardiology* 18(2): 129–138.

231. D) Immediate thrombolysis and then heparin

This young lady with a strong thromboembolic risk factor profile presents with chest pain, profound hypoxia, tachycardia, and hypotension, with a raised JVP and RV dysfunction on echocardiogram. This scenario is highly suggestive of a massive PE.

The lack of thrombus visualized in the pulmonary artery on echocardiography may go against this diagnosis, but it must be remembered that echo is not the most sensitive test for this and will fail to identify thrombus in the pulmonary artery or main branches in massive or sub-massive PE. Hence, the absence of thrombus in the pulmonary artery on echocardiography should *not* lead one to dismiss the diagnosis.

The management of suspected PE resides in treatment with heparins and CT pulmonary angiography (CTPA, the gold standard) or VQ scan to confirm the diagnosis, followed by oral anticoagulation. However, this is a case of massive PE with profound hypotension, and given that acute RV dysfunction has been demonstrated on echocardiography there is little doubt in the diagnosis. Thrombolysis is indicated, and there should not be any delay in administration in the absence of contraindications. CTPA should be arranged *after* the administration of thrombolysis, and once the patient is on heparin, to demonstrate massive or sub-massive PE. Indeed, the BTS states thrombolysis may be given without radiological confirmation if there is sufficient clinical suspicion and the patient is at immediate risk of cardiac arrest, which is clearly the case here. For this reason, giving just heparin alone, either before or after a CTPA, is not the correct choice.

Tutorial

High-risk PE (also termed 'massive PE') is characterized principally by arterial hypotension (SBP <90 mmHg, for >15 min), although RV dysfunction will also be present in this setting. Intermediate-risk PE (also termed 'sub-massive PE') is characterized by preserved blood pressure, but with evidence of RV dysfunction, myocardial necrosis (elevated troponin), or profound hypoxia. Despite anticoagulation, the mortality rate doubles for intermediate-risk PE patients and is even higher in patients who present with profound hypotension due to high-risk PE. Echocardiographic features indicating RV dysfunction are RV dilatation and/or RV systolic dysfunction (hypokinesis of RV free wall). Biochemical markers of RV dysfunction include: (1) elevated BNP; (2) elevated; or (3) elevated troponin. ECG markers of RV dysfunction include: (1) new complete or incomplete RBBB; (2) anteroseptal ST elevation or depression; and (3) anteroseptal T wave inversion

The definitive management of PE is anticoagulation. If PE is suspected, patients should be anticoagulated with LMWH, whilst the diagnostic investigations are in progress. Unfractionated heparin (UFH) can be used if thrombolysis is being contemplated in high-risk or intermediate-risk PE, where there is increased bleeding risk, or those with severe renal impairment. When the diagnosis is confirmed, this can be replaced with oral anticoagulants. The LMWH/UFH must be continued until the INR is in the therapeutic range (2–3) for two days. Patients with a first PE (or DVT) occurring in the setting of reversible risk factors such as immobilization, surgery, or trauma, should receive warfarin therapy for at least three months. In patients with idiopathic PE (or DVT), no differences in the rates of recurrence have been demonstrated in three vs six months—current recommendations are for anticoagulation for at least three months, with re-evaluation at that point. Warfarin treatment for longer than six months is indicated in patients with recurrent PE (or DVT) or in those in whom a continuing risk factor for venous thromboembolism exists, including malignancy, immobilization, or morbid obesity. Patients with pre-existing thrombophilic disorders, such as Factor V Leiden mutation, protein S, protein C, or antithrombin III deficiency, or the presence of antiphospholipid antibodies, should be placed on long-term anticoagulation.

Thrombolysis is indicated in patients with high-risk PEs. Its use in intermediate-risk PEs is still unclear, with many studies finding no difference in long-term outcomes but it should be considered on a case-by-case basis depending on patients' physiological state. Guidelines generally recommend evaluating the patient with intermediate-risk PE (normal BP but with RV dysfunction, elevated cardiac biomarkers, or profound hypoxia) for markers of severity that may indicate benefit of thrombolysis (Figure 11.7). If thrombolytic therapy is being considered, intravenous UFH is the recommended form of initial anticoagulation. The recombinant tissue-plasminogen activators, alteplase (t-PA) and reteplase (r-PA) that are administered over 1–2 hours, are superior to streptokinase (administered slowly over 12 hours). Streptokinase may further cause anaphylaxis, hypotension, and other adverse reactions, potentially leading to the cessation of therapy. Some centres are now beginning to offer catheter-directed treatment as an alternative to thrombolysis where contraindication to haemorrhage exist, or as a 'rescue' in those whom thrombolysis has failed, but this is not yet common practice in the UK.

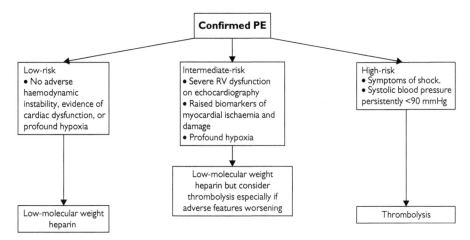

Figure 11.7 Treatment algorithm pulmonary emboli.

Further Reading

Howard L, Barden S, Condliffe R, et al. (2018). British Thoracic Society guideline for the initial outpatient management of pulmonary embolism (PE). *Thorax* 73(Suppl. 2): ii1–ii29.

Jaff M, McMurtry S, Archer S, et al. (2011). Management of massive and sub-massive pulmonary embolism, iliofemoral deep vein thrombosis, and chronic thromboembolic pulmonary hypertension: a scientific statement from the American Heart Association. *Circulation* 123: 1788–1830.

Konstantinides S, Meyer G, Becatinni C et al, 2019. The task force for the diagnosis and management of acute pulmonary embolism of the European Society of Cardiology (ESC). *European Respiratory Journal* 54(3): 1901647.

232. C) Legionella pneumonia

This patient presents with a febrile illness, preceded by prodromal symptoms with headaches and lethargy, followed by respiratory, gastrointestinal, and neurological symptoms. Laboratory investigations reveal, a leucocytosis with relative lymphopaenia, hyponatraemia, impaired renal function, deranged LFTs (hepatitis), hypocalcaemia, and hypophosphataemia. The most likely unifying diagnosis is Legionella pneumonia. A history of recent travel indicating a likely stay at a hotel (possible contamination of cooling systems by *Legionella pneumophilia*) is a supporting feature in the history.

Mycoplasma pneumonia may present with a similar clinical picture, but does not cause hypocalcaemia and hypophosphataemia, and usually does not produce such a low sodium. In the absence of other causes, hypophosphataemia is relatively specific to Legionella pneumonia. Streptococcal pneumonia may present with a similar picture and is often preceded by a prodromal viral illness. The cough is initially dry and non-productive, and is replaced by a productive cough with rusty-coloured sputum after 24–48 hours. Klebsiella pneumonia rarely occurs in otherwise healthy fit individuals and tends to occur in predisposed immunocompromised states, for example diabetes, alcoholism, HIV, prolonged hospitalization, severe illness, and following major surgery. It is associated with destructive changes in the lungs (abscess formation, cavitation, empyema, and pleural adhesions) with a predilection for the upper lobes. It is often associated with a productive cough with thick and blood-tinged sputum. Carcinoma of the lung is unlikely, given: (1) a short history of an acute febrile illness; (2) there are no risk factors for malignancy; and (3) absence of respiratory symptoms prior to this presentation.

Tutorial

Legionella pneumophila can cause two distinct clinical syndromes: (1) legionnaires disease (LD)—characterized by pneumonia and (2) Pontiac fever—a milder illness characterized by fever and myalgias without pneumonia that resolves without treatment. *Legionella* colonizes contaminated water-cooling systems, showers, or air-conditioning systems and can result in epidemic outbreaks of LD in fit, healthy individuals. LD can occur sporadically where predisposing factors include elderly age, debilitation, alcoholism, smoking, COPD, and immunodeficiency. The incubation period is 2–10 days. There is often a prodromal illness resembling a viral infection, with fever, headaches, and myalgia. Patients develop high-grade fevers and a dry non-productive cough. Gastrointestinal symptoms (watery diarrhoea, nausea and vomiting, and abdominal pain) occur in over 50% of patients. Neurological symptoms include headache, lethargy, encephalopathy, ataxia, and altered mental status (confusion, hallucinations, and memory defects). Altered mental status is the most common neurological symptom. Renal involvement is characterized by acute interstitial nephritis (haematuria is common and renal failure is rare). Other complications include hepatitis, pancreatitis, pericarditis, and myocarditis.

The laboratory investigations show normal or elevated WCC with neutrophilia and relative lymphopenia. Hyponatremia secondary to the SIADH (syndrome of inappropriate antidiuretic hormone secretion) is more common in LD than other pneumonias. Other contributors to hyponatraemia include acute interstitial nephritis and gastrointestinal loss of electrolytes. Hypophosphataemia is observed in LD, and can serve as a non-specific laboratory clue for LD. The CXR shows rapidly progressive asymmetrical infiltrates that are characteristic of LD, with predilection for the lower lobes. Pleural effusions are found in one third of patients; cavity and abscess formation is rare but can occur in immunocompromised patients. Diagnosis can be made using detection of Legionella antigen in the urine (present in 90% of cases in the first week of illness), Legionella serology or direct immunofluorescence, or PCR of respiratory specimens. Antibodies appear 7–10 days after the onset of symptoms, and for serological confirmation, comparison of acute and convalescent serum is required (separated by 2–3 weeks). In practice, all patients should have additional tests that include serology for mycoplasma and chlamydia that may present with a similar clinical picture.

Treatment is with macrolides (e.g. erythromycin, clarithromycin, or azithromycin) +/– oral rifampicin. Although erythromycin has been used historically, clarithromycin and azithromycin have greater *in vitro* activity and better intracellular penetration than erythromycin. Furthermore, the gastrointestinal manifestations of the disease added to the gastrointestinal adverse effects of erythromycin may be problematic. Other drugs that can be used include doxycycline, co-trimoxazole, tetracycline, and ciprofloxacin.

Further Reading

Cunha B (2006). Hypophosphatemia: diagnostic significance in Legionnaires' disease. 2006. *American Journal of Medicine* 119: e5–6.

Phin N, Parry-Ford F, Harrison T, et al. (2014). Epidemiology and clinical management of Legionnaires' disease. *Lancet Infectious Diseases* 14(10): 1011–1021.

233. B) Bronchiectasis

This patient's flow-volume loop is consistent with airflow obstruction. Causes of an obstructive pattern on spirometry include asthma, COPD, and bronchiectasis. This patient is clubbed, and the respiratory of causes of clubbing include bronchiectasis, empyema, interstitial lung disease, and carcinoma of the lung. Digital clubbing is present in approximately 2–3% of patients with bronchiectasis, and is more frequent in patients with moderate-to-severe disease. This patient has a *chronic* productive cough, which could be accounted for by bronchiectasis or carcinoma of the lung.

Carcinoma of the lung is possible on a background of COPD (that would account for the obstructive pattern on spirometry), but the CXR does not demonstrate any suspicious lesions. The unifying diagnosis is bronchiectasis. The CXR can often appear normal in patients with bronchiectasis, and many abnormal radiographic findings may be non-specific, and confirmation using HRCT scanning (gold standard) is required.

Tutorial

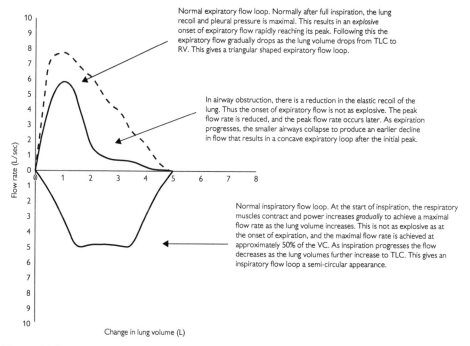

Figure 11.8 Annotated flow-volume loop demonstrating obstruction.

This patient's flow-volume loop demonstrates an obstructive pattern (Figure 11.8). The dotted expiratory flow loop represents a normal triangular-shaped flow expiratory flow loop. In airway obstruction, the amount of elastic recoil in the lung is reduced, and as expiration progresses, the smaller airways collapse to produce an earlier decline in flow that results in a concave expiratory loop after the initial peak.

Bronchiectasis is characterized by abnormal bronchial wall dilatation, destruction, and transmural inflammation. This abnormal dilatation of the proximal and medium sized bronchi (diameter >2 mm) is caused by destruction of the muscular and elastic components of the bronchial walls. This leads to inflammation, oedema, scarring, and ulceration of bronchial walls. Severely impaired clearance of secretions causes colonization and infection. This results in further bronchial damage, dilatation, impaired clearance of secretions, recurrent infections, and more bronchial damage (a vicious cycle). The causes of bronchiectasis are listed in Box 11.7. The most common respiratory pathogens in bronchiectasis are listed in Box 11.8. Smoking per se is not associated with bronchiectasis, and most patients with bronchiectasis have never smoked (55%). However, smoking is associated with COPD, and 30% of patients with COPD have evidence of bronchiectasis on CT.

The CXR may show increased bronchovascular markings from peri-bronchial fibrosis and intrabronchial secretions, tram lines (linear lucencies, and parallel markings radiating from the hila outlining dilated bronchi due to peri-bronchial inflammation and fibrosis), areas of honeycombing, or cystic areas with or without fluid levels. The CXR may be normal, especially those with mild-moderate disease. High-resolution CT scanning (resolution is 1–2 mm thickness compared to 10 mm thickness in standard CT) is the gold standard for diagnosing bronchiectasis, and has replaced bronchoscopy as the defining modality of bronchiectasis. The 'signet ring sign' is where the bronchial diameter is greater than adjacent vessel diameter. Pulmonary function tests may be normal. The most common abnormality is an obstructive pattern (FEV1: FVC <70%). The obstruction is not always reversible with bronchodilator therapy, though a small subgroup of patients may have airway hyper-reactivity that will respond to bronchodilators. In advanced disease, there may be a restrictive pattern (FEV1: FVC >70%) secondary to scarring and atelectasis. A restrictive pattern may also occur with underlying pulmonary fibrosis.

Complications of bronchiectasis include pneumonia, pneumothorax, empyema, lung collapse, metastatic cerebral abscess, respiratory failure, pulmonary hypertension, and amyloidosis. The goals of therapy are to improve symptoms, reduce complications, control exacerbations, and reduce overall morbidity and mortality. Recognition of any underlying predisposing condition is essential, which will require additional specific therapy. Antibiotics and chest physiotherapy are the mainstay treatment modalities. Others may include bronchodilators, corticosteroid therapy, dietary supplementation, supplementary oxygen, or surgical therapies. The management of bronchiectasis is outlined in Box 11.9.

1) Before starting antibiotics, a sputum sample should be sent off for culture. If there is no previous bacteriology to guide treatment, empirical antibiotics should be started as per local guidelines whilst awaiting sputum microbiology.

2) Inhaled or oral corticosteroids may be considered, especially if additionally there is underlying COPD. Current evidence does not support routine use of inhaled corticosteroids in bronchiectasis.

Box 11.7 Common causes of bronchiectasis

Respiratory childhood infections

- Pertussis
- Measles
- TB

Bronchial obstruction

- Foreign body
- Chronic aspiration
- Endobronchial tumour
- Lymph nodes (TB, sarcoidosis, and malignancy)
- Granulomas (TB, sarcoidosis, Chediak-Higashi syndrome)

Fibrosis

- Long-standing pulmonary fibrosis
- Fibrosis complicating TB and sarcoidosis
- Fibrosis complicating unresolved or suppurative pneumonia

Muco-ciliary clearance defects

- Cystic fibrosis
- Immotile cilia syndrome
- Kartagener's syndrome
- Young syndrome

Immunodeficiency

- Congenital and acquired hypogammaglobulinaemia
- Acquired immunodeficiency syndrome

Allergic bronchopulmonary aspergillosis

Autoimmune disease

- Rheumatoid arthritis (rheumatoid lung)
- Sjögren syndrome
- Inflammatory bowel disease (ulcerative colitis > Crohn's disease)

Congenital anatomical defects

- Bronchopulmonary sequestration
- William-Campbell syndrome
- Mounier-Kuhn syndrome
- Swyer-James syndrome
- Yellow-nail syndrome

Idiopathic

Box 11.8 Common respiratory pathogens in bronchiectasis

- *Staphylococcus aureus*
- *Haemophilus influenzae*
- *Pseudomonas aeruginosa*
- *Streptococcus pneumoniae*
- *Klebsiella pneumoniae*
- Aspergillus species

Box 11.9 Management of bronchiectasis

General measures

- Stop smoking
- Adequate nutritional intake and supplementation if necessary
- Immunizations for influenza and pneumococcal pneumonia
- Confirm immunity to measles, pertussis, and rubella
- Long-term oxygen therapy in advanced cases

Antibiotics

- Oral, parenteral, or nebulized antibiotics (depending on clinical situation)[1]
- Patients having ≥3 exacerbations per year requiring antibiotic therapy or exacerbations that are causing significant morbidity should be considered for long-term nebulized antibiotics
- Long-term nebulized antibiotics should be considered if chronically colonized with *P. aeruginosa*

Postural drainage and physiotherapy

- Postural drainage with percussion and vibration
- Other devices to help with mucous clearance include flutter devices and pneumatic compression devices
- Nebulized saline and mucolytics
- Maintaining good hydration reduces the viscosity of secretions

Bronchodilator therapy

Anti-inflammatory medication

- Inhaled or oral corticosteroids[2]

Surgery

- Surgical resection for localized bronchiectasis (poorly controlled by antibiotics)
- Bronchial artery embolization/surgery is first-line treatment for massive haemoptysis
- Foreign body or tumour removal

[1] Before starting antibiotics, a sputum sample should be sent off for culture. If there is no previous bacteriology to guide treatment, empirical antibiotics should be started as per local guidelines whilst awaiting sputum microbiology.
[2] Inhaled or oral corticosteroids may be considered, especially if additionally there is underlying COPD. Current evidence does not support routine use of inhaled corticosteroids in bronchiectasis.

Further Reading

Pasteur M, Bilton D, Hill T (2010). On behalf of the British Thoracic Society Bronchiectasis (non-CF) Guideline Group: a sub-group of the British Thoracic Society Standards of Care Committee. 2010. Guideline for non-CF Bronchiectasis. *Thorax* 65(1): i1–58.

234. B) Exacerbation of asthma

This patient's initial flow-volume loop demonstrates a concave expiratory flow loop that is consistent with airflow obstruction. The second flow-volume demonstrates a normal expiratory flow loop. Therefore this patient has *reversible* airflow obstruction, and thus asthma is the most likely diagnosis.

Whilst some degree of reversibility can be seen in patients with COPD, it will not be associated with complete normalization of the expiratory flow loop. Extrinsic allergic alveolitis is associated with a restrictive pattern on spirometry, but occasionally a mixed restrictive and obstructive pattern may be seen. Interstitial lung disease is associated with a restrictive pattern. In restrictive defects, the inspiratory and expiratory flow loops would resemble the shapes in normal subjects, but the lung volumes would be much smaller, with reduced FVC.

C) Graves' disease

The repeat flow-volume loop demonstrates a normal expiratory flow loop, but an abnormal inspiratory flow loop. The inspiratory flow loop is blunted with reduced flow rate. This flow-volume is characteristic of variable extrathoracic obstruction. Causes include vocal cord paralysis, tumour in the upper airways, lymphadenopathy, goitre, pharyngeal muscle weakness, and excess neck fat. This patient has diplopia and strabismus, along with a goitre. The unifying diagnosis is Graves' disease.

Myasthenia gravis can cause diplopia and there are rare reports that it can cause variable extrathoracic obstruction due to weakness of the bulbar and upper airway muscles. But this would not explain the goitre and the appearance of digital clubbing. Furthermore, bulbar and/ or pharyngeal muscle weakness would be associated with dysphonia and dysarthria. Botulism can cause diplopia, and whilst there may be recent history of diarrhoeal illness, other features of botulism, for example ptosis, bulbar weakness, descending paralysis, and autonomic dysfunction are not present. MEN2 is characterized by phaechromocytoma, primary hyperparathyroidism, and medullary carcinoma of the thyroid (goitre). However, the calcium and phosphate are normal, and MEN2 will not account for the diplopia. Carcinoma of the lung may rarely cause diplopia if associated with metastases, and may cause variable extrathoracic obstruction if complicated by vocal cord paralysis (malignant invasion of either the vagus or recurrent laryngeal nerve), but this would be associated with dysphonia.

Tutorial

To understand the mechanics of flow loops in large airway obstruction, remember, all intrathoracic airways lengthen and get wider with inspiration, while extrathoracic airways, because of a negative intraluminal pressure, get shorter and narrower. With expiration, intrathoracic airways get shorter and narrower while extrathoracic airways tend to get longer and wider.

In *variable extrathoracic airway obstruction*, the expiratory flow loop is normal, but the inspiratory flow is blunted and reaches a low plateau value. The high pressure in extrathoracic airways distends the airway, the obstruction is pushed outwards by the force of the expiration, resulting a normal expiratory flow loop. During inspiration the obstruction is sucked into the trachea with partial obstruction and flattening of the inspiratory part of the flow-volume loop—as seen in Figure 11.2 of the question. Variable extrathoracic large airway obstruction can be seen with any lesion occurring from the hypopharynx to the level of the sternal notch. Causes include vocal cord paralysis, tumour in the upper airways, lymphadenopathy, goitre, pharyngeal muscle weakness; laryngeal oedema, and neck fat. This is seen in Figure 11.3 of the question.

Thus, in *variable intrathoracic airway obstruction*, the opposite of variable extrathoracic airway obstruction occurs. During inspiration the obstructive lesion is pulled out, resulting in a normal inspiratory flow loop. During expiration the obstructive lesion is pushed into the airway with partial obstruction and consequent blunting of the expiratory flow loop. This pattern can be caused by any process which affects the trachea from approximately the level of the sternal notch to the carina. This pattern is more uncommon but can be caused by tumours, chondromalacia, Wegener's granulomatosis, infection, or compression of this segment of the trachea. This is shown in Figure 11.9.

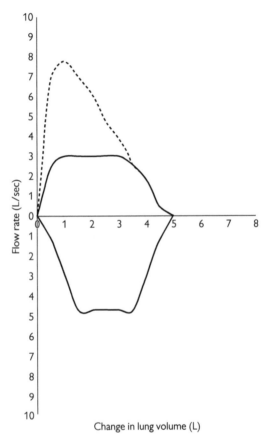

Figure 11.9 Variable intrathoracic airway obstruction. Dotted lines present normal flow loop patterns.

In *fixed extrathoracic and intrathoracic obstruction*, both the inspiratory and expiratory flow loops are blunted. If a process that causes obstruction fixes the airway wall so that it cannot vary with inspiration and expiration then the obstruction is 'fixed'. Causes include tracheal stenosis (complication of prolonged intubation), foreign body, or neoplasm. This is seen in Figure 11.10.

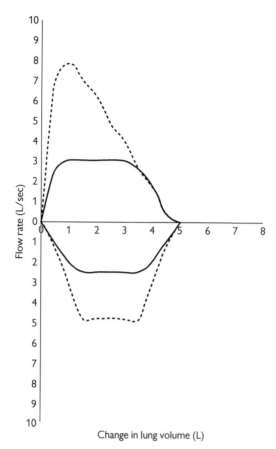

Figure 11.10 Fixed extra-thoracic or intrathoracic airway obstruction. Dotted lines present normal flow loop patterns.

Further Reading

Johnson J, Theurer W (2014). A stepwise approach to the interpretation of pulmonary function tests. *American Family Physician* 89(5): 359–366.

235. C) Outpatient patient treatment with oral amoxicillin

This question tests the candidate's knowledge of the revised and updated BTS guidelines for community acquired pneumonia (see Table 11.2). The CURB-65 criteria has been adopted for assessing the severity of community acquired pneumonia that dictates how patients are managed, but should be interpreted with clinical judgement. This patient's CURB-65 score is 1, placing her in the mild category. These patients can be managed as outpatients with oral amoxicillin. A decision to hospitalize patients without meeting any or just one of the CURB-65 criteria may still be appropriate and depends on clinical assessment. If the patient does not have severe symptoms, doesn't require supplementary oxygen or intravenous fluids to correct dehydration, is able to take oral medications, doesn't have other medical conditions which would warrant closer supervised hospital care, and has satisfactory social circumstances, the patient can be managed in the community.

Tutorial

The CURB-65 criteria is composed of five components, each of which score one point (confusion, urea, respiratory rate, blood pressure, and age). For the full score, please refer to the BTS guidelines (see Further Reading, Lim et al.).

The patient's score can be used to decide on subsequent management strategy. It is important to note that this score should be used in conjunction with clinical judgement. Patients managed in the community, should be advised to rest, to drink plenty of fluids and not to smoke. Review of patients in the community is recommended after 48 hours or earlier if clinically indicated (especially for a score of 1–2). Those who fail to improve after 48 hours of treatment should be considered for hospital admission. Regarding antibiotic choice, unless there are specific other local guidelines or the patient has a history of resistant organisms, amoxicillin is the first choice antibiotic and where a second agent is needed, it should be clarithromycin. These are discussed further in Table 11.2.

Table 11.2 Clinical management of community acquired pneumonia. Local antibiotic guidelines may vary and should be used if different.

CURB score	Severity (mortality)	Inpatient/out-patient treatment	Usual antibiotic recommendation
≤1	Low	Outpatient	PO amoxicillin
2	Moderate	Consider short inpatient treatment *or* hospital supervised outpatient treatment	PO amoxicillin + PO clarithromycin If oral administration not possible: IV amoxicillin/benzylpenicillin + IV clarithromycin
≥3	Severe	Inpatient	IV co-amoxiclav + IV clarithromycin

Data from British Thoracic Society community acquired pneumonia in adults guideline group. BTS guideline for the management of community acquired pneumonia in adults: update 2009. 2009. *Thorax* 64 (iii): 1–55.

Further Reading

British Thoracic Society Community Acquired Pneumonia in Adults Guideline Group (2009). BTS guideline for the management of community acquired pneumonia in adults: update 2009. *Thorax* 64 (iii): 1–55.

Lim W, van der Eerden M, Laing R, et al. (2003). Defining community acquired pneumonia severity on presentation to hospital: an international derivation and validation study. *Thorax* 58 (5): 377–382. doi:10.1136/thorax.58.5.377.

236. C) Hypersensitivity pneumonitis

The answer lies in close scrutiny of the history. This farmer has been developing breathlessness over a six-month period. However, his symptoms of a fevers, dry cough, and breathlessness have been present for a greater duration and are typically worse at the end of the day. The most likely diagnosis is hypersensitivity pneumonitis (extrinsic allergic alveolitis)—farmer's lung. The acute form represents a flu-like illness, breathlessness, and dry cough that typically occurs 3–9 hours after exposure to the sensitizing antigen (*Micropolyspora faenii*). In this case, the farmer would work throughout the day and develop the reaction to the antigen by the end of the day. Symptoms often resolve spontaneously within 12 hours to several days depending upon the cessation of exposure.

However, after a more prolonged exposure patients present with a type I respiratory failure, and spirometry demonstrates a restrictive lung defect (FEV1:FVC >70%) with a reduced transfer coefficient (KCO). Farmer's lung must be distinguished from febrile toxic reactions to inhaled mould dusts (organic dust toxic syndrome). Organic dust toxic syndrome is a non-infectious, non-immunologic febrile illness associated with chills, malaise, myalgia, a dry cough, breathlessness, headache, and nausea, which occurs after heavy organic dust exposure. It shares many clinical features with acute farmer's lung and other forms of hypersensitivity pneumonitis. However, organic dust toxic syndrome differs from acute hypersensitivity pneumonitis in that: (1) CXR does not show infiltrates; (2) severe hypoxia does not occur; (3) prior sensitization to antigens in the organic dust is not required; and (4) there are no known sequelae such as the recurrent attacks and the development pulmonary fibrosis which may be seen with chronic hypersensitivity pneumonitis. Organic dust toxic syndrome is thought to be much 30–50 times more common than farmer's lung. Symptoms are self-limiting, and treatment of fevers and myalgia is with paracetamol +/– NSAIDs. COPD would be associated with an obstructive lung defect (FEV$_1$:FVC <70%) and cannot explain the acute episodes of fever, dry cough, and breathlessness.

Pneumoconiosis is another occupational respiratory disease caused by inhalation of dusts which causes lung fibrosis. However, the difference here is that the dusts are inorganic (e.g. asbestosis, coal miner lung, silicosis) and these conditions don't present with the waxing-waning symptoms, rather symptoms are very slowly progressive. These conditions are also not due hypersensitivity reactions to organic dusts, but rather due to direct fibrogenic reaction within the lung. The clinical examination demonstrates features of pulmonary hypertension, a complication of chronic hypersensitivity pneumonitis. Whilst the presence of anterior Q waves on the ECG, previous history of heart failure, raised venous pressure, and cardiomegaly raise the suspicion of decompensated congestive cardiac failure, the CXR does not show pulmonary oedema. This patient is likely to have chronic heart failure (that has not decompensated), and the elevated venous pressure simply reflects cor pulmonale secondary to cardiorespiratory disease.

Tutorial

Hypersensitivity pneumonitis (extrinsic allergic alveolitis) refers to a group of disorders where inhaled organic antigens trigger a hypersensitivity reaction. Table 11.3 shows the different forms and their related antigens. A period of exposure (several weeks to months) is required before the attacks are actually noticed. The clinical presentation can be acute, subacute, or chronic:

- Acute: symptoms often commence 3–9 hours after exposure to the antigen, and often resolve spontaneously within 12 hours to several days depending on cessation of exposure. Patients abruptly develop flu-like symptoms (fever, chills, malaise, dry cough, chest tightness, headaches, and breathlessness).
- Subacute: gradual development of a dry cough, breathlessness, fatigue, anorexia, and weight loss. This may occur in patients who experience repeated acute attacks.
- Chronic: a history of acute episodes may not be present, with a gradual onset of a dry cough, progressive breathlessness, fatigue, and weight loss. Removing exposure to the antigen only results in partial improvement.

The initial diagnosis relies on the history and abnormal CXR findings. In acute hypersensitivity pneumonitis, diffuse micronodular shadowing (+/– ground-glass appearance) is seen in the mid-lower zones. In subacute hypersensitivity pneumonitis, micronodular or reticulonodular shadowing is seen most prominently in mid-upper zones. In chronic hypersensitivity pneumonitis, fibrotic changes (honeycomb appearance) with loss of lung volume can be seen particularly affecting the upper zones. Precipitating immunoglobulin G antibodies against potential antigens indicate prior exposure and sensitization, but do not necessarily represent disease. Many patients with clinical disease have no detectable antibodies, owing either to testing with an inappropriate antibody or to cessation of exposure. Furthermore, antibodies may be demonstrable in healthy individuals who have had exposure. A high-resolution CT scan will reveal the extent of parenchymal involvement. Spirometry demonstrates a restrictive defect. A severe restrictive or a mixed obstructive and restrictive defect is common in chronic hypersensitivity pneumonitis. A bronchoalveolar lavage may provide supportive information for the diagnosis. A marked lymphocytosis (>20%) is non-specific but helpful, as it helps to differentiate hypersensitivity pneumonitis from idiopathic pulmonary fibrosis (cryptogenic fibrosing alveolitis) where neutrophils predominate. However, an increase in $CD8^+$ T cells and a $CD4^+$:$CD8^+$ <1 is diagnostic. Abnormal bronchoalveolar lavage findings may be seen in asymptomatic individuals with antigen exposure. Transbronchial biopsies are rarely required to make the diagnosis, unless the cause of fibrosis is not clear. It remains the most sensitive way to differentiate between idiopathic pulmonary fibrosis, granulomatous disease, and hypersensitivity pneumonitis.

The management is primarily avoidance of antigen exposure. Corticosteroids are used for severely ill patients with all forms of hypersensitivity pneumonitis. They may accelerate the initial recovery in severe disease, but do not appear to affect long-term prognosis.

Table 11.3 Different forms of hypersensitivity pneumonitis

Disease	Source of exposure	Major antigen
Farmer's lung	Mouldy hay	*Saccharopolyspora rectivirgula* (*Micropolyspora faeni*)
Bagassosis	Mouldy sugar cane fibre	*Thermoactinomyces sacchari*
Grain handler's lung	Mouldy grain	*S. rectivirgula, Thermoactinomyces vulgaris*
Bird fancier's lung	Pigeons, parakeets, fowl, rodents	Avian or animal proteins
Cheese worker's lung	Cheese mould	*Penicillium caseifulvum*
Malt worker's lung	Mouldy malt	*Aspergillus clavatus*
Paprika splitter's lung	Paprika dust	*Mucor stolonifer*
Chemical worker's lung	Manufacture of plastics, polyurethane foam, rubber	Trimellitic anhydride, diisocyanate, methylene diisocyanate

Further Reading

Lacasse Y, Selman M, Costabel U, et al. (2003). Clinical diagnosis of hypersensitivity pneumonitis. *American Journal Respiratory and Critical Care Medicine* 168: 952–958.

237. B) Clarithromycin

This patient presents with a right middle lobe pneumonia with earache (bullous myringitis), maculopapular targetoid skin lesions (erythema multiforme), neurological involvement, deranged LFTs (hepatitis), SIADH, electrocardiographic and echocardiographic findings (indicating a myopericarditis), and an anaemia with evidence of RBC agglutination. The unifying diagnosis is mycoplasma pneumonia. *M. pneumoniae* is susceptible to macrolides and tetracyclines. Penicillins, sulphonamides, and trimethoprim are not effective due to the organism's lack of a cell wall. Oral erythromycin or one of the newer macrolides such as azithromycin or clarithromycin has been the established treatment for mycoplasma pneumonia. Clindamycin is also effective *in vitro*, but may not be active *in vivo* and therefore is not considered a first-line treatment. Fluoroquinolones are generally less potent than macrolides against *M. pneumoniae*. Their advantage lies in the fact that they are active against all classes of bacteria that produce clinically similar respiratory tract infections, including macrolide-resistant *S. pneumoniae*. Of the options given, erythromycin, clarithromycin, and doxycycline would be appropriate antibiotics. Macrolides are the antibiotics of choice for treating *M. pneumoniae* infections. The newer macrolides (clarithromycin and azithromycin) are better tolerated, require fewer doses, and have shorter treatment durations than older compounds. Thus the most appropriate answer is clarithromycin.

Tutorial

Mycoplasma is a well-recognized pathogen that colonizes mucosal surfaces of humans and animals. *M. pneumoniae* infects the upper and lower respiratory tracts, leading to a wide range of pulmonary and extra-pulmonary conditions. *M. pneumoniae* causes up to 40% of cases of community-acquired pneumonia. It can be transmitted by aerosol route from person to person. The incubation period varies from one to three weeks, although it is sometimes as short as four days. Upper respiratory tract symptoms include non-exudative sore throat, hoarseness, fever, dry cough, headache, chills, coryza, myalgias, earache (bullous myringitis), and general malaise. Infections of the lower respiratory tract generally manifest with a dry cough, sometimes with dyspnoea, lymphadenopathy, wheezing, and rarely, with respiratory failure. Although *M. pneumoniae* infections are usually mild, and many are asymptomatic, they are not always self-limiting. *M. pneumoniae* respiratory tract infections are also associated with a wide range of extra-pulmonary manifestations (seen in 25% of patients), including neurological, cardiac, dermatological, musculoskeletal, haematological, and gastrointestinal symptoms (Box 11.10). Extra-pulmonary manifestations can occur before, after, during, or in the absence of respiratory symptoms, but usually occur within three weeks after the onset of respiratory symptoms.

Laboratory investigations can reveal anaemia (autoimmune haemolytic anaemia-cold agglutinins), normal or mild leucocytosis, thrombocytopenia, SIADH, and hepatitis. Cold agglutinins are IgM antibodies directed to antigen 1 on erythrocytes. They are produced 1–2 weeks after infection in 50% of patients and may persist for several weeks. Abnormalities on chest radiographs often appear more severe than the clinical condition of the patient. Diffuse or interstitial infiltrates that involve the lower lobes are the most common radiographic abnormalities.

Box 11.10 Extra-pulmonary manifestations of mycoplasma pneumonia

Neurological

- Aseptic meningitis
- Encephalitis
- Transverse myelitis
- Guillain-Barré syndrome
- Cranial and peripheral neuropathy
- Bullous myringitis

Cardiac

- Myocarditis
- Pericarditis

Rheumatological

- Arthralgia
- Myalgia
- Myositis

Haematological

- Thrombocytopenia
- Cold autoimmune haemolytic anaemia
- Disseminated intravascular coagulation

Gastrointestinal

- Diarrhoea
- Vomiting
- Hepatitis
- Pancreatitis

Dermatological

- Erythema nodosum
- Erythema multiforme
- Steven-Johnson syndrome

Endocrine

- Syndrome of inappropriate ADH secretion (SIADH)

Renal

- Glomerulonephritis
- Interstitial nephritis

Diagnosis of *M. pneumoniae* infection is usually by isolation of organism from respiratory system (PCR methods to amplify specific mycoplasma DNA fragments) and serological methods (passive agglutination, complement fixation tests, and ELISA). Serological test for anti-*Mycoplasma* antibody is the most common method for retrospective diagnosis. A four-fold rise in complement fixation tests between acute and convalescent specimens or a single high anti-*Mycoplasma* complement fixation antibody titre of >1:128 indicates an acute infection. Detection of IgM antibodies is more sensitive, and can give positive results on a single specimen.

Further Reading

Cunha B (2006). The atypical pneumonias: clinical diagnosis and importance. *Clinical Microbiology and Infections* 12(3):12–24.

238. E) Serum α-1 antitrypsin

This young patient presents with progressive breathlessness. She has hyperinflated lungs, an obstructive defect (FEV1:FVC <70%), and reduced KCO. She has deranged LFTs suggestive of liver cirrhosis. This should raise the strong suspicion of α-1 antitrypsin deficiency. She is a smoker, which can lead to significantly earlier presentation in patients with α-1 antitrypsin deficiency (20–30 years earlier). The CXR demonstrates hyperlucent and oligaemic lungs fields consistent with this diagnosis.

There is a history of intensive dieting and use of appetite suppressants designed to mislead the candidate. Various appetite suppressants, for example fenfluramine have been linked with the development of primary pulmonary hypertension that may account for deranged LFTs, especially a cholestatic picture (as seen here) due to hepatic congestion. However, the clinical signs do not demonstrate elevated venous pressures and whilst primary pulmonary hypertension may result in a reduced KCO it will not result in a hyperinflated chest with evidence of airway obstruction on lung function tests. She has a budgerigar which raises the suspicion of hypersensitivity pneumonitis, but the history is not suggestive and this would cause a restrictive defect on lung function tests. The presence of hypoalbuminaemia and proteinuria on urinalysis may raise the suspicion of nephritic syndrome. However, the hypoalbuminaemia may be due to liver disease or poor appetite, and the proteinuria is not significant to make nephrotic syndrome the primary diagnosis. Furthermore, nephrotic syndrome would not account for the lung function tests and deranged LFTs. Whilst a liver biopsy may be useful in demonstrating cirrhosis, the findings on liver biopsy are not specific and will not make a definitive diagnosis.

Tutorial

α-1 antitrypsin deficiency is an autosomal dominant condition. The genetic defect is on chromosome 14, which encodes α-1 antitrypsin (*SERPINA1* gene). The primary function of this enzyme is to inhibit neutrophils proteases (trypsin, elastase, proteinase 3, cathepsin G). There are three main phenotypes of this enzyme, which can be characterized by their electrophoretic mobility: M (medium), S (slow), and Z (very slow)—Table 11.4. The most common form of α-1 antitrypsin deficiency is associated with allele Z, PiZZ. Other genotypes associated with severe alpha1-antitrypsin deficiency include PiSZ, PiZ/Null, and PiNull. The null gene is the least common of the known alleles associated with alpha1-antitrypsin deficiency. Patients with the null gene for α-1 antitrypsin will not produce any α-1 antitrypsin and are at high risk for developing emphysema (100% by the age of 30 years). Those with the null gene do not develop liver disease because of a lack of production, and thus the absence of accumulation of α-1 antitrypsin in the hepatocytes. The Pi ZZ genotype predisposes to the development of hepatocellular carcinoma. Serum levels >11 μmol/L appear to be protective, and emphysema usually develops with serum levels <9 μmol/L.

Hepatocytes synthesize α-1 antitrypsin, and release it into the serum. After its release, it circulates and diffuses into interstitial and alveolar fluids. The genetic defect results in alteration of the configuration of the α-1 antitrypsin molecule, which prevents its release from hepatocytes. As a result, the serum and alveolar concentrations of α-1 antitrypsin are low, leading to destruction of lung tissue by the neutrophil proteases. The pattern of lung damage is pan-acinar with a predilection for the lower lobes. Furthermore, the accumulation of α-1 antitrypsin in the hepatocytes leads to destruction of these cells, manifesting as chronic liver disease.

The initial symptoms are limited to the respiratory system and include cough and wheezing. Often, they present many times to physicians, and are diagnosed with asthma or COPD (of unknown aetiology). Patients may be treated with multiple courses of antibiotics and evaluated for sinusitis, postnasal drip, or gastroesophageal reflux. After the age of 30–35 years there is an accelerated decline in FEV_1 which is considerably worsened by cigarette smoking. In non-smokers, symptoms are generally seen at around 50 years of age, while smokers will be symptomatic by 30–40 years.

Diagnosis is based on checking serum α-1 antitrypsin levels and determining the phenotype with electromobility testing. The CXR often shows hyperlucent lung fields, often with a predilection for the bases. They may be described as oligaemic because they lack the normal pattern of branching blood vessels. High resolution CT scan of the chest can be used to demonstrate the extent of disease. In symptomatic patients at time of diagnosis, spirometry demonstrates moderate-to-severe airflow obstruction with an FEV_1 in the range of 30–40% of the predicted value. Lung volumes are increased secondary to air trapping. All patients with emphysema have reduced KCO, and KCO is significantly reduced (<50% of predicted value) in most symptomatic patients. The presentation of liver disease is highly variable and ranges from chronic hepatitis and cirrhosis to fulminant hepatic failure. The biochemical and histopathologic findings may be similar to those of adult alcoholic liver disease. Findings on liver biopsy are highly variable (giant cell transformation, lobular hepatitis, significant steatosis, fibrosis, hepatocellular necrosis, bile duct paucity, or bile duct proliferation). Periodic acid-Schiff (PAS) staining highlights the red 'globules' in hepatocytes. However, PAS-positive inclusions are not absolutely specific for α-1 antitrypsin deficiency. A liver biopsy is not necessary to establish the diagnosis, but can help to assess the degree of organ injury or disease progression.

Treatment consists of smoking cessation, enzyme replacement therapy (if levels <11 mmol/L), management of emphysema, lung transplantation (for severe emphysema), and liver transplantation (severe liver disease). Liver transplantation results in conversion to the genotype of the donor.

Table 11.4 The different phenotypes in α-1 antitrypsin deficiency

Phenotype	% normal serum α-1 antitrypsin levels	Risk of developing emphysema
Pi MM	100% (20–53 µmol/L)	General population
Pi MS	80%	Very low
Pi SS	60%	Low
Pi MZ	60%	Low
Pi SZ	40%	Moderate
Pi ZZ	10% (3–7 µmol/L)	High
Pi Z-null	<10% (<3 µmol/L)	Very high
Pi null-null	None	Very high

Further Reading

Kelly E, Greene C, Carroll T, McElvaney N, O'Neill S (2010). Alpha-1 antitrypsin deficiency. *Respiratory Medicine* 104: 763–772.

239. C) Full blood count

This patient has a history of hereditary haemorrhagic telangiectasia (HHT). He presents with progressive breathlessness. Physical examination is normal. The CXR and ABG demonstrate no abnormality. The spirometry demonstrates normal lung volumes, but the only abnormality is a reduced KCO. The primary cause of a reduced KCO with otherwise normal spirometry is anaemia or pulmonary arteriovenous malformation (PAVM). PAVMs are common in HHT (approximately 70% of PAVMs are associated with HHT, and 15–30% of patients with HHT have a PAVM), which would be diagnosed using a contrast-enhanced CT scan of the chest or CT pulmonary angiography. PAVMs result in an abnormal communication between the pulmonary artery and pulmonary vein, thus lead to a right-to-left shunt. This is often associated with the finding of a pulmonary nodule on CXR, and in symptomatic patients, this is associated with hypoxia and cyanosis. Thus the diagnosis of PAVM is unlikely. In this case, anaemia could be due to gastrointestinal blood loss in the context of HHT, and is the most likely cause for breathlessness in this patient. Thus the most appropriate initial test is a full blood count.

The history, examination, and investigations are not suggestive of heart failure or pulmonary hypertension. Heart failure is unlikely given a normal ECG, absence of cardiomegaly on CXR, and clear lung fields. The CXR in pulmonary hypertension will demonstrate prominent pulmonary vasculature at the hila, and may produce a restrictive lung defect. Breathlessness in a young smoker raises the possibility of α-1 antitrypsin deficiency. In α-1 antitrypsin deficiency, symptomatic patients at presentation would demonstrate an obstructive lung defect, with a reduced FEV_1 and increased TLC. Liver function tests may demonstrate liver involvement but would not be diagnostic for this condition.

Tutorial

The diffusing capacity is a measure of the conductance of the CO molecule from the alveolar gas to haemoglobin in the pulmonary capillary blood. The terms often used are DLCO or TLCO, also known as the transfer factor of the lung for CO (TLCO). This is a measurement of the ease of transfer for CO molecules from alveolar gas to the haemoglobin of the red blood cells in the pulmonary circulation. The transfer of the CO molecule is limited by both perfusion and diffusion. CO (and oxygen) must pass through the alveolar epithelium, tissue interstitium, capillary endothelium, blood plasma, and red cell membrane and cytoplasm before attaching to the haemoglobin molecule. An abnormal haemoglobin level can affect the diffusing capacity and, if known, should be used to mathematically correct the measured diffusing capacity to normal haemoglobin. Anaemia will reduce TLCO and polycythaemia will increase TLCO. When the TLCO is divided by the alveolar volume (V_A), this gives KCO, which corrects for different lung volumes. On this basis, both asthma and COPD will result in a reduced TLCO, but the KCO is reduced in COPD, due to increase in V_A, but is normal or increased in asthma. Pleural thickening results in smaller lung volumes, thus can result in increased KCO (despite a normal TLCO). The causes of reduced and increased KCO are listed in Boxes 11.11 and 11.12 respectively.

Box 11.11 Causes of a reduced KCO

- Interstitial lung disease
- COPD
- Pulmonary oedema
- Thromboembolic disease
- Primary pulmonary hypertension
- Right-to-left shunt
- Anaemia
- Lymphangitis carcinomatosa

Box 11.12 Causes of increased KCO

- Left-to-right shunts
- Pulmonary haemorrhage
- Thoracic cage abnormalities, for example kyphoscoliosis
- Lung resection (lobectomy/pneumonectomy)
- Asthma
- Polycythaemia
- Pleural thickening
- Following exercise

Further Reading

Olitsky S (20100. Hereditary hemorrhagic telangiectasia: diagnosis and management. *American Family Physician* 82(7): 785–790.

240. D) Histoplasmosis

This young smoker presented eight months earlier, after a caving holiday, with an acute febrile illness, arthralgia, erythema nodosum, and dry cough. This is highly suggestive of acute histoplasmosis. *Histoplasma capsulatum* is found in bird and bat excreta, and a history of dust inhalation from a cave with bats, as in this case, or a bird-house, is often found in patients with acute histoplasmosis. He now presents with protracted symptoms of fevers, dry cough, and breathlessness. The CXR demonstrates a solitary nodule with ipsilateral hilar adenopathy, consistent with this diagnosis. Investigations reveal a pancytopaenia, raised inflammatory markers, deranged LFTs, and raised LDH, indicating chronic disseminated disease (bone marrow and liver involvement).

An elevated serum ACE with a high-normal calcium may suggest sarcoidosis, but this is rare in young Caucasian males and CXR would usually show bilateral versus unilateral hilar adenopathy. A raised serum ACE is not specific for sarcoidosis (Box 11.13), and hypercalcaemia can be seen in disseminated disease. Coccidioidomycosis has a similar presentation, and remains an important differential diagnosis for histoplasmosis. *Coccidioides immitis* is found in soil, geographically confined to Southwestern USA, northern Mexico, and areas of Central and South America, and given the absence of travel to these endemic areas, histoplasmosis is more likely. Carcinoma of the lung is an important differential for a solitary pulmonary nodule with ipsilateral hilar adenopathy in a smoker with chronic respiratory symptoms and weight loss—the pancytopenia could be explained by bone marrow infiltration and hepatomegaly by metastases. However, a primary lung carcinoma with disseminated metastases is unlikely in a young man of this age and he would be far more symptomatic and cachexic. Given this man's occupation, a hypersensitivity pneumonitis is possible due to inhalation of various antigens in the plastics industry (trimellitic anhydride and methylene diisocyanate). However, this is likely to affect both lungs and produce a restrictive pattern on spirometry.

Tutorial

Histoplasma capsulatum is a dimorphic fungus that remains in a mycelial form at ambient temperatures and grows as yeast at body temperature in mammals. It is predominantly found in river valleys in North and Central America, Eastern and Southern Europe. Soil containing large amounts of bird or bat excreta supports growth of *H. capsulatum*. Caves can be highly contaminated by *H. capsulatum* that thrives on the bat excreta. Most individuals with histoplasmosis are asymptomatic. Those who develop clinical manifestations are usually immunocompromised or are exposed to a high quantity of inoculum. There are three main syndromes caused by histoplasmosis:

Acute pulmonary histoplasmosis

Symptoms often develop 3–14 days after exposure, but most patients are asymptomatic. Fever, headaches, malaise, and myalgia are common. Erythema nodosum and erythema multiforme are the most common skin manifestations. Acute severe pulmonary infection also occurs when a person is exposed to a large inoculum of *H. capsulatum*. CXR may show a patchy infiltrates with a predilection for the lower lobes, enlarged hilar and mediastinal lymph nodes, or diffuse reticulonodular infiltrates. As the infiltrates resolve, the remaining nodules often calcify, leaving the appearance of 'buckshot' throughout the lung fields. Histoplasmomas are healed pulmonary lesions that appear as residual nodules on CXR, usually 1–4 cm in diameter. This infection is self-limiting, and many patients will recover without treatment, but severe disease should always be treated, because respiratory compromise can occur and recovery without antifungal therapy is slow.

Chronic pulmonary histoplasmosis

This occurs in older patients with underlying pulmonary disease and is associated with fever, weight loss, cough, breathlessness, and fatigue. It often involves the apical lung segments near emphysematous bullae. Pleural thickening is often seen. Cavitation of lung lesions can result in haemoptysis. CXR will often show cavitations predominantly in the upper lobes; calcified nodes from prior healed infections; and fibrotic changes in long-standing disease; but hilar lymphadenopathy is rare.

Disseminated histoplasmosis

This occurs mostly in immunocompromised patients. Symptoms vary depending on duration of illness. The acute form may produce fever, cough, weight loss, malaise, and breathlessness with

CNS involvement in 5–20% of cases. The subacute form is associated with a wide spectrum of symptoms depending on the organs involved. Gastrointestinal involvement may produce diarrhoea and abdominal pain. Cardiac involvement results in pericarditis, pericardial effusions, and endocarditis, with sequelae of valvular disease. CNS involvement may produce headaches, visual disturbances, confusion, and seizures. Haematological involvement results in bone marrow infiltration with pancytopaenia, hepatosplenomegaly, and lymphadenopathy. The chronic form is associated with constitutional symptoms. Oropharyngeal mucous membrane lesions are common in disseminated histoplasmosis. In acute disseminated histoplasmosis, pancytopaenia occurs in 70–90% of patients, but may occur in chronic disseminated histoplasmosis. Hypercalcaemia and raised lactate dehydrogenase levels may be seen in disseminated disease.

Blood and sputum cultures are often negative. Antibody tests play an important role in the diagnosis. The standard assays are the complement fixation test and the immunodiffusion assay. Diagnosis is based on a four-fold rise in complement fixation antibody titre; a single titre of ≥1:32 is suggestive but not diagnostic. Complement fixation antibodies persist for years after infection; thus, the presence of a single low titre means previous exposure to *H. capsulatum*. The complement fixation test appears to be less specific than the immunodiffusion assay- cross-reactions that occur with other fungal infections and other granulomatous diseases, including TB and sarcoidosis. A rising complement fixation titre confirms the diagnosis. The immunodiffusion assay tests for the presence of M and H precipitin bands. An M band develops with acute infection, is often present in chronic forms of histoplasmosis, and persists for months to years after the infection has resolved. An H band is much less common, is rarely, if ever, found without an M band, and is indicative of chronic or severe acute forms of histoplasmosis. Urinary antigen detection is useful in individuals who are immunocompromised when antibody production may be impaired. Other fungal infections, for example blastomycosis, coccidioidomycosis, and penicilliosis may cause false-positive urinary antigen results.

Treatment with anti-fungal therapy is indicated in acute severe histoplasmosis, chronic cavitatory pulmonary disease, and disseminated disease. Amphotericin B and itraconazole are the recommended agents.

Box 11.13 Causes of increased serum ACE

- Sarcoidosis
- TB
- Asbestosis
- Berylliosis
- Silicosis
- Histoplasmosis
- Hyperthyroidism
- Lymphoma
- Gaucher's disease
- Primary biliary cirrhosis
- Scleroderma
- Hepatitis
- Leprosy
- Amyloidosis
- Diabetes

Further Reading

Kauffman C (2007). Histoplasmosis: a clinical and laboratory update. *Clinical Microbiology Reviews* 20: 115–132.

Kauffman C (2009). Histoplasmosis. *Clinic in Chest Medicine* 30: 217–225.

241. A) Histiocytosis X

This patient has a history of spontaneous pneumothorax, and now presents with chronic respiratory symptoms and weight loss. There is a history of polyuria and polydipsia (suggestive of diabetes insipidus). The CXR demonstrates upper-mid zone interstitial changes. The spirometry demonstrates a mixed obstructive and restrictive with a reduced KCO. Of the choices given, histiocytosis X is the unifying diagnosis. A history of a cough and arthralgia in patient with raised serum ACE and a high normal calcium may raise the suspicion of sarcoidosis. Furthermore, pituitary infiltration leading to diabetes insipidus is recognized in sarcoidosis. Whilst the CXR may be in keeping with sarcoidosis, the absence of hilar lymphadenopathy is against this, and spirometry often demonstrates a restrictive lung defect, although mixed patterns may be seen in a small proportion of patients.

A raised serum ACE is not specific to sarcoidosis and may be seen in histiocytosis X. The high calcium and raised alkaline phosphatase seen in this case may indicate lytic bone lesions in histiocytosis X. The occupational history raises the possibility of hypersensitivity pneumonitis or occupational asthma. Hypersensitivity pneumonitis is often associated with a restrictive defect, whilst asthma would be associated with an obstructive defect. Furthermore they would not account for other features in the history. Lymphangioleiomyomatosis (LAM) is a rare disorder characterized by proliferation of an immature smooth muscle cell (LAM cell) in the lung and kidney, typically occurring in premenopausal women. This may lead to airflow obstruction, air trapping, formation of bullae, and pneumothoraces. Obstruction of lymphatics may result in chylothorax, chyluria, and chylous ascites. Obstruction of venules may result in haemosiderosis and haemoptysis. Excessive proteolytic activity, associated with LAM cells, may lead to lung destruction and formation of cystic lesions. Patients often present with cough and breathlessness. Other complications include alveolar haemorrhage, pericardial effusion, pneumoperitoneum, and lymphoedema.

Tutorial

Histiocytosis X (also known as eosinophilic granuloma) is an uncommon interstitial lung disease that predominantly affects young adults, primarily occurring in the third or fourth decades of life. It is characterized by parenchymal infiltration of the lungs by activated Langerhans cells. It is epidemiologically related to tobacco smoking, and accumulation of Langerhans cells in the lungs is hypothesized to occur in response to exposure to cigarette smoke. Cigarette smoking worsens morbidity and mortality, and smoking cessation frequently stabilizes the disease and sometimes leads to its regression.

Symptoms include fever, dry cough, breathlessness, fatigue, weight loss, and atypical chest pains. Spontaneous pneumothorax, which may be recurrent, is seen in 10–20% of patients. Cystic bone lesions may be painful and may predispose to pathologic fractures. Common sites of bone lesions include the skull, vertebra, rib, mandible, femur, ilium, and scapula. Infiltration in hands and feet is unusual. When skull lesions extend they may cause otitis media by destruction of the temporal and mastoid bones, proptosis secondary to orbital masses, loose teeth from infiltration of the mandibles, or pituitary stalk dysfunction (diabetes insipidus) due to involvement of the sella turcica. Most cases of established diabetes insipidus are irreversible at the time of presentation. Cutaneous manifestations include petechiae and yellow-brown papules topped with scale and crust. Hepatosplenomegaly and lymphadenopathy can be seen in 50% of cases. The triad of diabetes insipidus, exophthalmos, and lytic bone lesions is known as the Hand-Schüller-Christian syndrome.

The CXR characteristically shows bilateral, symmetrical, poorly-defined nodules and reticulonodular infiltrates with a predilection for the upper zones. As the disease progresses, cystic lesions appear. Mediastinal or hilar lymphadenopathy is rare and should prompt the suspicion of sarcoidosis or malignancy. A high resolution CT scan of the chest may be diagnostic. Pathognomonic findings include nodules and cysts, predominantly in the mid and upper lung zones, with sparing of the costophrenic regions. The nodules may be cavitatory and variable in size. Likewise, the cysts may be of various diameters and wall thicknesses. If nodules are an isolated finding, then other granulomatous disorders cannot be excluded. If cysts are an isolated finding, then LAM must be considered. In LAM, the cysts are uniformly distributed throughout the lungs, and sparing of the costophrenic angles is supportive of histiocytosis X. Spirometry demonstrates an obstructive, restrictive or mixed defect. Bronchoalveolar lavage fluid demonstrating a greater than 5% increase in the number of Langerhans cells is supportive of the diagnosis. Histological demonstration of Langerhans cells in affected tissues (bone, lung, or skin biopsy) is the most sensitive and specific test. Langerhans cells demonstrate the characteristic intracytoplasmic Birbeck granules.

Smoking cessation is the most important therapeutic intervention. Corticosteroids may be considered in patients with persistent respiratory or constitutional symptoms, but are not indicated in patients with normal lung function. Many cytotoxic drugs including etoposide, mercaptopurine, vinblastine, cyclophosphamide, and arabinoside may be useful in selected cases. Lytic bone lesions can be treated with surgical curettage, corticosteroid injection, irradiation, bisphosphonates, or NSAIDs. Diabetes insipidus can be treated with desmopressin therapy.

Further Reading

Herwig M, Wojno T, Zhang Q, Grossniklaus H (2013). Langerhans cell histiocytosis of the orbit: five clinicopathologic cases and review of the literature. *Survey of Ophthalmology* 58(4): 330–340.

242. C) Repeat arterial blood gas

The arterial blood gas gives a pH of 7.2, indicating acidosis. However, the pCO_2 and HCO_3^- are normal. Furthermore, the anion gap ($[Na^+ + K^+] - [HCO_3^- + Cl^-] = 10.1$) is normal. This should raise the strong suspicion that there has been a laboratory error. The most appropriate next step is to repeat the arterial blood gas. There are many confounders in the history to distract the candidate. In the context of COPD, a respiratory acidosis should prompt the need for non-invasive ventilation. A metabolic acidosis with an increased anion gap should prompt the consideration of lactic acidosis in a patient on metformin therapy.

Tutorial

The acidity of body fluids is measured by the pH, where $pH = -\log[H+]$. The relationship between $[H^+]$ and $HCO_3^- CO_2$ buffering system can be provided by the modified Henderson-Hasselbalch equation:

Given that $pH = -\log[H+]$, this equation can be re-arranged to give the following:

Thus the $HCO3^-$:pCO_2 ratio determines the pH. Thus an increase in $HCO3^-$ or decrease in pCO_2 will increase pH (alkalosis), and similarly, a decrease in $HCO3^-$ or increase in pCO_2 will reduce pH (acidosis). In the given question, this ratio is normal, and should at once prompt the suspicion of a laboratory error.

Further Reading

Hall J (2015). Respiratory insufficiency—pathophysiology, diagnosis, oxygen therapy. In *Guyton and Hall Textbook of Medical Physiology*, Thirteenth Edition. Saunders Elsevier, Philadelphia, USA.

243. C) Replace oxygen with 24% venturi mask

This patient presents with acute type II respiratory failure. The arterial blood gas demonstrates an adequate pO_2, but profound hypercapnia on high-flow oxygen. This patient is likely to have chronic hypercapnia, given the elevated HCO_3^-, indicating metabolic compensation. However, a fall in pH indicates acute respiratory acidosis. The confusion in this patient reflects the hypercapnia. The first and foremost thing to do is to deliver controlled oxygen via a 24% venturi mask. Often this, in conjunction with nebulized bronchodilators, will result in an improvement. If, however, reducing the supplementary oxygen results in significant hypoxia, or does not result in an improvement of the acid-base status, then non-invasive ventilation or intubation should be considered. Hudson face masks are less precise than venturi masks, and can worsen the hypercapnia if flow rate <5 L/min due to re-breathing of CO_2. Whilst aminophylline is a bronchodilator and can act as respiratory stimulant, its use should be considered in exacerbations of COPD, only after establishing a poor response to nebulized bronchodilator therapy.

Tutorial

Some patients with COPD are very sensitive to uncontrolled oxygen therapy and easily develop type II respiratory failure. The consequences of the increased pCO_2 are respiratory acidosis, tachycardia, seizures, coma, respiratory arrest, and death. The major processes which contribute to worsening hypercapnia in the setting of administration of supplementary uncontrolled oxygen to patients with COPD are:

(1) Worsened ventilation-perfusion matching due to attenuation of hypoxic pulmonary vasoconstriction—increased perfusion of diseased alveoli compared to less-diseased alveoli. Thus, a larger fraction of blood passes through parts of the lung that are poorly-ventilated, with a resultant increase in the pCO_2.

(2) Decreased binding affinity of haemoglobin for carbon dioxide.

(3) A reduction in the 'hypoxic drive'—CO_2 narcosis. When CO_2 levels are chronically elevated, the respiratory centres becomes less sensitive to CO_2 as a respiratory stimulant—in such cases, it is the PO_2 that provides the primary stimulus for respiration. Thus excess supplemental oxygen can potentially suppress the respiratory centre, further increasing pCO_2.

Paramedics are unable to deliver controlled oxygen therapy and this is responsible for considerable mortality and morbidity in the COPD population. However, in the absence of controlled oxygen, it is essential to administer oxygen to patients with significant hypoxia to avoid the potentially life-threatening complications of a low pO_2. Chronic hypercapnia is common in patients with COPD and a raised HCO_3^-, demonstrating metabolic compensation, should indicate this. However, when the pH falls, this indicates acute respiratory acidosis (type II respiratory failure). The first and foremost thing to do in this setting is to establish the clinical status of the patient and determine whether this is not due to uncontrolled supplementary oxygen. Often administering controlled oxygen therapy and bronchodilators will result in an improvement. However, if reducing the supplementary oxygen will result in a significant drop in pO_2, then non-invasive ventilation should be considered.

Further Reading

National Institute for Clinical Excellence (2019). Chronic obstructive pulmonary disease in over 16s: diagnosis and management. (NG115). Dec 2018, updated July 2019. Available at: https://www.nice.org.uk/guidance/ng115

244. C) A long-acting muscarinic antagonist inhaler

This patient has a long-standing history of smoking. She presents with progressive breathlessness. CXR demonstrates hyperinflated lung fields. Spirometry demonstrates an obstructive pattern with an FEV_1 of 48%. The diagnosis is COPD-the FEV_1 indicates moderate severity. She is currently on a short-acting β_2-agonist inhaler, but is still symptomatic. According to the current NICE guidelines, increasing inhaled therapy is indicated. The FEV1 in this setting dictates the use of different therapies. If the FEV1 $\geq$50%, then one should consider the addition of a long-acting β_2-agonist or long-acting muscarinic antagonist inhaler. If the FEV1<50%, then one should consider long-acting β_2-agonist inhaler plus an inhaled corticosteroid (in a combined inhaler) or a long-acting muscarinic antagonist inhaler. This patient has an FEV <50%, and from the options provided, a long-acting muscarinic antagonist inhaler is the next most appropriate management step.

Tutorial

COPD is defined as progressive and irreversible (or partially reversible—30% of patients demonstrate an increase in FEV_1 by 15% or more after bronchodilator therapy) airflow obstruction due to chronic bronchitis or emphysema. Air flow obstruction is defined as FEV_1 <80% predicted *and* FEV_1: FVC <70%. Chronic bronchitis is a clinical diagnosis defined as cough productive of sputum on most days for three months during two consecutive years. Emphysema is a pathological diagnosis defined as abnormal and permanent enlargement of air spaces distal to the terminal bronchioles. The traditional difference between emphysema and chronic bronchitis is describing patients as either a 'pink-puffer' or a 'blue bloater' (see Table 11.5). This classification is not used in clinical practice, as often patients have a combination of emphysema and bronchitis. When emphysema is more predominant, loss of elastic recoil rather than bronchiolar inflammation is the mechanism of airflow limitation. When bronchitis is more predominant, bronchiolar inflammation is more responsible for airflow limitation. The severity of COPD can be defined on spirometry parameters (Table 11.6).

The typical CXR findings include: hyper-inflated lung fields with flattened hemidiaphragms; long narrow heart shadow; hyper-lucency of lung fields; bullae; increased retrosternal airspace in lateral films; and prominent hilar pulmonary vasculature (if pulmonary hypertension is present). Spirometry will show FEV_1 <80% predicted AND FEV_1: FVC <70% (airflow obstruction), ↑ TLC, FRC and RV, ↓ VC, ↓ T_LCO, and KCO (decreased in proportion to severity of COPD).

The general management of chronic COPD comprises smoking cessation, immunizations for influenza and pneumococcal pneumonia, and prompt treatment of respiratory infections (antibiotics and steroids). The current treatment algorithm for the use of inhaled bronchodilators and corticosteroids can be found in the most recent NICE COPD guideline, a summary of which can be found at: https://www.nice.org.uk/guidance/ng115/resources/visual-summary-treatment-algorithm-pdf-6604261741. Long-term oral steroids are not usually recommended in COPD. Some patients with advanced COPD may require maintenance oral steroids when they cannot be withdrawn following an exacerbation. Mucolytic therapy may be considered in patients with chronic productive cough and continued if there is symptomatic improvement. Inappropriate oxygen therapy in patients with COPD may cause hypercapnia and respiratory depression; therefore patients are selected carefully using specific criteria (see tutorial for question 243).

Table 11.5 Differences between chronic bronchitis and emphysema

Feature	Chronic bronchitis	Emphysema
Diagnosis	**A** clinical diagnosis	**A** pathological diagnosis
Appearance	'Blue bloater'	'Pink puffer'
Cyanosis	Prominent	Absent
Hyper-inflation	+	++
Dyspnoea	+	++
Cor pulmonale	++	+
Inspiratory drive	Reduced	Present

Table 11.6 Classifying severity of COPD based on spirometry

	Severity	FEV1: FVC	FEV1 (% predicted)
Stage 1	Mild	<70%	≥80%
Stage 2	Moderate	<70%	50–79%
Stage 3	Severe	<70%	30–49%
Stage 4	Very severe	<70%	<30% [A]

[A] Or FEV_1 <50% with respiratory failure.

Further Reading

National Institute for Clinical Excellence (2019). Chronic obstructive pulmonary disease in over 16s: diagnosis and management. (NG115). Dec 2018, updated July 2019. Available at: https://www.nice.org.uk/guidance/ng115

245. E) Spurious hypoxaemia

This patient has CML with significant leucocytosis, and presented with a DVT. He has no respiratory symptoms. The CXR is normal. Given the absence of respiratory symptoms, normal oxygen saturations on pulse oximetry, and absence of tachycardia, the pre-test probability for PE is low and the VQ scan is negative for PE. However, the pO_2 is very low on the arterial blood gas sample, and this may lead the candidate to think of many diagnoses. CT pulmonary angiography remains the gold standard to diagnose PE, so candidates may still consider this given the low pO_2 but this would cause low peripheral oxygen saturations and also cause symptoms. For similar reasons, pulmonary leucostasis which can cause hypoxaemia in patients with profound leucocytosis, is also incorrect.

There are no features in the history to suggest methaemoglobinaemia, in which patients are cyanosed with normal pO_2 and reduced oxygen saturations on pulse oximetry. Intra-cardiac shunts are unlikely, as in the context of a low pO_2 one would expect low oxygen saturations on pulse oximetry, cyanosis, and the CXR would show prominent pulmonary vasculature with plethoric lung fields. The RBBB on the ECG can be a normal finding in individuals, especially in the context of a normal axis, and the ECG showing RBBB in this question may distract the candidate to make the diagnosis of atrial septal defect. The crucial point here is that there is a discrepancy between oxygen saturation as measured by pulse oximetry and pO_2 on arterial blood gas analysis, in an otherwise well patient with no respiratory symptoms and normal CXR. The most likely explanation is 'leucocyte larceny', a phenomenon where spurious hypoxaemia results on arterial blood gas analysis in patients with profound leucocytosis or thrombocytosis.

Tutorial

Patients with profound leucocytosis in the setting of acute myeloid or lymphoblastic leukaemia or those with chronic leukaemias in the accelerated phase are at risk for both true and spurious hypoxemia. This can also occur in patients with significant thrombocytosis. Spurious hypoxemia may occur for a number of reasons, including improper sampling (venous blood), delay in transport with failure to cool the specimen, presence of air bubbles in the sample, leucocytosis or thrombocytosis. In the presence of leucocytosis or thrombocytosis, spuriously low levels of pO_2 are believed to reflect a metabolic consumption of dissolved oxygen from the arterial blood gas specimen, a phenomenon sometimes referred to as 'leucocyte larceny'. This results in a low pO_2 and can increase pCO_2 in the sample. White blood cells have a comparatively high metabolic rate and thus are an important source of oxygen consumption, monocytes having the highest rate of oxygen consumption. Pulse oximetry is generally viewed as the most accurate way of assessing oxygenation in patients with profound leucocytosis or thrombocytosis. An arterial blood gas sample should be analysed immediately and transported on ice to slow the metabolism of leucocytes and platelets. It has been suggested that adding sodium fluoride or potassium cyanide to the arterial blood sample can inhibit leucocyte metabolism and prevent oxygen uptake within the blood sample.

Further Reading

Lele A, Mirski M, Stevens R (2005). Spurious hypoxemia. *Critical Care Medicine* 33: 1854–1856.

246. E) Urgent anaesthetic review and ventilation

This patient presents with an infective exacerbation of COPD with type II respiratory failure and respiratory acidosis. In such a setting, patients should be given non-invasive ventilation. However, he is hypotensive and haemodynamically unstable, so non-invasive ventilation is contraindicated. This patient needs urgent intubation and ventilation. Whilst nebulizers, antibiotics, and steroids are important in the acute management of infective exacerbation of COPD, the single most important intervention for this patient is intubation and ventilation.

Tutorial

Patients with COPD and type II respiratory failure with respiratory acidosis, require respiratory support. This can be delivered either through (1) non-invasive ventilation through a fitted face mask or (2) intubation and ventilation. Whilst non-invasive ventilation can prevent the need for intubation and ventilation, and has been shown to reduce morbidity, mortality, and length of hospital stay compared to intubation, it is important to be aware of its limitations.

The criteria for using non-invasive ventilation are: (1) able to protect airway; (2) conscious and cooperative; (3) no excessive respiratory secretions; (4) potential for recovery to quality of life acceptable to the patient; and (5) patient's wishes considered. However, non-invasive ventilation may be considered if the patient is unconscious and endotracheal intubation is deemed inappropriate or it is to be provided in an intensive care setting.

Contraindications to the use of non-invasive ventilation include: facial trauma/burns; recent facial, upper airway, or upper gastrointestinal tract surgery; fixed upper airway obstruction; inability to protect airway; life-threatening hypoxaemia; haemodynamic instability; severe co-morbidity; and impaired consciousness (confusion/agitation); undrained pneumothorax; vomiting; copious respiratory secretions; or against the patient's wishes.

Further Reading

Royal College of Physicians/British Thoracic Society (2008). Non-invasive ventilation in chronic obstructive pulmonary disease: management of acute type 2 respiratory failure. Available at: http://www.brit-thoracic.org.uk

247. D) Psittacosis

This question has many confounding factors designed to distract the candidate. This cattle and sheep farmer presents with an acute febrile illness with dry cough and breathlessness. The clinical history and CXR finding are consistent with left basal consolidation. There is leucocytosis, raised inflammatory markers, and deranged LFTs. He is a farmer, with intermittent symptoms over the previous six months, suggestive of a hypersensitivity pneumonitis (extrinsic allergic alveolitis). Positive precipitins for *Micropolyspora faeni* suggest farmer's lung. However, positive precipitins only confirm exposure and are not diagnostic. Furthermore, CXR findings are often bilateral, confined to the mid-upper zones, and do not include consolidation. Similarly, he has recently started to keep budgerigars, and positive precipitins for avian proteins may raise the suspicion of bird fancier's lung—another form of hypersensitivity pneumonitis. But again, positive precipitins only confirm exposure and are not diagnostic. The CXR findings would be similar to those seen in farmer's lung, and thus cannot account for this presentation.

This patient has an acute pneumonia, and the most likely pathogen is *Chlamydia psittaci*, an obligate intracellular bacterium from birds. Q fever is a zoonosis caused by *Coxiella burnetii*, that infects different hosts, including humans, ruminant livestock (cattle, sheep, goats), and pets. A history of acute febrile illness in a livestock farmer may lead to the consideration of acute Q fever. Acute Q fever may present in a similar fashion with fever, headaches, dry cough, pneumonia, and deranged LFTs. However, the full blood count in acute Q fever often shows a normal WCC with mild thrombocytopenia.

Tutorial

Psittacosis is an infection caused by the obligatory intracellular bacterium, *Chlamydia psittaci* that can infect parrots, parakeets, canaries, and other avian species (e.g. turkeys, pigeons, and ducks). It is an occupational disease of zoo and pet-shop employees, poultry farmers, and ranchers. Human-to-human transmission is rare. Transmission is via the respiratory route, and infection develops after organisms from aerosolized dried avian excreta or respiratory secretions from sick birds are inhaled. The incubation period is generally 5–14 days. Patients often present with fever, malaise, dry cough, and breathlessness. Other symptoms include headache, photophobia, pharyngitis, and epistaxis. Gastrointestinal symptoms are rare. Skin manifestations include Horder spots (macular rashes resembling the rose spots in typhoid fever but appearing on the face), erythema nodosum, and erythema multiforme. Splenomegaly occurs in up to 70% of patients, and, when present in a patient with pneumonia, should prompt the diagnosis of psittacosis. Complications include reactive arthritis, glomerulonephritis, tubulointerstitial nephritis, meningoencephalitis, seizures, and GBS, haemolysis and disseminated intravascular coagulation. The chest X-Ray often shows unilateral, lower-lobe consolidation, but may show bilateral, nodular, miliary, or interstitial patterns. Serology remains the mainstay of diagnosis: a four-fold or greater rise in the antibody titre between acute and convalescent serum (two weeks) confirms the diagnosis. However, PCR techniques offer a rapid and specific alternative. Doxycycline remains the drug of choice.

Further Reading

Sforza G, Marinou A (2017). Hypersensitivity pneumonitis: a complex lung disease. *Clinical and Molecular Allergy* 15: 6.

248. E) *Staphylococcus aureus*

The patient in this case presents with classic symptoms of a community acquired pneumonia with a preceding history of a flu-like illness, most likely influenza. *Staphylococcus aureus*, whilst not a common causative organism for community acquired pneumonia, does classically present as a secondary infection following a flu infection. This is likely as a result of breakdown of mucosa in the respiratory tract resulting in translocation of nosocomial *S. aureus* (e.g. from nasopharynx).

Klebsiella pneumonia is an increasingly common cause of cavitating lung infections but is primarily due to aspiration. Aspergillus, whilst it does infect pre-existing lung cavities causing aspergillomas from which patients can become very unwell, is not cavitating in itself. Furthermore, there is no previous history of TB that may have resulted in a pre-existing pulmonary cavity in this patient. TB remains an important cause of caveating lung lesions, but the clinical course of the disease is usually much more protracted and patients with TB often do not develop an overwhelming inflammatory response as seen here. Indeed a cavitating lung lesion with an otherwise mild biochemical and haematological inflammatory response would actually point to TB as the diagnosis. Lobar adenocarcinoma may also present in this manner, and may even have a superimposed bacterial infection. However, the patient's younger age, sparse smoking history, and lack of constitutional symptoms such as weight loss and anorexia all point against this. In any case, clinically this patient would require a follow-up chest X-ray after treatment to ensure the changes seen were improving. If they weren't, further radiological imaging such as a CT and referral to respiratory clinical would be warranted.

Tutorial

With the advent of more detailed radiological imaging, cavitating pneumonias are becoming increasingly prevalent. Klebsiella pneumonia is classically seen in alcoholics and patients intubated in intensive care settings, but is increasingly being seen as a cause of hospital acquired pneumonias in immunosuppressed patients and those with an impaired swallow reflex. For similar reasons, many anaerobic bacteria, including *E. coli*, can also cause cavitating lung lesions. *Staphylococcus aureus* is also commonly considered a cause of a cavitating pneumonia. Classically, patients with this fall into one of two categories. Either, they have developed a superimposed post-influenzae *Staph. aureus* infection, or it is due to bacteraemia spread most commonly from right heart endocarditis, which is seen in patients with venous lines or intravenous drug users. It is worth noting that whilst *Streptococcus pneumoniae* and *Haemophilus influenzae* are not classically characterized as cavitating pathogens, given that they are such a common cause of bacterial pneumonias, they do actually represent a significant fraction of cavitating pneumonias, especially when there is evidence of bacteraemia, thus representing high disease burden. *Mycobacterium tuberculosis* is also a common cause of a cavitating lung lesion but, unlike other bacterial infections, patients can have little evidence both clinically and biochemically of an inflammatory response. It is worth noting, however, that whilst the patient themselves many not be 'very unwell' a cavitating lesion represents a very high mycobacterial burden and these patients are highly infectious. The various causes of cavitating lung lesions are discussed further in Table 11.7.

Table 11.7 Causes of cavitating lung lesions

Common bacterial causes:	• *Klebsiella pneumoniae* • *Staphylococcus aureus* • *Mycobacterium tuberculosis* • *Streptococcus pneumoniae* • *Haemophilus influenzae* • Anaerobic bacteria • Endocarditis associated organisms causing septic emboli
Common bacterial causes worldwide (rare in UK):	• Nocardia • Salmonella (non-typhoid) • *Burkholderia pseudomallei* • *Histoplasma capsulatum* • Echinococcus
Bacterial causes in the immuno-suppressed:	• Non-tuberculous mycobacteria (immuno-suppressed) • *Penicillium marneffei* • *Cryptococcus spp.* • *Coccidioides immitis*
Non-infectious causes of cavitating lung lesions:	• Malignancy • Granulomatous polyangiitis • PE • Rheumatoid nodules

Further Reading

Gadkowski L, Stout J (2008). Cavitary pulmonary disease. *Clinical Microbiology Reviews* 21(2): 305–333.

249. B) Fat embolism

This patient has developed type I respiratory failure, confusion, and skin petechiae 48 hours following a right hip replacement for a fractured neck of femur. Whilst PE is an important differential in a post-operative patient, the above triad of respiratory, cerebral, and skin changes within the first 72 hours following a fracture +/− orthopaedic surgery should raise the strong suspicion of fat embolism. Blood tests demonstrate anaemia, thrombocytopenia, and hypofibrinogenemia; and the CXR demonstrates diffuse bilateral pulmonary infiltrates, all of which are consistent with this diagnosis. PE may produce similar CXR changes if it is complicated by acute respiratory distress syndrome (ARDS), which is very rare. Pneumonia is unlikely given the absence of consolidation on the CXR. Disseminated intravascular coagulation would be associated with increased PT and APTT. Thrombotic thrombocytopenic purpura results in neurological dysfunction, anaemia, or thrombocytopaenia (with petechiae). Respiratory manifestations are not a feature of this condition. The unifying diagnosis is fat embolism.

Tutorial

Fat embolism syndrome (FES) is commonly associated with traumatic fracture of femur, pelvis, and tibia, and, post-operatively, after intramedullary nailing and pelvic and knee arthroplasty. The other forms include massive soft tissue injury, severe burns, bone marrow biopsy, bone marrow transplant, cardiopulmonary resuscitation, liposuction, and median sternotomy. The non-traumatic associations are acute pancreatitis, fatty liver, corticosteroid therapy, diabetes, decompression sickness, and sickle cell crisis. The mechanical theory states that large fat droplets are released into the venous system that are deposited in the pulmonary capillary beds and reach the brain via arteriovenous shunts. The biochemical theory states that trauma induces systemic release of free fatty acids as chylomicrons that coalesce, followed by the above pulmonary and cerebral sequelae.

FES is a clinical diagnosis, and the clinical triad includes respiratory failure, cerebral dysfunction, and skin petechiae, often developing within 24–72 hours after trauma. Respiratory symptoms include tachypnoea, dyspnoea, and cyanosis. Cerebral manifestations are non-specific, ranging from acute confusion to drowsiness, rigidity, convulsions, or coma. Cerebral oedema contributes to the neurological deterioration. The skin dysfunction is manifested as reddish-brown non-palpable petechiae on the chest, axilla, conjunctiva, and neck that appears within 24–36 hours and disappears. These occur in only 20–50% of patients and resolve quickly, but may aid diagnosis in the correct clinical setting. The particular distribution of the rash is related to the fact that the fat particles float in the aortic arch like oil in water with subsequent embolization to the non-dependent areas of the body. Renal manifestations may include lipuria, oliguria, or anuria. Jaundice may be seen with hepatic involvement. Retinal changes include exudates, oedema, haemorrhage, or intravascular fat globules. Arterial blood gas analysis will show type I respiratory failure. Thrombocytopaenia, anaemia, hypofibrinogenaemia are seen, but are non-specific findings. A decrease in haematocrit should raise the suspicion of pulmonary haemorrhage. Cytological examination of urine may reveal fat globules, but this is neither sensitive nor specific for diagnosis. Fat globules in the urine are common after trauma. The CXR will show diffuse bilateral pulmonary infiltrates. Ventilation-perfusion imaging of the lungs may be performed for suspicion of pulmonary embolus—the findings may be normal or may demonstrate subsegmental perfusion defects. CT pulmonary angiography may be normal, as the embolic particles are lodged in the capillary beds. Parenchymal changes consistent with acute lung injury may be seen. Nodular or ground glass opacities in the setting of trauma suggest fat embolism.

Treatment of FES is supportive: ensuring adequate oxygenation and intravascular volume repletion as needed. Albumin has been recommended for volume resuscitation in addition to balanced electrolyte solution, because it also binds fatty acids and may limit lung injury. Mechanical ventilation may be necessary.

Further Reading

Kwaitt M, Seamon M (2013). Fat embolism syndrome. *International Journal of Critical Illness and Injury Science* 3(1): 64–68.

250. C) Initiate long-term oxygen therapy

This question tests the candidate's knowledge of the current BTS guidelines for the use of long-term oxygen therapy in patients with COPD, and the commonly used inhaler therapies for patients with COPD. This patient has severe COPD with a FEV_1 of 30%. Physical examination reveals signs of pulmonary hypertension and cor pulmonale. The full blood count demonstrates a high haemoglobin, suggestive of secondary polycythaemia. He is on the appropriate inhalers that comprise a short-acting β_2-agonist (salbutamol), long-acting muscarinic antagonist (tiotropium), and combination long-acting β_2-agonist *and* corticosteroid inhaler (seretide). The pO_2 is 7.8, and in the presence of cor pulmonale and polycythaemia, he fulfils the criteria for long-term oxygen therapy. Long-term oral steroids are not usually recommended in COPD. However, some patients with advanced COPD may require maintenance oral steroids when they cannot be withdrawn following an exacerbation. Mucolytics can be used as adjunctive therapy for symptom relief, but there is no history of increased sputum production. Spironolactone would be indicated in left ventricular systolic function. This is unlikely given the absence of cardiomegaly and pulmonary congestion on the CXR.

Tutorial

The current BTS guidelines indicate that assessment for long-term oxygen therapy (LTOT) should be carried out when there is evidence of any of the following: (1) very severe airflow obstruction (FEV_1 <30% predicted); (2) cyanosis; (3) polycythaemia; (4) peripheral oedema; (5) a raised jugular venous pressure; or (6) S_aO_2 ≤92% (on air). It may also be considered for patients with severe airflow obstruction (FEV_1 30–49% predicted). Assessment should be made by measuring arterial blood gases on two occasions at least three weeks apart in people with confirmed, stable COPD who are receiving optimum medical management. Thus, assessment should not follow a recent exacerbation, as this will impact on the measured pO_2 (generally a six-week period after an exacerbation is acceptable). Patients *must* not be smoking; otherwise they do not qualify for LTOT. LTOT can be offered to patients if the pO_2 <7.3, or pO_2 = 7.3–8.0 and one of following: (1) secondary polycythaemia; (2) pulmonary hypertension; (3) peripheral oedema (cor pulmonale); or (4) nocturnal hypoxaemia (S_aO_2 <90% for >30% of the time).

This question also tests the candidate's knowledge of commonly used inhalers, their constituents, and their brand names. Failure to recognize inhalers in questions will cause problems in deciding how to escalate therapy. Table 11.8 lists the commonly used inhalers, which the candidate should be familiar with.

Table 11.8 Commonly used inhalers in COPD and their brand names

Inhaler type	Mechanisms	Generic name	Brand name(s)
Short-acting bronchodilators	β_2-agonist	Salbutamol	Airomir®, Asmasal®, Salamol®, Salbulin®, Pulvinal Salbutamol® and Ventolin®
	Anti-muscarinic	Terbutaline	Bricanyl®
		Ipratropium	Atrovent®).
Long-acting bronchodilator	β_2-agonist	Formoterol	Atimos®, Foradil®, and Oxis®
		Salmeterol	Serevent®
	Anti-muscarinic	Tiotropium	Spiriva®
Corticosteroids	Beclometasone		Asmabec®, Beclazone®, Becodisks®Clenil Modulite®, Pulvinal Beclometasone® and Qvar®
	Budesonide		Budesonide®, Novolizer Budesonide® and Pulmicort®
	Fluticasone		Flixotide®
Combination inhalers	Long-acting β_2-agonist + corticosteroid	Formoterol and beclometasone	Fostair®
		Salmeterol and fluticasone	Seretide®
		Formoterol and budesonide	Symbicort®

Further Reading

British Thoracic Society (2015). BTS guidelines for home oxygen use in adults. *Thorax* 70(1): 1–43.

National Institute for Clinical Excellence (2019). Chronic obstructive pulmonary disease in over 16s: diagnosis and management. (NG115). Dec 2018, updated July 2019. Available at: https://www.nice.org.uk/guidance/ng115

251. D) Lung malignancy

This patient with a long-standing history of smoking presents with productive cough, haemoptysis, and weight loss. He is clubbed. The respiratory causes for clubbing and productive cough include bronchiectasis, empyema, TB, and lung malignancy. Investigations reveal hypolabuminaemia and proteinuria, suggestive of nephrotic syndrome. The differential diagnoses for nephrotic syndrome, given the history, may include bronchiectasis with secondary amyloidosis or malignancy complicated by (most commonly) membranous glomerulonephritis. The key to the answer is the interpretation of the calcium. Often the calcium provided in examinations is corrected for the serum albumin. If the 'total calcium' is provided, then this should prompt the candidate to calculate the corrected calcium. The corrected calcium (mmol/L) = measured total calcium (mmol/L) + 0.02 (40—serum albumin [g/L]), where 40 represents the average albumin level in g/L. In light of this the corrected calcium is 2.88 mmol/L. This patient has hypercalcaemia with a low-normal phosphate. The most likely unifying diagnosis for the history, and clinical and laboratory findings is lung malignancy—squamous cell carcinoma amongst all lung malignancies is most commonly associated with hypercalcaemia. Hypercalcaemia in malignancy can be caused by: (1) metastatic bone involvement (elevated ALP) and/or (2) secretion of parathyroid hormone-related peptide (PTHrP) and resultant osteoclastic bone resorption. Hypercalcaemia secondary to PTHrP secretion is often seen in squamous cell carcinomas.

Whilst long-standing advanced pulmonary TB may result in clubbing, it is not associated with hypercalcaemia. A positive Mantoux test indicates previous exposure to *M. tuberculosis* and with the given information, one cannot differentiate between previous infection, active infection, or previous BCG vaccination. Interstitial lung disease and extrinsic allergic alveolitis often affect the lungs bilaterally and are associated with a dry cough; hypercalcaemia is not a feature.

Tutorial

There are two broad classifications for lung carcinomas: small cell lung carcinoma (SCLC) or NSCLC. SCLC account for 20% of lung cancers and are the most aggressive and rapidly growing of all lung cancers. They arise from Kulchitsky cells (members of APUD system) and secrete many polypeptide hormones. It is often considered a systemic disease. About 60–70% of patients have disseminated disease at presentation.

NSCLC are the most common, accounting for 80%, of all lung cancers. They can be further classified based on the cells that make up the tumour: (1) adenocarcinoma—most common type, accounting for 50% of NSCLC, occurs in non-smokers as well as smokers, often in outer or peripheral lung areas; (2) bronchoalveolar carcinoma—a subtype of adenocarcinoma that develops at multiple sites and spreads along the pre-existing alveolar walls; (3) squamous cell carcinoma (also known as epidermoid carcinomas)—account for 30% of NSCLC, is associated with cavitating lesions; and (4) large cell carcinoma (also known as undifferentiated carcinomas)—the least common type.

Paraneoplastic syndromes are defined as clinical syndromes involving non-metastatic systemic effects that accompany malignant disease. There are many paraneoplastic manifestations of lung carcinomas. Hypercalcaemia secondary to PTHrP secretion is often seen in squamous cell carcinomas. Hypertrophic pulmonary osteoarthropathy is seen in NSCLC, particularly adenocarcinoma. Different endocrine syndromes (SIADH and ectopic ACTH production) and neurological syndromes (Lambert-Eaton syndrome, paraneoplastic cerebellar degeneration, and paraneoplastic limbic encephalitis) are seen with SCLC. Whilst clubbing can be seen with all types of lung carcinoma, it is commonly associated with squamous cell carcinoma and adenocarcinoma.

The normal functions of PTHrP include the regulation of bone development, mammary gland formation, smooth muscle function, and tooth eruption. The cellular targets for PTHrP and PTH are broadly similar and result in hypercalcaemia and hypophosphataemia, but PTHrP has a much broader spectrum of effects as it also binds to several other receptors. The hypercalcaemia secondary to PTHrP will be associated with an appropriate suppression of PTH and 1,25 $(OH)_2$-D levels, as opposed to primary hyperparathyroidism where PTH and 1,25 $(OH)_2$-D levels will be elevated.

Further Reading

Wysolmerski J, Broadus A (1994). Hypercalcemia of malignancy: the central role of parathyroid hormone-related protein. *Annual Review of Medicine* 45: 189–200.

252. C) Intubation and ventilation

This patient presents with features of life-threatening asthma. The CXR demonstrates clear lung fields and no evidence of pneumothorax. The arterial blood gas shows a respiratory acidosis with type II respiratory failure. In acute asthma, typically a type I respiratory failure pattern is seen with a low pO_2 and low pCO_2. A normal or rising pCO_2 indicates fatigue and life-threatening or near fatal asthma, and should prompt an urgent anaesthetic opinion. The single most important therapy for this patient is intubation and ventilation, and whilst intravenous magnesium and aminophylline may be appropriate in the setting of acute severe asthma, they should delay intubation. Non-invasive ventilation has not been recommended in acute severe asthma. This patient does not have COPD, thus the administration of controlled oxygen followed by repeat blood gas analysis is not appropriate.

Tutorial

The clinical features of acute severe asthma include: (1) PEFR 33–50% of best or predicted; (2) respiratory rate ≥25/min; (3) heart rate ≥110/min; and (4) inability to complete sentences in one breath.

In a patient with severe asthma any one of the following makes a diagnosis of life-threatening asthma: (1) PEFR <33% best or predicted; (2) S_aO_2<92%; (3) pO_2<8 kPa (without oxygen supplementation); (4) normal pCO_2; (5) silent chest; (6) cyanosis; (7) poor respiratory effort; (8) arrhythmia; and (9) exhaustion (altered consciousness). In a patient with severe asthma, a raised pCO_2 makes a diagnosis of near fatal asthma.

The initial management of acute asthma comprises delivery of high-flow oxygen to maintain S_aO_2 between 94–98%, nebulized β_2-agonist bronchodilator therapy, and oral (or intravenous if oral intake not possible) corticosteroids. A single dose of intravenous magnesium sulphate can be given to those with acute severe asthma who have not responded to bronchodilator therapy or those with life-threatening or near fatal asthma. Nebulized ipratropium bromide can be added to those with acute severe asthma or life-threatening asthma and those who have responded poorly to nebulized β_2-agonist bronchodilator therapy. Patients with signs of life-threatening or near fatal asthma should be immediately referred for an anaesthetic opinion.

Further Reading

British Thoracic Society (2016). British guidelines for the management of asthma. September 2016. Available at: http://www.brit-thoracic.org.uk

253. D) Granulomatosis with polyangiitis (GPA, formerly Wegner's granulomatosis)

This patient presents with frank haemoptysis. Investigations demonstrate anaemia, renal impairment, type I respiratory failure, and compensated metabolic acidosis. The CXR demonstrates diffuse bilateral alveolar shadowing which could be consistent with pulmonary oedema, alveolar haemorrhage, or acute lung injury. The differential diagnosis of pulmonary-renal syndromes is listed in Box 11.14, and of these, the options given include Goodpasture's syndrome, GPA (formerly Wegner's granulomatosis), and legionnaire's disease. Legionnaire's disease remains a possibility, given a recent history of travel and exposure to environments with air conditioning, but pulmonary haemorrhage is not a feature. Pulmonary haemorrhage can occur in both Goodpasture's syndrome and GPA, and may present with similar pulmonary-renal manifestations. However, Goodpasture's syndrome is a much less common disorder. The occupational history suggests contact with birds, and possible exposure to *H. capsulatum* found in bird excreta (acute histoplasmosis) or avian antigens (acute hypersensitivity pneumonitis), but these conditions are not associated with pulmonary haemorrhage.

Tutorial

The differential diagnoses for pulmonary-renal syndromes and pulmonary haemorrhage are listed in Boxes 11.14 and 11.15 respectively. Some patients may present with severe acute respiratory distress, but fever, cough, and breathlessness are the common initial symptoms. Haemoptysis may be absent at the time of presentation in up to a third of patients because the total alveolar volume is large and can absorb large amounts of blood, without extending more proximally into the airways. Haemoptysis must be differentiated from haematemesis or pseudohaemoptysis (alveolar fluid that resembles blood, as in *Serratia marcescens* pneumonia, in which the reddish hue of the infecting organism can create the impression of alveolar bleeding). It is important to obtain a careful history as this will help identify the cause. A recent infection suggests Henoch-Schönlein purpura or cryoglobulinaemic vasculitis, as infection greatly increases the risk of pulmonary haemorrhage in these conditions. If asthma and eosinophilia are present, consideration should be given to EGPA (formerly Churg-Strauss syndrome). If there is upper airway involvement, GPA should be considered. In a young smoker with glomerulonephritis and pulmonary haemorrhage, Goodpasture's syndrome should be considered.

The CXR findings include coalescent alveolar infiltrates or consolidation with air bronchograms. The distribution of the infiltrates is mainly perihilar or predominates in the middle and lower pulmonary fields. The apices and costophrenic angles are often spared. The presence of Kerley B lines should prompt the suspicion of pulmonary venous congestion. As blood in the lungs can absorb inhaled carbon monoxide, the TLCO will be increased, and serial increases in the TLCO may indicate progressive alveolar haemorrhage. However, the clinical instability of patients often precludes performing the TLCO measurements in the acute setting. Recurrent episodes of pulmonary haemorrhage can lead to interstitial fibrosis that may result in restrictive changes on spirometry. Significant anaemia may result from persistent intrapulmonary bleeding. When a pulmonary-renal syndrome is suggested by accompanying haematuria or renal dysfunction, anti-GBM and ANCA levels should be checked as a matter of urgency. Other tests, for example complement fractions C3 and C4, anti-dsDNA, and antiphospholipid antibodies should be ordered if an underlying condition such as SLE or antiphospholipid antibody syndrome are suspected. Circulating ANCA antibodies are detected in the majority of patients presenting with pulmonary haemorrhage. ANCA positivity leads to the differential diagnosis of three major systemic syndromes: GPA, microscopic polyangiitis, and EGPA. ANCA are directed against specific antigens present in the cytoplasm of neutrophils. Perinuclear (p-ANCA) are reactive with myeloperoxidase (anti-MPO subset), and elastase, lactoferrin, lysozyme, and cathepsin G (non-specific subset). p-ANCA (anti-MPO subset) is associated with microscopic polyangiitis, idiopathic cresenteric glomerulonephritis, and Churg-Strauss syndrome, whilst p-ANCA (non-specific subset) is associated with SLE, primary sclerosing cholangitis, ulcerative colitis, chronic active hepatitis, and drug-induced vasculitis. Cytoplasmic (c-ANCA) are reactive with proteinase-3, and are associated with GPA but also microscopic polyangiitis.

GPA is characterized by systemic necrotizing vasculitis, necrotizing granulomatous inflammation of the upper and lower respiratory tract, and necrotizing glomerulonephritis. The upper respiratory tract manifestations include chronic sinusitis, crusting rhinitis, epistaxis, and saddle nose deformity (collapse of nasal support). Purulent or sanguineous nasal discharge, or serous otitis media and hearing loss are common presenting features. Lower respiratory tract manifestations include cough, breathlessness, haemoptysis, and alveolar haemorrhage. Renal disease manifests as cresenteric necrotizing glomerulonephritis. Ocular findings include scleritis, keratitis, uveitis, episcleritis, and conjunctivitis. Proptosis indicates a retrobulbar granulomatous mass. Peripheral nervous system manifestations include mononeuritis multiplex, sensorimotor polyneuropathy, and cranial nerve palsies. Central nervous system manifestations include vasculitis of small-to-medium-sized vessels of the brain or spinal cord and granulomatous masses that involve the orbit, optic nerve, meninges, or brain. Cutaneous findings are variable and non-specific and usually affect the lower extremities. Palpable purpura, papules, subcutaneous nodules, and ulcerations (resembling pyoderma gangrenosum) are the most common findings. Musculoskeletal symptoms are common, with polyarticular and symmetric arthritis usually affecting both small and large joints. Though c-ANCA is more specific for GPA, some patients do express p-ANCA (anti-MPO subset). Common findings on CXR include single or multiple diffuse nodules and masses, and approximately half are cavitated, or pulmonary haemorrhage.

Goodpasture's syndrome comprises a triad of pulmonary haemorrhage, rapidly progressive glomerulonephritis, and circulating anti-GBM antibodies. These autoantibodies mediate the tissue injury by binding to antigens in the basement membranes. Under normal conditions, the alveolar endothelium prevents anti-GBM binding to the basement membrane. However, with increased vascular permeability, antibody occurs in the alveoli resulting in lung injury and pulmonary haemorrhage. Predisposing factors include: association with HLA-DR2, exposure to organic solvents, hydrocarbons or metal dusts, smoking, respiratory infection, and cocaine inhalation. Most patients have features of pulmonary and renal disease, whilst a smaller proportion may have disease limited to either the pulmonary or renal system. Haemoptysis is the presenting symptom when the disease affects the lungs. Whilst anti-GBM antibodies are specific for this condition, as many as one third of patients with Goodpasture's syndrome have circulating ANCA in addition to anti-GBM antibody.

Supportive therapies for pulmonary haemorrhage include supplemental oxygen, bronchodilators, reversal of any coagulopathy, intubation with bronchial tamponade, and mechanical ventilation. Specific therapy for pulmonary haemorrhage consists of treating both the autoimmune destruction of the alveolar capillary membrane and the underlying condition. Corticosteroids and immunosuppressive agents remain the gold standard for most patients, especially if associated with systemic or pulmonary vasculitis, Goodpasture's syndrome, and connective tissue disease. Intravenous methylprednisolone is recommended, followed by a gradual taper to maintenance doses of oral steroids. Intravenous cyclophosphamide is generally the preferred adjunctive immunosuppressive drug though occasionally other agents have been used depending on treatment response such as rituximab. Plasmapheresis is indicated for pulmonary haemorrhage associated with Goodpasture's syndrome or with other vasculitic processes in which the titres of pathogenic immunoglobulins are very high, for example ANCA-associated vasculitis.

Box 11.14 Differential diagnosis of pulmonary haemorrhage

Conditions with vasculitis or capillaritis:

- Goodpasture's syndrome
- Granulomatosis with polyangiitis
- Microscopic polyangiitis
- Anti-phospholipid syndrome
- Systemic lupus erythematosus
- Pauci-immune pulmonary capillaritis
- Henoch-Schönlein purpura
- Mixed cryoglobulinaemia
- Behçet syndrome

Conditions without vasculitis or capillaritis:

- Mitral stenosis
- Pulmonary veno-occlusive disease
- Infections:
  - Invasive aspergillosis
  - Hantavirus
  - Leptospirosis
- Toxins:
  - Trimellitic anhydride
  - Isocyanates
  - Crack cocaine
  - Pesticides
- Drugs:
  - Propylthiouracil
  - Amiodarone
  - Nitrofurantoin
  - Methotrexate
  - Bleomycin
  - Infliximab
  - Montelukast
  - D-penicillamine
- Bleeding diatheses:
  - Anticoagulants
  - Disseminated intravascular coagulation
  - Profound thrombocytopenia
  - Haemophilia

Box 11.15 Differential diagnosis of pulmonary-renal syndromes

Autoimmune conditions:

- Granulomatosis with polyangiitis
- Goodpasture's syndrome
- Microscopic polyangiitis
- Pauci-immune pulmonary capillaritis
- Behçet's syndrome
- Eosinophilic granulomatosis with polyangiitis
- Mixed cryoglobulinaemia
- Henoch-Schönlein purpura
- Systemic lupus erythematosus
- Rheumatoid arthritis
- Systemic sclerosis
- Dermatomyositis
- Polymyositis

Non-autoimmune conditions:

- Infections
  - Legionella
  - Mycoplasma
  - Human immunodeficiency virus
  - Hantavirus
  - Leptospirosis
- Drugs:
  - Propylthiouracil
  - D-penicillamine
  - Hydralazine
  - Allopurinol
  - Sulphasalazine
- Sarcoidosis
- Lung malignancy with secondary glomerulonephritis
- Renal vein thrombosis with subsequent PE
- Any cause of renal failure with fluid overload (pulmonary congestion)

Further Reading

Martínez-Martínez M, Oostdam D, Abud-Mendoza C (2017). Diffuse alveolar hemorrhage in autoimmune diseases. *Current Rheumatology Reports* 19(5): 27.

254. D) Re-activation of tuberculosis

This patient has a history of asthma and TB. He presents with respiratory symptoms and postural dizziness, which correlate with physical signs and CXR appearances of a cavitating apical lung lesion. Laboratory investigations show a low sodium with a high-normal potassium, which may suggest a diagnosis of hypoadrenalism. The most likely unifying diagnosis is reactivation of TB with adrenalitis (the original Addison's disease) which remains an important cause of hypoadrenalism worldwide.

A urinary dipstick positive for blood and protein might suggest a diagnosis of GPA with renal involvement, but this would not explain the hypoadrenalism. In this patient, the haematuria may indeed be explained by renal calculi or even renal TB. An eosinophilia with positive precipitins for A. fumigatus may raise the suspicion of aspergilloma, which has developed in an old tuberculous cavity. Whilst this is possible, it would not explain the hypoadrenalism. Positive precipitins for A. fumigatus are present in more than 90% of patients with aspergilloma, but are not diagnostic, as they only indicate exposure to the antigen. A mild eosinophilia is indeed often seen with an adrenalitis. The adrenals are a common site for lung metastases. These are often unilateral, and although bilateral adrenal metastases have been described, they almost never result in hypoadrenalism as enough of the glands remains intact.

Tutorial

TB is a multisystem disease with multiple presentations that depend on the organs involved, and is caused by *Mycobacterium tuberculosis*. Its spread is primarily airborne and thus pulmonary involvement is the most common. Classical symptoms associated with active TB include cough, weight loss, fever, night sweats, and haemoptysis. The most common sites of extrapulmonary disease are: mediastinal, retroperitoneal, and cervical (scrofula) lymph nodes; bone; adrenals; meninges; skin; and gastrointestinal and genitourinary tracts. Advanced cases of tuberculous lymphadenitis may suppurate and form a draining sinus. Tuberculous meningitis may present with a headache that is either intermittent or persistent for 2–3 weeks, with subtle mental status changes that may progress to coma over a period of days to weeks. Fever may be low-grade or absent. The most common site for bone involvement is the spine (Potts disease). Patients present with back pain or stiffness and paraplegia occurs in up to half of patients with undiagnosed Potts disease. Tuberculous arthritis usually involves a single joint—the hips and knees are most commonly affected, followed by the ankle, elbow, wrist, and shoulder. Pain may precede radiographic changes by weeks to months. Any site along the gastrointestinal tract may become infected and symptoms of gastrointestinal TB depend on site of infection. Ocular manifestations include keratitis, iridocyclitis, uveitis, retinitis, scleritis, choroidal tubercles, choroiditis, and orbital abscess. Genitourinary symptoms include dysuria, haematuria, and urinary frequency. In men, painful scrotal mass, prostatitis, orchitis, and epididymitis may occur. Cardiac manifestations include pericarditis and pericardial effusion.

Risk factors for active disease include HIV infection, intravenous drug abuse, diabetes, alcoholism, immunosuppressive therapy, malignancy, end-stage renal disease, silicosis, intestinal bypass surgery or gastrectomy, travel to or emigration from a TB endemic area, and homelessness. Anti-TNFα therapy (rheumatoid arthritis, inflammatory bowel disease, and psoriasis) has been associated with a significantly increased risk for TB.

The diagnosis is based on identifying the organism. Ziehl-Neelsen staining of sputum is a quick and simple method, and whilst it is highly specific for mycobacteria it is relatively insensitive and detection requires at least 10,000 organisms/mL. A more sensitive stain is auramine-rhodamine fluorescent stain (auramine O). Routine culture uses a non-selective egg medium (Lowenstein-Jensen) and can take 6–8 weeks to grow because of the 22-hour doubling time of the organism. If the Ziehl-Neelsen staining of the sputum is negative, then the diagnosis can be made quickly using PCR techniques to detect the organism in clinical specimens, for example sputum, allowing identification within 24 hours. Patients suspected of having TB should submit sputum for smear and culture. Sputum should be collected in the early morning on three consecutive days. Approximately 35% of culture-positive specimens are associated with a negative smear result. The CXR may show a patchy or nodular infiltrate and upper-lobe involvement is most common. Cavity formation is seen with advanced infection and a high bacterial load. Non-calcified round infiltrates may be confused with lung carcinoma. Tuberculomas are homogeneously calcified nodules that represent old infection rather than active disease. Miliary TB is characterized by the appearance of numerous small, nodular lesions that resemble millet seeds.

The primary screening for TB infection (active or latent) is the tuberculin skin test (Mantoux test) with purified protein derivative (PPD). An intradermal injection of PPD is given and reaction noted 72 hours after administration. The results of this test must be interpreted in the context of the patient's history and risk factors (Table 11.9). A positive result indicates TB exposure, and cannot differentiate active infection, latent infection, or previous BCG vaccination. Anergy refers to a lack of reaction and thus the tuberculin reaction occurs weakly. This can potentially compromise the value of Mantoux testing and can be seen in HIV, sarcoidosis, and malignancy. Interferon-gamma (IFN-γ) release assays (IGRAs) are based on the ability of the *Mycobacterium tuberculosis* antigens (early secretory antigen target 6, ESAT-6, and culture filtrate protein 10, CFP-10) to stimulate host CD4 lymphocyte production of IFN-γ. If an individual has been exposed to TB, these memory CD4 cells should react with ESAT-6 and CFP-10 to produce IFN-γ, which can be measured. Because these antigens are not present in non-tuberculous mycobacteria or in any BCG vaccine variant, these tests can help distinguish latent TB infection. IGRAs are particularly useful in contact screening.

The standard treatment regimen for pulmonary, bone, lymph node, pericardial, or miliary disease is isoniazid and rifampicin (six months) plus pyrazinamide and ethambutol (first two months). In patients with meningeal disease, isoniazid and rifampicin should be continued for 12 months. Patients with meningeal or pericardial disease should also receive adjunctive corticosteroid therapy. Once a patient has been diagnosed with active TB it is important to assess individuals who have come into close contact with the patient. Contacts require a CXR and Mantoux test ± interferon gamma test. Those with evidence of disease should be fully treated, whereas those with evidence of infection but no evidence of disease should receive treatment for latent infection with isoniazid for six months or rifampicin and isoniazid for three months. BCG vaccination cannot be used as evidence of immunity in individuals with HIV infection. Similarly, a negative interferon-gamma test does not exclude TB infection in immunocompromised individuals.

Table 11.9 Interpretation of the Mantoux test

Positive if ≥5 mm	Positive if ≥10 mm	Positive if ≥15 mm
• HIV positive • Recent contacts with active TB • Immunosuppressed • CXR demonstrating old healed TB	• Intravenous drug users • Residents and employees of high-risk settings, for example prisons, nursing homes, hospitals, homeless shelters • Recent arrivals (less than 5 years) from high-prevalence countries	• Persons with no known risk factors for TB

Further Reading

Ai J, Ruan Q, Liu Q, Zhang W (2016). Updates on the risk factors for latent tuberculosis reactivation and their managements. *Emerging Microbes and Infections* 5(2): e10.

National Institute for Clinical Excellence (2019). Tuberculosis [NG23]. January 2016, updated September 2019. Available at: https://www.nice.org.uk/guidance/ng33

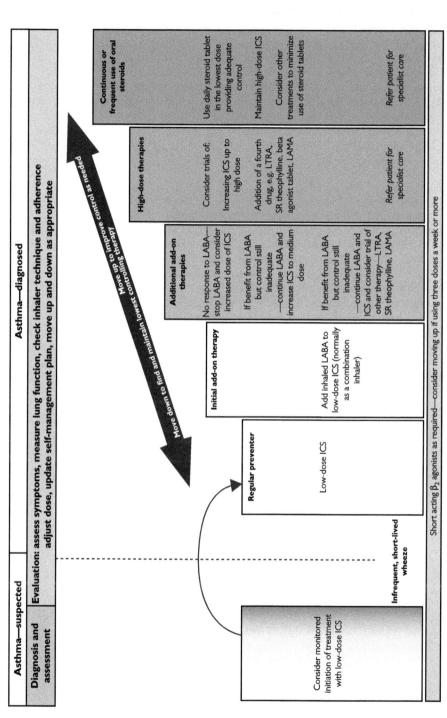

Figure 11.11 BTS guidelines 2009 for the stepwise management of asthma.

Reproduced from: British Thoracic Society and Scottish Intercollegiate Guidelines Network. (SIGN). British Guidelines for the Management of Asthma. Edinburgh: SIGN; 2019. (SIGN publication no. 153). Available at: http://www.sign.ac.uk and http://www.brit-thoracic.org.uk. With permission from Scottish Intercollegiate Guidelines Network and British Thoracic Society

255. B) Replace low-dose with high-dose inhaled steroid therapy

This question tests the candidate's knowledge of the BTS guidelines for the management of asthma. It is important to be aware of the different inhalers (and their brand names) that are commonly used in clinical practice (see Table 11.8). This patient is currently on a short-acting β_2-agonist inhaler, a low-dose steroid inhaler, a long-acting β_2-agonist inhaler. She is currently on STEP 3 of the BTS management algorithm. She had initially responded to long-acting β_2-agonist inhaler, but the control is still inadequate. The next most appropriate step would be to continue the long-acting β_2-agonist inhaler and initiate high-dose inhaled steroids. If she had no response to the long-acting β_2-agonist inhaler, then it would be appropriate to stop long-acting β_2-agonist inhaler and initiate high-dose inhaled steroids. If the control was still inadequate, then trials of leukotriene receptor antagonist or aminophylline might be considered.

Tutorial

The aim of asthma management is to control the disease, where control is defined as: (1) no daytime symptoms; (2) no night-time awakening due to asthma; (3) no need for rescue medication; (4) no limitation on activity or exercise tolerance; (5) PEFR >80% of best or predicted; and (6) no side effects of therapy. The BTS guidelines for the stepwise management of asthma are summarized in Figure 11.11. Patients should start treatment at the step most appropriate to the initial severity of their asthma. Control should be achieved early, and maintained either by stepping up therapy if response is poor or stepping down therapy if control is good. It is important to review patients regularly during step down of therapy. Before stepping up therapy, it is important to check compliance to therapy and inhaler technique, and eliminate potential triggers. Patients should be maintained at the lowest possible dose of inhaler steroid therapy, and reduction should be considered every three months. Reduction in steroid dose should be slow, aiming to decrease dose by 25–50% each time. Patients with exercise-induced asthma are likely to have poorly controlled asthma, and require review of their regular therapy. If exercise is a specific problem, despite inhaled steroid therapy, then consider leukotriene receptor antagonists, long-acting β_2-agonist inhaler, chromoglycates, oral β_2-agonists, or theophyllines.

Further Reading

British Thoracic Society (2016). British guidelines for the management of asthma. September 2016. Available at: http://www.brit-thoracic.org.uk

256. A 47-year-old female with a three-year history of rheumatoid arthritis (RA) attended clinic for review. Six months previously her disease activity scale (DAS) showed that her arthritis was highly active (DAS 7.12). Hydroxychloroquine was stopped and etanercept commenced. At her current review, she reported one or two minor flares in the preceding four months; she had ongoing pains in her knees, hands, and wrists.

Her drug list included etanercept 25 mg twice weekly, methotrexate 25 mg weekly, folic acid 5 mg weekly, and prednisolone 5 mg daily. She took calcium and vitamin D for bone protection. On examination 12 out of 28 joints were tender and mildly swollen. A patient global health visual analogue scale gave a reading of 64 mm. Her DAS score was 6.09 (still highly active).

```
Investigations:
  Hb                   106 g/L
  WBC                  4.1 × 10⁹/L
  Plts                 280 × 10⁹/L
  CRP                  33.5 mg/L
  ESR                  26 mm/hr
  ANA                  negative
  Vitamin D            72 nmol/L
  Rheumatoid factor    67 iU/mL
  Anti-CCP antibody    35 iU/mL
```

Which treatment option is most recommended?

A. Administer a depot injection of steroids and continue current treatment

B. Change to tocilizumab (anti-IL-6) and continue methotrexate

C. Restart the hydroxychloroquine and continue current treatment

D. Start rituximab (anti-CD20) and continue methotrexate

E. Switch to an alternative anti-TNF and continue methotrexate

257. **A 24-year-old female Caucasian non-smoker presented with an aching right arm. She had no past medical history. She reported an eight-month history of lethargy and some general aches and pains. She occasionally felt feverish. She had no history of joint swelling but described that her right arm tired quickly and ached. She was struggling to cope with normal housework and caring for her infant child. She reported no other focal symptoms.**

On examination, she had no evidence of synovitis or point tenderness. She had no rash. Her pulse was regular and 76 beats per minute on the left arm, but was not palpable on the right. Blood pressure was 156/88 mmHg. The right neck was tender and there was an audible bruit over the right carotid artery. The rest of the pulses were palpable. Lung fields were clear. The abdominal and neurological examinations were unremarkable.

```
Investigations:
  Hb                     106 g/L
  WBC                    10.1 × 10⁹/L
  Platelet count         390 × 10⁹/L
  Neutrophils            6.8 × 10⁹/L
  Lymphocytes            3.0 × 10⁹/L
  CRP                    33.5 mg/L
  ESR                    43 mm/hr
  CK                     62 IU/L
  Creatinine             55 µmol/L
  Urea                   4.1 mmol/L
  Sodium                 141 mmol/L
  Potassium              4.0 mmol/L
  ANA                    1:80
  ANCA                   negative
  ENA                    negative
  C3                     1.78 g/L (0.8–1.6 g/L)
  C4                     0.6 g/L (0.16–0.48 gL)
  Anti-cardiolipin Ab    negative IgG and IgM
  Lupus anticoagulant    not detected
```

What is the most likely diagnosis?

A. Atherosclerotic disease

B. Buerger's disease (thromboangiitis obliterans)

C. Cervical rib

D. Systemic lupus erythematosus

E. Takayasu's arteritis

258. **A 78-year-old Caucasian female presented with a four-day history of sudden onset pain in her left shoulder. She had known nodal osteoarthritis and often suffered from a few scattered aches and pains. The pain had come on over 24 hours and was more severe than her usual symptoms. There was no history of injury. Over the preceding four days her shoulder had become hot, red, and tender. She had previously experienced acute episodes of similar severe pain in the knee which usually settled after a few weeks. She was otherwise in reasonable health. She was known to have hypertension and had recently had an uncomplicated partial parathyroidectomy for a benign lump. She was a non-smoker and was fully independent. She drank ten units of alcohol per week.**

```
Investigations:
  Hb                        126 g/L
  WCC                       11.1 × 10⁹/L
  Platelets                 290 × 10⁹/L
  Neutrophils               8.6 × 10⁹/L
  Lymphocytes               3.0 × 10⁹/L
  CRP                       20 mg/L
  ESR                       45 mm/hr
  Creatinine                95 µmol/L
  Urea                      10.8 mmol/L
  Sodium                    138 mmol/L
  Potassium                 4.2 mmol/L
  Uric acid                 230 µmol/L
  Corrected calcium         2.15 mmol/L
  Phosphate                 1.11 mmol/L
  Shoulder X-ray:           patient unable to tolerate
                            positioning.

  Knee X-rays:              see Figure 12.1
```

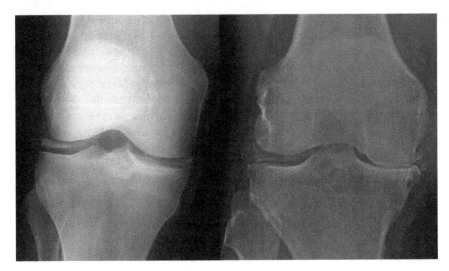

Figure 12.1 Bilateral knee X-rays.

Reproduced with permission from *Oxford Textbook of Osteoarthritis and Crystal Arthropathy*, Third Edition, edited by Doherty M, Hunter D, Bijlsma H, Arden N, Dalbeth N, Fig. 51.2, p. 479, Oxford University Press, Oxford, UK, Copyright © 2016.

What is the likely diagnosis?

A. Gout

B. Osteoarthritis

C. Polymyalgia rheumatica

D. Pseudogout

E. Septic arthritis

259. **A 36-year-old Caucasian hospital porter presented with acute right knee pain and swelling. He denied any rashes, red eyes, or genitourinary issues; there was no history of trauma or previous joint issues. He had hypertension, type II diabetes, and weighed 108 kg. He had had a few female sexual partners recently. He was a non-smoker but drank 2–3 pints every night after work.**

On examination he had a hot, swollen, tender right knee joint with marked erythema of the overlying skin. There were no skin wounds, bites, or cuts. Around 40 ml of opaque yellow and cloudy fluid was aspirated from the knee and sent for microscopy and culture.

```
Investigations:
  Hb                       126 g/L
  WCC                      15.7 × 10⁹/L
  Platelets                330 × 10⁹/L
  Neutrophils              8.82 × 10⁹/L
  Lymphocytes              0.92 × 10⁹/L
  CRP                      154.5 mg/L
  ESR                      104 mm/hr
  Creatinine               85 µmol/L
  Sodium                   143 mmol/L
  Potassium                4.2 mmol/L
  Uric acid                385 µmol/L
  Rheumatoid factor        negative
  Anti-CCP Ab              negative
  Urethral swab            no growth on culture
Synovial aspirate:
  Microscopy:              no organisms seen on direct
                           microscopy. Neutrophils predominate.
                           Slit lamp examination pending.
Synovial culture: sterile at 48 hours
```

What is the likely diagnosis?

A. Acute gout

B. Gonococcal arthritis

C. Psoriatic arthritis

D. Reactive arthritis

E. Septic arthritis

260. **A 21-year-old Asian student was referred with right wrist pain. Three months previously, she had fractured her wrist. She suffered no tendon or neurovascular damage. However, since the injury she had kept her arm in a sling and felt that even very light touch to the skin was painful. Over the preceding week her wrist had become swollen and purple. She gave a history of chronic pain and joint hypermobility had been diagnosed when she was 13. She had missed school due to pain and related depression. She denied easy bruising and had no history of heart disease. She had a normal height and weight.**

   Generalized joint hypermobility was confirmed on examination. She had no striae or bruises. The affected forearm had reduced hair growth and was cool to touch. There was swelling over and surrounding the joint. There was slight purple discolouration but no erythema. Light touch to the skin was perceived as painful but there was no numbness over any part of the hand. X-rays suggested some soft tissue swelling and mild osteopenia. Blood tests including auto-antibody screening were normal.

   What is the likely cause of this patient's wrist pain?

   A. Atypical carpal tunnel syndrome
   B. Complex regional pain syndrome (reflex sympathetic dystrophy)
   C. Marfan syndrome
   D. Occult radial fracture
   E. Takayasu's arteritis with stenosis of the radial artery

261. **A 55-year-old Caucasian accountant presented with a three-month history of fevers and weight loss, with two weeks of worsening breathlessness. He complained of muscular aches, lethargy, and abdominal pain. He had no history of foreign travel, infectious contacts, or drug use. He took no regular medications but his GP had given him two courses of antibiotics in the previous fortnight without improvement.**

Examination revealed a normal respiratory and cardiovascular systems and he was haemodynamically stable. His abdomen was mildly tender generally but otherwise normal. He had a palpable, non-tender purpuric rash on his shins. Two of his toes showed a purple discolouration.

```
Investigations:
   Hb                        106 g/dL
   WCC                       12.1 × 10⁹/L
   Platelets                 450 × 10⁹/L
   Neutrophils               9.8 × 10⁹/L
   Lymphocytes               0.4 × 10⁹/L
   Eosinophils               0.1 × 10⁹/L
   CRP                       153 mg/L
   ESR                       112 mm/hr
   Sodium                    137 mmol/L
   Potassium                 4.2 mmol/L
   Creatinine                178 µmol/L
   Urea                      19 mmol/
   ANA                       negative
   Rheumatoid factor         81 iU/mL
   Anti-CCP antibody         negative
   ANCA                      cANCA pattern on indirect
immunofluorescence; negative PR3 on ELISA
   C3                        0.98 g/L (0.8–1.6 g/L)
   C4                        0.1 g/L (0.16–0.48 g/L)
   Lupus anticoagulant       not detected
   Anti-GBM                  not detected
   HBsAg                     not detected
   Anti-HBcore               not detected
   Anti-HBsurface            >100
   Anti-HCV                  detected
   Blood cultures            sterile to date
   Urine dipstick            blood ++ protein ++
```

What is the most likely diagnosis?

A. Cryoglobulinaemia
B. Eosinophilic granulomatosis with polyangiitis (Churg-Strauss syndrome)
C. Granulomatosis with polyangiitis (Wegener's granulomatosis)
D. Polyarteritis nodosa
E. Subacute bacterial endocarditis

262. **A 50-year-old male was referred with 5 kg weight loss in the preceding two months. For a few months he had experienced various symptoms including joint pains, red eyes, a sore nose, and red painful ears. These had not responded to analgesia or antibiotics.**

On examination, he was febrile (temperature 38°C) but haemodynamically stable. He had an audible inspiratory wheeze. Musculoskeletal assessment revealed active synovitis of the elbows and knees. Head and neck exam showed erythema and tenderness over the pinna of both ears. The rest of the systems examination was unremarkable.

```
Investigations:
   Hb                        146 g/L
   WCC                       5.7 × 10⁹/L
   Platelets                 287 × 10⁹/L
   Neutrophils               4.31 × 10⁹/L
   Lymphocytes               1.32 × 10⁹/L
   Eosiniophils              0.44 × 10⁹/L
   C-reactive protein        26.5 mg/L (0.0-10.0)
   ESR                       25 mm/hr (0-20)
   Creatinine                76 µmol/L
   Sodium                    140 mmol/L
   Potassium                 3.7 mmol/L
   Rheumatoid factor         negative
   Anti-CCP Ab               negative
   Urethral swab             no growth on culture
   ANA                       1:80
   ANCA                      negative
   Urine dip                 no abnormalities detected
```

What is the likely diagnosis?

A. Behçet's syndrome

B. Eosinophilic granulomatosis with polyangiitis (Churg-Strauss syndrome)

C. Granulomatosis with polyangiitis (Wegener's granulomatosis)

D. Marfan syndrome

E. Relapsing polychondritis

263. A 34-year-old Afro-Caribbean female with known SLE presented with central chest pain not related to breathing or position. It had occurred twice in the preceding two weeks: once when climbing three flights of stairs and again when rushing for the bus. She had a 15-year history of SLE, which manifested as lupus nephritis (class IV), serositis, arthralgias, and a photosensitive rash. She was known to have positive serology for ANA, anti-Ro, anti-La, and anti-cardiolipin antibodies, with a prior history of high double-stranded DNA antibodies and low complement levels. Although she was currently well controlled, she had had previous treatment with high dose steroids and cyclophosphamide.

Other medical history included fibromyalgia, migraine, and depression. She smoked ten cigarettes a day but did not drink. Her current medications were mycophenolate mofetil 1.5 g bd, prednisolone 15 mg od, amitriptyline 25 mg on, enalapril 10 mg od, lansoprazole 15 mg od, and the oral contraceptive pill. Her examination revealed multiple diffuse tender trigger points consistent with her known fibromyalgia. Blood pressure was 144/88 mmHg and respiratory and cardiovascular examination was unremarkable.

What is the likely cause of the new reported pain?

A. Costochondritis
B. Fibromyalgia
C. Ischaemic heart disease
D. Pericarditis
E. Serositis

264. **A 45-year-old Caucasian male was referred with swelling, stiffness, and pain in his metacarpophalangeal and metatarsal joints, wrists, and knees. The joints were symmetrically involved and he reported that stiffness was especially problematic in the mornings. His symptoms had been on-going for two months, during which time he felt fatigued and lost 4 kg. He was a current smoker (40 pack-year history) and worked as a waiter, although he had had to take sick leave due to pain over the previous month. On review of symptoms he reported dry eyes. He had been taking ibuprofen tablets with some relief. He mentioned that a cousin had 'some sort of arthritis'.**

A full examination revealed several swollen tender joints, but was otherwise normal. The GP had arranged a chest X-ray and blood tests, the results of which the patient brought to the consultation.

```
Investigations:
  Hb                        111 g/dL
  WCC                       8.2 × 10⁹/L
  Platelets                 267 × 10⁹/L
  Neutrophils               5.4 × 10⁹/L
  Lymphocytes               2.00 × 10⁹/L
  C-reactive protein        43.5 mg/L
  ESR                       36 mm/hr
  Creatinine                76 µmol/L
  Sodium                    140 mmol/L
  Potassium                 3.7 mmol/L
  Rheumatoid Ffactor        44 iU/mL
  ANA                       1:160
  ANCA                      negative
  ENA                       anti-Ro/SSA positive
  Chest X-ray               good inspiratory effort; clear
                            lung fields
```

How should he be managed?

A. Administer an IM Depo-Medrone steroid injection and commence methotrexate and etanercept

B. Commence etanercept

C. Commence high-dose prednisolone with gastro- and bone protection

D. Commence methotrexate and prednisolone

E. Complete a disease activity score (DAS) survey, refer for urgent OT and PT input and review in 4–6 weeks to discuss pharmacological management options

265. **A 26-year-old Greek banker presented to A&E with an acutely sore and swollen right calf. He was a social smoker and had recently taken a short flight to Spain for work. He had no previous medical diagnoses apart from uveitis diagnosed 12 months previously. On systems review he reported that he almost always had a few mouth ulcers, particularly when run down. He reported having some acne spots on his chest and arms. He suffered from some occasional irritable bowel-like symptoms, headaches, and fatigue, which he attributed to the stress of his job. He had seen his GP for these symptoms, who had recommended yoga. He took ibuprofen frequently for his headaches. Blood tests, including clotting and autoimmune screen, were arranged and were unremarkable. A lower limb doppler study showed a proximal right sided thrombus in the popliteal vein.**

What unifying diagnosis should be considered in this clinical context?

A. Antiphospholipid syndrome
B. Behçet's syndrome
C. Familial Mediterranean fever
D. Sickle cell disease
E. Systemic lupus erythematosus (SLE)

266. **A 28-year-old Caucasian postal worker presented with swelling of her hands and tightness of the skin over the hands and forearms. She also reported some mild dyspepsia. She was married with two young children and had been well until six months previously. During the winter she had found it increasingly difficult to work because of cold and the tightness in her hands.**

Examination revealed nailfold capillary changes with thickened skin over her fingers and wrists extending to her mid-forearms. Her skin was also tight and thickened on the chest wall. Her blood pressure was 145/80 mmHg and her examination was otherwise unremarkable.

```
Investigations:
   Hb                          114 g/L
   WCC                         6.1 × 10⁹/L
   Platelets                   267 × 10⁹/L
   C-reactive protein          24.5 mg/L
   ESR                         36 mm/hr
   Creatinine                  84 µmol/L
   Sodium                      143 mmol/L
   Potassium                   4.3 mmol/L
   ANA                         positive, speckled pattern
   ENA                         positive
   Scl-70 Ab                   positive
   Rheumatoid factor           negative
   Anti-CCP antibody           negative
   Urine dipstick              Blood - Protein +
```

What is the most likely diagnosis?

A. Diffuse cutaneous systemic sclerosis

B. Limited cutaneous systemic sclerosis

C. Mixed connective tissue disorder

D. Scleroderma renal crisis

E. Systemic lupus erythematosus

267. **A 55-year-old Caucasian typist presented with mild pain and moderate weakness in her shoulders. She found it difficult to raise her hands above her head and to stand from sitting. Her symptoms had been worsening over the preceding six months. She was an ex-smoker (60 pack-year history). On systems review, she complained of lethargy and possibly some low-grade fevers at night. She had lost 3 kg of weight. She denied any respiratory or gastrointestinal symptoms.**

On examination, she was pale but apyrexial and normotensive. There was symmetrical proximal muscle weakness with power of 4/5 bilaterally. There were no fasciculations and reflexes and sensation were normal. There was no lymphadenopathy. There were some papules over the knuckles and elbows; a purple rash with oedema was noticed on the eyelids.

```
Investigations:
   Hb                      102 g/L
   MCV                     78.9 fL
   WBC                     8.8 × 10⁹/L
   Platelet count          234 × 10⁹/L
   CRP                     13 mg/L
   ESR                     25 mm/hr
   Creatinine Kinase       780 IU/L
   Creatinine              66 µmol/L
   Urea                    3.9 mmol/L
   Sodium                  144 mmol/L
   Potassium               4.8 mmol/L
   ANA                     positive
   Anti-Jo                 negative
   Anti-Mi2                positive
```

What is the likely diagnosis?

A. Dermatomyositis

B. Inclusion body myositis

C. Lambert-Eaton syndrome

D. Polymyalgia rheumatica

E. Polymyositis

268. **A 27-year-old Caucasian software programmer presented with lower back pain radiating to the buttocks which had been present for one year. His pain was worse in the morning and overnight; however, exercise improved the pain and stiffness. He had been taking ibuprofen, diclofenac, and naproxen regularly for the previous two months with some improvement in symptoms but no resolution. He had a family history of psoriasis and inflammatory bowel disease. His only medical history was recurrent red eyes for which he took steroid drops. He had no history of bowel or genitourinary symptoms and had no infectious illnesses prior to the onset of his condition.**

    On examination he had no nail pitting and no evidence of psoriasis. He was noted to have lower back muscle spasm with a loss of lumbar lordosis. He had moderate limitation of movement of the lumbar spine in both sagittal and frontal planes. His systems examination was otherwise normal. An X-ray of the pelvis showed moderate sacroiliitis with erosions and sclerosis bilaterally

    Which of the following treatments would you recommend?

    A. Commence anti-TNF therapy and refer for physiotherapy
    B. Commence methotrexate and refer for physiotherapy
    C. Commence sulphasalazine and refer for physiotherapy
    D. Continue NSAIDS, add further pain killers, and refer for physiotherapy
    E. Give a tapering dose of steroids, commence methotrexate, and refer for physiotherapy

269. **A 76-year-old was admitted for investigation of night sweats and 6 kg weight loss over two months. She had a 60 pack-year smoking history but had no specific symptoms apart from some generalized aching. She had had a chronic morning productive cough for many years. She had no gastrointestinal symptoms or infectious contacts although she did look after her toddler grandson every week. She had no foreign travel. On specific questioning regarding her generalized aching, she described muscular aching and prolonged early morning stiffness that particularly affected her shoulders, arms, and thighs. She had no visual symptoms, jaw claudication, or cardiovascular symptoms. Musculoskeletal examination revealed some osteoarthritic changes in her hands but no evidence of any active synovitis.**

```
Investigations:
   Hb                      116 g/L
   MCV                     86.9 fL
   WCC                     8.8 × 10⁹/L
   Neutrophils             5.7 × 10⁹/L
   Lymphocytes             2.0 × 10⁹/L
   Platelet count          580 × 10⁹/L
   CRP                     78 mg/L
   ESR                     96 mm/hr
   Creatinine              66 µmol/L
   Urea                    3.9 mmol/L
   Sodium                  144 mmol/L
   Potassium               4.8 mmol/L
   AST                     25 iU/L
   ALT                     35 iU/L
   ALP                     130 iU/L
   Bilirubin               13 µmol/L
   Albumin                 42 g/L
   ANA                     negative
   Anti-CCP antibody       negative
   ENA                     negative
   ANCA                    nuclear and cytoplasmic
                           immunofluorescence detected, PR3
                           and MPO negative
   Chest X-ray             unremarkable
```

What is the most likely underlying diagnosis?

A. ANCA vasculitis

B. Gastrointestinal malignancy

C. Giant cell arteritis

D. Lung cancer

E. Rheumatoid arthritis

270. **A 29-year-old photographer was referred with a two-month history of high fevers which occurred in the mornings and late afternoons. He also complained of joint pains affecting his knuckles, wrists, and knees with generalized muscle aches. His symptoms were severe when febrile, but he felt relatively well between episodes. He had lost 8 kg over the preceding two months. He recalled that he had had a sore throat a few weeks before becoming unwell. He had travelled to Spain four months previously but did not remember any insect bites or stings. He had a long-term girlfriend and denied any other sexual relationships. He had had no infectious contacts. There was no resolution of symptoms despite numerous courses of antibiotics.**

On examination he appeared unwell. He had a fever of 39.8°C with pulse of 88 bpm and blood pressure 110/70 mmHg. He had cervical lymphadenopathy and moderate hepatosplenomegaly. His wrists and knees were swollen. There was a salmon-coloured non-itchy macular rash on his torso.

```
Investigations:
    Hb                      106 g/L
    WCC                     14.8 × 10⁹/L
    Neutrophils             11.9 × 10⁹/L
    Lymphocytes             1.9 × 10⁹/L
    Platelet count          265 × 10⁹/L
    CRP                     188 mg/L
    ESR                     86 mm/hr
    Creatinine kinase       156 iU/L
    Creatinine              82 µmol/L
    Urea                    6.5 mmol/L
    Sodium                  142 mmol/L
    Potassium               4.4 mmol/L
    AST                     75 iU/L
    ALT                     88 iU/L
    ALP                     169 iU/L
    Bilirubin               48 µmol/L
    Albumin                 28 g/L
    ANA                     negative
    ANCA                    negative
    ENA                     negative
    Rheumatoid factor       negative
    Anti-CCP antibody       negative
    Mantoux                 negative
    Chest X-ray             normal
    Lymph node biopsy       reactive changes
Skin biopsy non-specific perivascular mononuclear cell
    infiltrate
```

What is the likely diagnosis?

A. Adult-onset Still's disease

B. Hodgkin's disease

C. Periodic fever syndrome (Muckle Wells syndrome)

D. Sarcoidosis

E. TB

256. D) Start rituximab (anti-CD20) and continue methotrexate

Glucocorticoids are effective in suppressing the symptoms of RA but are unsuitable for long-term use due to their multiple side effects. However, as active RA may lead to irreversible joint damage early in the disease process, treatment with disease-modifying anti-rheumatic drugs (DMARDs) should not be delayed. An IM steroid injection might improve the patient's immediate symptoms, but as she has already had six months' treatment with an anti-TNF agent, then it is highly unlikely that any improvement will be maintained without a change in treatment and therefore the synovitis will continue unchecked for longer. Hydroxychloroquine would be a step backwards in terms of strength of treatment and so also wouldn't be an option here.

Tutorial

The major traditional DMARDs used in RA include methotrexate, hydroxychloroquine, sulphasalazine, leflunomide, azathioprine, gold, and ciclosporin. Methotrexate is the cornerstone of therapy and can potentiate the effects of biological agents. All patients on methotrexate should be on supplemental folic acid; patients on azathioprine should have their baseline thiopurine methyltransferase (TPMT) status assessed; and patients on hydroxychloroquine should have baseline formal ophthalmology examinations.

New DMARDs are appearing on the market every year for the treatment of RA. The ones discussed here are the ones that NICE have approved and listed, but you should be aware that oral agents will be imminently available that show similar efficacy to the anti-TNF agents (e.g. JAK-inhibitors). Tocilizumab is an agent that targets anti-IL6, a cytokine that is pro-inflammatory and stimulates the liver to produce C-reactive protein. Rituximab is an anti-CD20 agent that targets mature (but not memory) B cells.

NICE give very clear evidence-based and best practice guidelines for the management of RA. The key message is to treat RA early and aggressively. NICE recommend commencing standard DMARD therapy (commencing two DMARDs, one to be methotrexate) with short-term glucocorticoids immediately upon diagnosis. Measures of response to treatment should be calculated at every clinic visit using scoring systems: the American College of Rheumatology (ACR) response criteria are favoured in North America; in Europe, the disease activity score (DAS28) is used instead.

The DAS is a composite measure that reflects the number of tender joints, swollen joints, ESR, or CRP, and an evaluation of general health made by patient self-assessment. A score of ≥5.1 reflects high disease activity; 3.2–5.1 represents moderate disease activity; and ≤3.2 indicates low disease activity. If the DAS is >5.1 on two occasions more than one month apart, and if the patient has undergone two six-month trials of DMARDs including methotrexate, then the recommendation from NICE is to commence the cheapest of the following biological therapies: adalimumab, certolizumab, etanercept, golimumab, infliximab, or tocilizumab. Methotrexate should be continued. If these therapies are tolerated for six months but disease is still active, then rituximab with methotrexate is the next line of therapy.

Further Reading

Haraoui B, Bokarewa M, Kallmeyer I, Bykerk V, RESET Investigators (2011). Safety and effectiveness of rituximab in patients with rheumatoid arthritis following an inadequate response to 1 prior tumor necrosis factor inhibitor: the RESET Trial. *Journal of Rheumatology* 38(12): 2548–2556.

National Institute for Clinical Excellence (2018). Rheumatoid arthritis in adults: management [NG100]. July 2015, updated 2018. Available at: https://www.nice.org.uk/guidance/ng100

257. E) Takayasu's arteritis

A cervical rib could explain the symptoms of claudication but would not account for the raised inflammatory markers. SLE is associated with thrombosis, especially in the setting of having a secondary anti-phospholipid syndrome. Thrombosis could lead to claudication symptoms. However, this patient has an ANA which is not significantly positive, and normal complement levels and negative screen for APLS make the diagnosis unlikely. Atherosclerotic disease can eventually lead to stenosis with resultant bruits. However, this lady is young and has no conventional risk factors, making this highly unlikely. Buerger's disease (thromboangiitis obliterans) is a rare thrombo-occlusive vasculopathy of medium and small arteries, characteristically occurring in young male smokers who present with distal leg ischaemia. The diagnosis should be considered in all young smokers with distal lower limb ischaemia. The condition is strongly associated with heavy smoking, and is more common in Ashkenazi Jews. Systemic symptoms are uncommon in this condition. Claudication of the foot and the development of rest pain are typical. Patients may have upper limb involvement and superficial thrombophlebitis. CRP and ESR should be normal, or only mildly elevated, and serology should be negative.

Tutorial

Takayasu's arteritis is a rare large vessel vasculitis, usually presenting in young females. It is also known as pulseless disease. It is an autoimmune granulomatous disease.

Onset is usually non-specific and insidious which may lead to a significant delay in diagnosis. Symptoms include general constitutional symptoms (low grade fevers, weight loss, fatigue, lethargy); claudication symptoms (e.g. exertional limb pain); and carotidynia (tenderness over carotids which is rare but very characteristic). When arterial stenosis eventually develops the disease may be picked up because of bruits or missing pulses, visual disturbances, TIAs, or strokes. Hypertension may be present and renal artery stenosis is common. Occasionally the disease is picked up at an earlier stage when, for example, PET imaging is used to search for a possible malignancy in people presenting with constitutional symptoms. There is usually a high ESR and CRP and a mild anaemia. Other auto-antibodies should be negative (patients may have an anti-endothelial antibody but this does not form part of the usual panel currently). Due to the rarity of the disease, there are no trials to guide treatment. Though widespread practice is to treat with immunosuppression, namely steroids (though increasingly anti-TNF drugs are being used), it remains unclear as to the extent treatment actually alters the progression of the disease. Evidence suggests that by the time patients are diagnosed with pre-existing stenotic lesions that aren't visible on PET-CT, the disease has already passed its inflammatory stage.

Further Reading

Direskeneli H, Aydin S, Merkel P (2011). Assessment of disease activity and progression in Takayasu's arteritis. *Clinical and Experimental Rheumatology* 29(1 Suppl. 64): S86–91.

Mason J (2010). Takayasu arteritis—advances in diagnosis and management. *Nature Reviews Rheumatology* 6(7): 406–415.

Mukhtyar C, Guillevin L, Cid M, et al. (2009) European Vasculitis Study Group. EULAR recommendations for the management of large vessel vasculitis. *Annals of the Rheumatic Diseases* 68(3): 318–323. Epub 2008.

258. D) Pseudogout

This patient's story is typical for an inflammatory mono/oligoarthritis. The acute nature of the acute onset makes osteoarthritis an unlikely principal diagnosis in this case, although the patient may also have some baseline osteoarthritis in the background. Gout is a possibility but she is not a typical patient, this would not be a typical joint, and her uric acid is within normal limits. Polymyalgia presents with bilateral proximal stiffness and pain, but the monoarthritis seen here is not typical. Septic arthritis should always be considered, and it can be difficult to differentiate from acute pseudogout as they both activate inflammatory pathways (in particular via IL-1). It is therefore not uncommon to find an elevated neutrophil count, leukocytosis, and low-grade temperature in both diagnoses and it is always worthwhile to obtain synovial fluid to confirm a diagnosis and exclude infection. Given her knee X-ray shows chondrocalcinosis and she has had a recent parathyroidectomy, which no doubt has altered her calcium homeostasis precipitating a flare, pseudogout is the most likely answer.

Tutorial

Deposition of basic calcium crystals in the cartilage of joints is common and incidence increases with age. Basic calcium crystals are implicated in osteoarthritis and one subtype, calcium pyrophosphate crystals (CPP), is implicated in calcium pyrophosphate disease (CPPD).

CPPD may present as isolated chondrocalcinosis which may be asymptomatic and manifests as visible calcium deposits seen in cartilage on X-rays, or as acute or chronic disease. The acute form is also known as 'pseudogout'. The main risk factor is ageing in the context of nodal osteoarthritis, as in this patient. In younger individuals (under 50 years) it is important to consider the associations with other diseases: haemochromatosis, hypothyroidism, Wilson's disease, hyperparathyroidism, hypomagnesaemia, hypophosphataemia, hypercalcaemia, and diabetes mellitus.

Pseudogout is typically monoarticular, particularly in early disease. Pain is acute in onset, and is associated with swelling and erythema. It may mimic gout or septic arthritis. The knee, wrist, shoulder, and elbows are the most commonly affected joints. Attacks are usually self-limiting but tend to be more prolonged than gout. Fever with malaise may occur. Precipitants include inter-current illness, trauma, and surgery. Elderly patients can present with systemic malaise; the pain may also be so intense as to present as a sort of delirium. Flares of pseudogout after parathyroidectomy have been particularly noted and may reflect abrupt reduction in serum calcium levels during the post-operative period.

Treatment of pseudogout is mainly supportive. Symptomatic control is often achieved with NSAIDs which will also help reduce inflammation, though should always be used with caution in the elderly to prevent risk of gastric or renal complications. Steroids, either intra-articular or oral, can also be used for severe flares. If patients get recurrent flares, they can sometimes be started on prophylactic colchicine long term to reduce the number of flares.

Further reading

Doherty M, Dieppe P (1988). Clinical aspects of calcium pyrophosphate dihydrate crystal deposition. *Rheumatic Disease Clinics of North America* 14(2): 395–414.

Molloy E, McCarthy G (2006). Calcium crystal deposition diseases: update on pathogenesis and manifestations. *Rheumatic Disease Clinics of North America* 32(2): 383–400, vii.

259. A) Acute gout

The history of an acute attack of monoarthritis in an obese patient who consumes excess alcohol is classic for gout. He likely has metabolic syndrome, which is present in 75% of cases of gout. In almost half of the cases of gout the uric acid level is not raised; conversely, hyperuricaemia can occur without gout. Uric acid is a negative inflammatory marker so is often reduced in the acute phase. Needle-shaped negatively birefringent urate crystals on slit lamp examination are the definitive finding. Non-infectious inflammatory aspirates can contain high concentrations of neutrophils. Skin overlying a gouty joint may be mistaken as cellulitic as it may become intensely red during the acute attack. Septic arthritis should be considered, but it is reassuring that both direct microscopy and a 48-hour culture revealed no organisms, and the history points more strongly to gout.

Neisseria gonorrhoeae causes migratory monoarticular joint involvement in sexually active young adults with a ratio of men to women of 1:3. Knees, wrists, ankles, and finger joints are the most commonly affected sites. It is usually asymmetrical, may be severe and may be associated with fever and a skin rash. Synovial microscopy and culture is likely to reveal Gram negative diplococci in about 50% of the cases and blood cultures are positive in about the same number of patients. Cultures of the mucosa of the genital tract have a greater yield (80% positivity).

Psoriatic arthritis may present with a monoarthritis of the knee, but there is usually a hint towards the correct diagnosis with either skin psoriasis or pitting of the nails.

Tutorial

NICE guidelines recommend starting NSAIDs with proton-pump inhibitor (PPI) cover as first-line treatment for acute gout; if NSAIDs are contraindicated, colchicine and systemic corticosteroids are second- and third-line options respectively. Patients should be given lifestyle advice to reduce the risk of recurrent attacks. If the patient has had two or more attacks within the year or has risk factors for recurrence, xanthine oxidase inhibitors, which reduce endogenous production of uric acid, such as allopurinol or febuxostat, should be prescribed. Uricosuric agents such as probenecid are alternative prophylactic agents. When commenced, colchicine or an alternative therapy should be co-prescribed for the first 3–6 months to prevent precipitating an acute attack. Novel agents such as IL-1b inhibitors (canakinumab) or IL-1 receptor antagonists (anakinra) have been recommended for acute attacks of gout in the latest British Society for Rheumatology guideline but have not yet been licensed by NICE.

Further Reading

Jordan, Kelsey M (2012). Up-to-date management of gout. *Current Opinion in Rheumatology* 24(2): 145–151.

Zhang W, Doherty M, Pascual E, et al., EULAR Standing Committee for International Clinical Studies Including Therapeutics (2006). EULAR evidence based recommendations for gout. Part I: Diagnosis. Report of a task force of the Standing Committee for International Clinical Studies Including Therapeutics (ESCISIT). *Annals of the Rheumatic Diseases* 65(10): 1301–1311.

Zhang W, Doherty M, Bardin T, et al., EULAR Standing Committee for International Clinical Studies Including Therapeutics (2006). EULAR evidence based recommendations for gout. Part II: Management. Report of a task force of the EULAR Standing Committee for International Clinical Studies Including Therapeutics (ESCISIT). *Annals of the Rheumatic Diseases* 65(10): 1312–1324.

260. B) Complex regional pain syndrome (reflex sympathetic dystrophy)

The clinical history or examination does not fit with any of the options other than complex regional pain syndrome. This is discussed in more detail in the tutorial.

Tutorial

Complex regional pain syndrome (CRPS) was first described in wounded soldiers in the US civil war in the late 1800s. Although earlier studies suggested an association with psychosocial co-morbidities and personality traits, this is now more controversial as this has not been borne out in subsequent research.

Typically, following a noxious event or immobilization, spontaneous pain evolves at the injured site that is disproportionate in time and degree to the initiating event. The pain is regional but does not follow a specific nerve territory or dermatome. There is a predilection for distal limbs. It can occur at any age (seventh decade commonest) and is more common in females (2–4:1). The onset of symptoms is usually within 4–6 weeks of the precipitating event. The commonest clinical findings are of colour and temperature asymmetry, swelling, spontaneous pain, hyperaesthesia, sweating asymmetry, and altered skin/nail/hair appearances. There can be patchy bone demineralization. CRPS can evolve over time.

Two subtypes of CRPS have been recognized; however, the underlying pathophysiology and clinical relevance of making such distinctions is unclear:

- Type I: also known as reflex sympathetic dystrophy. No evidence of peripheral nerve injury; approximately 90% of cases.
- Type II: also known as causalgia. Peripheral nerve injury present.

There is no 'gold standard' investigation; however, X-rays of both limbs for comparison, repetitive skin temperature measurements, and three-phase bone scintigraphy have been advocated as adjuncts. The Budapest diagnostic criteria are used by current consensus and require: disproportionate pain; at least one symptom in three of four categories, and one sign in two of four categories (sensory/vasomotor/sudomotor/motor or trophic); and the lack of a better-fitting diagnosis.

The best treatment for CRPS is prevention. A meta-analysis of four studies suggested that supplemental vitamin C following fracture or surgery decreased the risk of developing CRPS. For those patients who develop CRPS, a multidisciplinary approach is essential and should include physiotherapy, occupational therapy, and a clinical psychologist. Possible pharmacological options include NSAIDs, anti-neuropathic agents (e.g. gabapentin, amitriptyline), bisphosphonates, and topical agents like lidocaine or capsaicin creams. Interventions such as trigger point injections, regional sympathetic nerve block, and epidurals have varying efficacy. The prognosis is highly variable in different studies; recurrence is relatively common, with rates of up to 30%, especially in younger patients.

Further Reading

Harden R, Bruehl S, Stanton-Hicks M, Wilson P (2007). Proposed new diagnostic criteria for complex regional pain syndrome. *Pain Medicine* 8(4): 326–331.

Marinus J, Moseley G, Birklein F, et al. (2011). Clinical features and pathophysiology of complex regional pain syndrome. *Lancet Neurology* 10(7): 637–648.

Turner-Stokes L, Goebel A (2011). Guideline Development Group. Complex regional pain syndrome in adults: concise guidance. *Clinical Medicine* 11(6): 596–600. Review.

261. A) Cryoglobulinaemia

This patient has symptoms suggestive of a systemic disorder: fever, weight loss, and arthralgias. On clinical examination he has a palpable purpuric rash with evidence of ischaemia in his peripheries, with blood and protein in urine. This clinical picture alone points to cryoglobulinaemic vasculitis and is confirmed by test results which show renal impairment, a strongly positive rheumatoid factor, and low C4. The positive hepatitis C test points to an underlying cause.

There is a positive c-ANCA on immunofluorescence, but this is likely a non-specific positive result given the PR3 is negative. Given the presence of a purpuric rash and negative PR3, GPA is unlikely. Given the predominant absence of significant respiratory symptoms and examination findings, as well as a normal eosinophil count and negative P-ANCA, ePGA is unlikely. It also worth noting that eGPA seldom causes renal involvement. Polyarteritis nodosa is a rare medium-vessel necrotizing arteritis which primarily affects the skin, nerves, gut, and kidney. A secondary cause can be found in 30% of patients, such as hepatitis B or C, SLE, RA, Sjögren's, or hairy cell leukaemia; 70% of cases are idiopathic. There is no glomerular inflammation, but haematuria can occur due to uncontrolled secondary hypertension. It does not, however, cause a low complement or purpuric rash. Renal dysfunction in bacterial endocarditis is classically attributed to immune-complex glomerulonephritis which would cause microscopic haemoproteinuria and low complement. However, one would expect a murmur and positive blood cultures to consider endocarditis.

Tutorial

Cryoglobulins are proteins that precipitate from serum and plasma at temperatures lower than 37°C and re-dissolve upon warming. Cryoglobulinaemia refers to the systemic inflammatory syndrome caused by circulating cryoglobulins causing tissue damage. Clinically significant cryoglobulinaemia is estimated to be around 1:100,000; it is strongly associated with hepatitis C and is more common in women. Cryoglobulins can be present in otherwise healthy people: prognosis depends on both disease activity and associations. Renal disease is associated with a poorer outcome. 'Meltzer's triad' of palpable purpura, arthralgia, and myalgia was first described in the 1960s and is associated with polyclonal cryoglobulins.

Type I cryoglobulinaemia is defined by the presence of a monoclonal immunoglobulin, most commonly IgM, but IgG, IgA, and light chains, in that order of frequency, can also be causal. Type I is associated with lymphoproliferative disorders such as multiple myeloma, lymphoma, and Waldenström's macroglobulinaemia. It accounts for 20% of cases. Type I cryoglobulins cause damage via hyperviscosity due to high levels of monoclonal immunoglobulins, which form cold-induced precipitates. Hyperviscosity manifests as acrocyanosis, retinal occlusions, and other neurological manifestations, Raynaud's syndrome, digital ulceration, livedo reticularis, purpura, and arterial and venous thrombosis.

Type II cryoglobulinaemia (mixed essential cryoglobulinaemia) involves a monoclonal immunoglobulin (IgM or IgA) which binds the Fc component of polyclonal IgG, thus causing large immunocomplexes which precipitate in the cold. It is the commonest type of cryoglobulinaemia, accounting for 50–60% of cases. Rheumatoid factor, by definition, is an antibody against the Fc receptor of IgG. Thus all type II patients will be rheumatoid factor positive. Everyone has a small amount of circulating rheumatoid factor which is thought to have a physiological role in dampening the immune response and clearing out antibodies. Raised levels can be associated with many autoimmune conditions (e.g. rheumatoid factor, SLE, Sjögrens) or infections such as HCV, HIV, HBV, or syphilis. It remains unclear, however, why some people with these conditions have high titre immune complexes to precipitate and cause cryoglobulin formation, whilst others do not. Similarly, it remains unclear why HCV seems to cause cryoglobulinaemia far more readily than other infections.

Type III cryoglobulinaemia is a polyclonal IgM directed against IgG. Unlike type II, there is no monoclonal component. It is also associated with autoimmune diseases and viral infections. It may evolve into type II with time.

Type II and type III cryoglobulins cause systemic inflammation and present with constitutional and non-specific symptoms. The classical 'Meltzer's triad' of purpura, arthralgia, and weakness occurs in only 25–30% of patients. Cutaneous manifestations occur in almost all patients and may precede extracutaneous features by decades. Arthralgias and myalgias are common (around 70%) but frank inflammation is rare. Neuropathy and pulmonary manifestations are more common than in type I. Renal disease occurs early in up to 60% of cases and usually presents as nephritic syndrome with an AKI. It is due to immune complex disease and biopsy reveals an MCGN.

Management involves treating the underlying condition (e.g. direct acting antivirals for HCV) and then immunosuppression with agents such as steroids and cyclophosphamide. Plasma exchange is used in cases of hyperviscosity or severe disease such as rapidly progressive AKI.

Further Reading

Gibelin A, Maldini C, Mahr A (2011). Epidemiology and etiology of Wegener granulomatosis, microscopic polyangiitis, Churg-Strauss syndrome and Goodpasture syndrome: vasculitides with frequent lung involvement. *Seminars on Respiratory Critical Care Medicine* 32(3): 264–273.

Ramos-Casals M, Stone J, Cid M, Bosch X (2012). The cryoglobulinaemias. *Lancet* 379: 348.

262. E) Relapsing polychondritis

EGPA and GPA are both ANCA-associated vasculitides and one would expect to see positive serology and blood and protein on the urine dip. Mucosal ulcers are more characteristic in Behçet's syndrome, which tends to occur in patients who live in countries which contained the old silk road from eastern Asia to the Mediterranean. All three of these conditions can co-exist with relapsing polychondritis and may represent an underlying predisposition to autoimmune disease. Marfan syndrome, whilst termed a connective tissue disorder, is not an inflammatory condition and does not cause synovitis.

Tutorial

Relapsing polychondritis is a rare condition characterized by recurrent episodes of inflammation and destruction of cartilage. Males and females are affected equally and the disease appears to be most prevalent in Caucasians with peak age of onset at 40–60 years. Approximately 30% of cases occur in association with another disease such as systemic vasculitis, connective tissue disorder, or myelodysplastic syndrome.

The most common feature is auricular chondritis (90% of patients); other features include non-erosive seronegative inflammatory polyarthritis, nasal chondritis, inflammation of ocular structures (conjunctivitis, keratitis, scleritis, episcleritis, uveitis), and chondritis of the respiratory tract involving laryngeal and/or tracheal cartilage (which can lead to dyspnoea with stridor, i.e. an inspiratory rather than an expiratory 'wheeze'). Cochlear and vestibular damage is relatively uncommon at presentation but develops in 30% of patients; it may lead to sensorineural hearing loss, tinnitus, and vertigo. Nasal and ocular involvement occurs in 20% of patients at presentation and 60% over the course of the disease. Clinically significant aortic or mitral valvular disease occurs in approximately 10% of patients and in some cases can manifest up to ten years from the onset of the disease. Renal, skin, gut, and neurological involvement has been reported. Non-specific constitutional symptoms may also be present.

Abnormal lab results are non-specific: they can include anaemia, eosinophilia (10%), and raised inflammatory markers. Homogenous ANA pattern can occur in 22–66% of patients but is non-specific. Anti-type II collagen antibodies have also been recorded in <50%: these lack disease specificity and their role in pathogenesis is unknown.

There is significant variability in the course of the disease between patients: some have a benign self-resolving illness; others have episodic disease flares; and in some, there can be a fulminant deterioration that ends in death.

For patients with chondritis but no visceral involvement, initial treatment with an NSAID is recommended, progressing to treatment with dapsone or prednisolone if there is no response within one week. Most patients will respond with this treatment within two weeks. If there is visceral involvement or lack of adequate response, then treatment with anti-inflammatory or immunomodulatory drugs, including newer biological therapies, is suggested. Data to support the use of one agent over another is scarce: cyclophosphamide is the preferred treatment due to greater clinical experience with the drug and its proven value in systemic necrotizing vasculitis. Other therapies include methotrexate, ciclosporin, TNFα antagonists, and tocilizumab (anti-IL-6 receptor antibody).

Further Reading

Chopra R, Chaudhary N, Kay J (2013). Relapsing polychondritis. *Rheumatic Disease Clinics of North America* 39(2): 263–276.

Kent P, Michet C Jr, Luthra H (2004). Relapsing polychondritis. *Current Opinions in Rheumatology* 16(1): 56–61.

Mohammad A, Ambrose N, Tuohy M (2008). Relapsing polychondritis: reversible airway obstruction or asthma. *Clinical and Experimental Rheumatology* 26(5): 938–940.

263. C) Ischaemic heart disease

This patient has many traditional and non-traditional risk factors for cardiovascular disease. She has had severe SLE with nephritis for a long duration, she is anti-cardiolipin IgG Ab positive, her cumulative steroid dose appears to be high, and she also smokes and has hypertension. She is not taking hydroxychloroquine, aspirin, or a statin. Therefore her risk is high and a history of any exertional pains or breathing difficulties makes cardiac causes, despite her young age, very high.

Tutorial

Many studies have demonstrated that, with all other risk factors being equal, the incidence of coronary artery disease in women with SLE is 5–9 times higher compared to controls. Even more striking is the finding that in pre-menopausal women—an age group normally protected against CVD—having SLE increases the likelihood of suffering from myocardial infarction by 50 times compared to their non-SLE pre-menopausal counterparts. All of these studies indicate that both classical and non-classical risk factors play a pivotal role in SLE-accelerated atherosclerosis.

Disease-specific risk factors include: the presence of lupus anticoagulant antibody or anti-cardiolipin IgG antibodies, being on the combined oral contraceptive pill, cumulative glucocorticoid dose, a history of nephritis, and a high disease activity and long disease duration. The conventional risk factors of hypertension, diabetes, hypercholesterolaemia, obesity, and smoking are also relevant and are common in SLE, possibly due to the side effects of steroids. Atherosclerosis is increasingly being recognized as an inflammatory disease and in SLE it is likely that an interplay between conventional and disease specific risk factors accounts for the increased risk.

Non-coronary cardiac manifestations of SLE include valvular, pericardial, and myocardial disease. Overall the prevalence of cardiac disease in SLE is around 50%. Non-bacterial thrombotic endocarditis (Libman-Sacks) is associated with antiphospholipid antibodies and should be treated with systemic anticoagulation for those who develop systemic emboli. It should also be remembered that pregnant women with SLE are at increased risk of congenital heart block developing in the foetus due to anti-Ro/SSA and anti-LA/SSB antibodies crossing the placenta.

Further Reading

Manzi S, Meilahn E, Rairie J, et al. (1997). Age-specific incidence rates of myocardial infarction and angina in women with systemic lupus erythematosus: comparison with the Framingham Study. *American Journal of Epidemiology* 145: 408–415.

Moder K, Miller T, Tazelaar H (1999). Cardiac involvement in systemic lupus erythematosus. *Mayo Clinic Proceedings* 74: 275.

Salmon J, Roman M (2001). Accelerated atherosclerosis in systemic lupus erythematosus: implications for patient management. *Current Opinion in Rheumatology* 13: 341–344.

264. A) Administer an IM Depo-Medrone steroid injection and commence methotrexate and etanercept

Several studies have shown that early aggressive intervention makes a long-term difference to the course of RA, and the advantage of receiving early treatment is maintained over years. Therefore, it is imperative to get the patient immediately immunosuppressed with steroids and commence him on DMARDs as soon as possible. Current NICE guidelines recommend starting two DMARDS (one to be methotrexate) at the time of diagnosis, ideally within three months of the onset of persistent symptoms. Later, if disease is well controlled, one can consider removing an agent. Short-term glucocorticoids (oral, intramuscular, or intra-articular) can be used to rapidly improve symptoms.

Tutorial

This patient has antibody positive new onset RA. He has all the classic findings and several poor prognostic markers—antibody positive and a smoker, which make him likely to develop severe erosive disease without treatment. The diagnosis can be made on this visit, and so while imaging, further blood tests, and an assessment of disease activity are useful to get at baseline, what he needs urgently today is to be treated.

Systemic features (weight loss, fevers) are commonly reported in active connective tissue diseases including RA. The complaint of dry eyes together with the presence of anti-Ro antibodies suggests that this patient has Sjögren's features overlapping with his RA, which is also relatively common among RA patients. While primary Sjögren's syndrome may also be associated with a positive rheumatoid factor, the history here is classic for RA and treatment should be commenced without delay.

Conventional DMARDs include methotrexate, sulphasalazine, and hydroxychloroquine. Biologics include anti-TNFα agents (e.g. etanercept), the IL-1 receptor antagonist anakinra, and the IL-6 receptor antagonist tocilizumab. Under current NICE guidance, anakinra is not recommended for use in the treatment of RA and combinations of anti-TNFα agents with anakinra should not be used.

Once sustained and satisfactory levels of disease control have been achieved, drug doses should be cautiously reduced to minimal levels required to maintain disease control. The patient should be under close and regular review when weaning off or stopping DMARDs.

Further Reading

Lard L, Visser H, Speyer I, et al. (2001). Early versus delayed treatment in patients with recent-onset rheumatoid arthritis: comparison of two cohorts who received different treatment strategies. *American Journal of Medicine* 111(6): 446–451.

National Institute for Clinical Excellence (2015). Rheumatoid arthritis in adults: management [NG100]. July 2015. Available at: https://www.nice.org.uk/guidance/ng100.

Smolen J, Aletaha D, Bijlsma J, et al. (2010). Treating rheumatoid arthritis to target: recommendations of an international task force. *Annals of the Rheumatic Diseases* 69: 631–637.

265. B) Behçet's syndrome

The diagnosis of Behçet's syndrome is made clinically as there are no characteristic lab findings. Inflammatory markers may be raised or within normal limits; auto-antibodies are used to exclude other diseases. As oral ulcers are relatively common, suspicion should be raised in patients who have recurrent ulcerations together with characteristic systemic manifestations, especially if they come from an endemic country. The International Study Group criteria suggest that the diagnosis should be made in patients who have:

- Recurrent oral ulcers (at least three times in a year) in addition to two of the following features:
- Recurrent genital ulcers (aphthous ulceration or scarring)
- Eye lesions
- Skin lesions
- Positive pathergy test

Reprinted from *The Lancet*, 335, 8697, International Study Group for Behçet's Disease, Criteria for diagnosis of Behçet's disease, pp. 1078–1080, Copyright 1990, with permission from Elsevier.

In this scenario, making the diagnosis of Behçet's will alter management, as the focus of therapy will be anti-inflammatory or immunosuppressive drugs rather than short-term anticoagulation.

Familial Mediterranean fever (FMF) is characterized by recurrent febrile episodes lasting 24–72 hours accompanied by serositis, rash, and arthralgias. It is an autosomal recessive condition most frequently found in Ashkenazi Jews, Armenians, Arabs, or Turks. Between attacks patients are asymptomatic. Inflammatory markers are often raised but auto-antibodies should be negative and complement is normal.

While SLE and the antiphospholipid syndrome are associated with clotting, and the former with oral ulcers, scrotal ulcerations are not a feature. ANA and auto-antibody screening is usually positive, and the APTT is prolonged, suggesting the presence of a lupus anticoagulant. Sickle cell is unlikely here as the patient has no evidence of anaemia and the presentation is not typical.

Tutorial

Behçet's syndrome is a multi-systemic inflammatory condition of unknown aetiology characterized by painful aphthous ulcers, genital sores, uveitis, and arthritis. Most of the clinical manifestations are thought to be due to vasculitis; Behçet's is unusual for its ability to involve blood vessels of all sizes on both the arterial and venous aspects of the circulation. The prevalence and severity of the disease reflects the route of the ancient silk road from the Mediterranean to east Asia. The highest incidence is in Turkey. It is more common in young adults aged 20–40 years. Most cases are sporadic, although familial clustering and genetic anticipation have been reported.

The common feature is recurrent and painful mucocutaneous ulcers that occur in the mouth, the skin, or the genitals. Genital ulcers (usually scrotal or vulval) are the most specific for Behçet's and occur in 75% of cases. Cutaneous manifestations include pseudofolliculitis, erythema nodosum, pyoderma gangrenosum, or erythema multiforme-type lesions, papulopustular lesions, and acneiform spots. Pathergy and dermatographism are also associated features. Uveitis occurs in 25–75% of patients and is typically bilateral; it is more common in males. An asymmetrical medium-joint arthritis occurs in approximately 50% of cases. Venous involvement is more common than arterial and can cause Budd-Chiari syndrome, dural sinus thrombosis, and other occlusive disease in addition to the more common superficial and deep vein thrombosis. Arterial involvement can manifest as aneurysms or stenosis. Neurological, renal, cardiac, and gut involvement can also occur.

Further Reading

Hatemi G (2008). EULAR recommendations for the management of Behçet disease. *Annals of the Rheumatic Diseases* 67: 1656–1662.

Sakane T, Takeno M, Suzuki N, Inaba G (1999). Behçet's Disease. *New England Journal of Medicine* 341: 1284–1291.

266. A) Diffuse cutaneous systemic sclerosis

Systemic sclerosis (SSc) is categorized into diffuse cutaneous (dcSSc) and limited cutaneous (lcSSc) disease on the basis of the extent and distribution of skin involvement (in this case, 'limited' does not mean that disease is limited to the skin, but rather the disease is limited to the acral area—hands, feet, face, nape). The former is associated strongly with the auto-antibody anti-Scl70, whilst the latter is strongly associated with the anti-centromere antibody. Lupus does not present with sclerodermal skin features and you would not expect a positive anti-Scl70 antibody. Mixed connective tissue diseases can share many features of systemic sclerosis, as well as other autoimmune conditions such as lupus, dermatomyositis (DM), and RA. A speckled ANA is often seen but the hallmark is the presence of anti-ribonucleoprotein antibodies (anti-U1-RNP). Whilst this patient has evidence of mild proteinuria, she does not have a deranged renal function, hypertension, or blood on her urinary dipstick suggestive of renal crisis.

Tutorial

The classification of systemic sclerosis and the relevance of auto-antibodies can be a confusing area. Scleroderma is the term for hardened and thickened skin. Scleroderma can exist as an isolated disorder of the skin, but if it is associated with visceral organ involvement then the disease is called systemic sclerosis. The manifestations of the disease are variable and can involve multiple systems, most commonly the skin, vasculature, gastrointestinal, pulmonary, renal, and cardiac. This autoimmune disorder is characterized by inflammation, fibrosis, and vasomotor abnormalities and is most common in women aged 30–40 years.

In patients with lcSSc, skin sclerosis is restricted to the hands, distal forearms, and, to a lesser extent, the face and neck. There is a tendency towards prominent vascular manifestations, including severe Raynaud's phenomenon and cutaneous telangiectasia. Many patients with lcSSc have aspects of the CREST syndrome (calcinosis cutis, Raynaud's phenomenon, oesophageal dysmotility, sclerodactyly, and telangiectasia). Anti-centromere antibodies are typical.

Skin sclerosis in patients with dcSS extends to the chest, abdomen, or upper arms, and shoulders. This group is more likely to have significant organ damage due to ischaemic injury or fibrosis than the lcSSc group. Reynaud's phenomenon in this group usually occurs at the same time, or after, the other manifestations of the disease, in comparison with lcSSc where Reynaud's may precede the other features by years. Anti-Scl-70 and anti-RNP antibodies are characteristic.

Reynaud's is the most classical sign of vascular dysfunction but it can also manifest as gastric antral vascular ectasia (GAVE), pulmonary arterial hypertension, scleroderma renal crisis, an increased risk of thromboembolic disease, and digital ulcers.

Pulmonary involvement may manifest as interstitial lung disease or pulmonary vascular disease. Anti-Scl 70 is associated with severe interstitial lung disease in dcSSc; in contrast, pulmonary vascular disease is usually a late manifestation of lcSSc. Although 50% of patients have no GI symptoms, 90% with either subtype have evidence of gut involvement from anywhere from the mouth to the anus. Chronic reflux and micro-aspiration can exacerbate interstitial lung disease.

Renal disease and scleroderma renal crisis is far more common in dcSSc, especially in the early stages of the disease. Although microalbuminuria, a mild elevation in creatinine, and/or hypertension are observed in up to 50% of patients, most do not progress to chronic kidney disease. Scleroderma renal crisis describes a syndrome of AKI and accelerated hypertension in the setting of SSc. It is the first presentation of the disease in 20% of patients. Urine is often surprisingly bland but there are usually features of MAHA on blood tests. Treatment with an ACE-inhibitor significantly reduces mortality (from 80% to 15%) but there is no evidence for a prophylactic role.

Further Reading

Barnes J, Mayes M (2012). Epidemiology of systemic sclerosis: incidence, prevalence, survival, risk factors, malignancy and environmental triggers. *Current Opinion in Rheumatology* 24: 165–170.

Tan A, Denton C, Mikhailidis D, Seifalian A, (2011). Recent advances in the diagnosis and treatment of interstitial lung disease in systemic sclerosis (scleroderma): a review. *Clinical and Experimental Rheumatology* 29(2 Suppl. 65): S66–74.

267. A) Dermatomyositis

A detailed discussion of the options given is found in the tutorial section.

Tutorial

DM and polymyositis (PM) are rare idiopathic inflammatory myopathies characterized by muscle inflammation and symmetrical proximal muscle weakness; dermatomyositis has typical cutaneous features. It is most common in females over 40. The disease is thought to be an immune-mediated micro-angiopathy affecting skin and muscle. Muscle damage probably occurs from ischaemia secondary to capillary damage. Symptoms can start insidiously and muscle weakness (rather than pain) is the dominant symptom. Most patients have fatigue and some constitutional features. Cutaneous features include: Gottron papules (raised violaceous papules and plaques over MCP/PIP joints of the hands); Gottron's sign (erythematous and violaceous macules or patches over elbows and knees); a heliotrope rash (violaceous rash on eyelids, sometimes with associated oedema); and an erythematous rash on the face and neck (shawl sign). Calcinosis of the skin or muscle may occur in juvenile DM. There is an increased risk of malignancy in patients with DM.

Laboratory findings include anaemia, thrombocytosis, and a raised CK. ANA is positive in 80%. Anti-Jo-1 antibodies (against histidyl-tRNA synthetase) are the most common specific antibody found in PM (65%) and in the anti-synthetase syndrome (myositis, interstitial lung disease, arthritis, mechanic's hands, and Raynaud's phenomenon). Anti-Mi-2 is directed against the helicase family of proteins, though only present in 20% of DM, and is quite specific. They are associated with a relatively acute onset of disease; patients often have a shawl sign and respond well to treatment. Anti-SRP antibodies are present in 5% of patients and almost exclusively in a histological subtype of PM which shows a necrotic and fibrotic picture rather than inflammatory infiltrate. DM and PM can respond to steroids but some patients will require steroid-sparing agents for long-term treatment.

Inclusion body myositis occurs in people over 50, typically Caucasian males. There is an insidious onset of muscle weakness and the mean time from symptom onset to diagnosis is six years. Weakness involves both proximal and distal muscles and is typically asymmetrical and painless. Falls are a common presenting feature. Loss of manual dexterity is typical. Dysphagia eventually occurs in 60%. CK is mildly elevated or normal. Auto-antibodies are negative. Steroids do not tend to improve symptoms.

Lambert-Eaton myaesthenic syndrome (LEMS) is strongly associated with small cell lung cancer and manifests as slowly progressive proximal muscle weakness, especially in the legs. Reflexes are typically flattened or absent. Autonomic dysfunction is also present. Antibodies against the voltage-gated calcium channel at the neuromuscular junction decrease the release of acetylcholine. Symptomatic treatments such as pyridostigmine can increase the amount of acetylcholine available in the neuromuscular junction; immunosuppressive agents target the auto-antibodies.

Polymyalgia rheumatica (PMR) is a disease of the over 65s, with aching and stiffness in proximal muscles and the hip girdle as the presenting feature. Weakness is not a feature of PMR and should lead one away from this diagnosis. It is associated with giant cell (temporal) arteritis. There is a raised ESR but CK is normal. Symptoms normally resolve with steroids.

Further Reading

Dalakas M. Inflammatory muscle diseases (2015). *New England Journal of Medicine* 372: 1734–1747.

Choy E, Isenberg D (2002). Treatment of dermatomyositis and polymyositis. *Rheumatology* 41 (1): 7–13.

268. A) Commence anti-TNF therapy and refer for physiotherapy

The clinical history, examination, and radiological findings are consistent with a diagnosis of ankylosing spondylitis (AS). NICE guidelines currently recommend anti-TNF therapies like adalimumab or etanercept as treatment options for adults with severe active ankylosing spondylitis if they have failed to respond to conventional treatment with two or more NSAIDs for four weeks. This patient has been on multiple NSAIDs for nearly a year. Response to treatment should be assessed at 12 weeks. DMARDs such as methotrexate and sulphasalazine used to be the standard of treatment but studies have shown that they have minimal effect on disease activity. Whilst intra-articular steroids can provide symptomatic relieve, systemic glucocorticoid treatment is ineffective in seronegative spondyloarthropathies.

Tutorial

AS has a prevalence of 1% in Caucasians and is strongly linked to HLA-B27. The clinical hallmark of AS is inflammatory spinal pain and stiffness. Inflammatory back pain tends to get better after exercise and worse after rest and has an insidious onset before the age of 40 years. NSAIDS tend to help more than simple analgesics. AS classically progresses from sacroiliitis and ascends the spine leading to ankylosis and kyphosis which can manifest within the first ten years of the disease. Peripheral arthritis affecting the ankles, hips, knees, and shoulders, and dactylitis can also occur.

Extra-articular manifestations include anterior uveitis, inflammatory bowel disease, psoriasis, and cardiovascular and pulmonary disease. Aortic regurgitation and conduction disturbances are increased in patients with ankylosing spondylitis compared to the normal population. In long-standing disease, complications include spinal fracture and atlantoaxial subluxation. Renal involvement is rare.

Imaging can be used to guide the diagnosis. The degree of involvement is given a grade in keeping the modified New York criteria: there is radiological evidence of sacroiliitis if the score is grade 2 or above bilaterally or grade 2 or above unilaterally:

- Grade 0: normal
- Grade 1: suspicious but not definite changes
- Grade 2: minimal abnormality: small localized areas with erosions or sclerosis without alteration in the joint width
- Grade 3: unequivocal abnormality, moderate or advanced sacroiliitis with one of more of the following: erosions, sclerosis, joint space widening, narrowing or partial ankylosis
- Grade 4: total ankylosis of joints

If there are no radiological features but the patient has typical features and is HLA-B27 positive, then they can be diagnosed as having non-radiological axial spondyloarthritis. If the diagnosis is still unclear, then an MRI is a helpful adjunct.

NSAIDs provide effective relief of symptoms in 70–80% of patients. There was inadequate evidence in a recent Cochrane review to support methotrexate use in AS. There is some evidence for sulphasalazine in AS with peripheral arthritis, although its impact on the spine and peripheral enthesopathy is minimal. Steroids are not of significant use in AS.

Most patients with mild disease are able to continue with their normal lives. However, some patients do develop severe skeletal disease that restricts movement or life-threatening extra-articular complications. Disease activity can wax and wane in individuals over decades. Only about 1% of patients have long-term remission. It has been suggested that the early use of TNF inhibitors may be more effect in controlling inflammation or may reduce radiographic progression.

Further Reading

Fendler C (2011). Glucocorticoid treatment in spondyloarthritis. *Clinical and Experimental Rheumatology* 29(5): 139–142.

Van der Heijde D (2011). Update of international recommendations for the use of anti-TNF agents in patients with axial spondyloarthritis. *Annals of Rheumatic Diseases* 70 (6): 905–908.

269. C) Giant cell arteritis

This patient presents with quite a non-specific history of weight loss, fevers, and myalgias. The differential is actually quite wide. However, the specific symptoms of girdle weakness (symptoms of PMR) in the mornings along with raised ESR and CRP provides a strong clue towards the diagnosis of GCA. Raised ALP is also often seen with GCA for reasons that are not entirely clear.

The patient has an extensive smoking history and whilst a normal CXR doesn't exclude lung cancer, it does make it less likely. Lung cancer also doesn't present with night sweats and it is likely her chronic cough represents a degree of COPD. Whilst the patient is rheumatoid factor positive, this is not a specific test and indeed is often found in patients with GCA. She also has no examination findings consistent with RA. Similarly, whilst she has a non-specific pattern of immunofluorescence positivity from her ANCA test, she is PR3 and MPO negative. Studies have shown ANCA positivity can occur in up to 5% of the general population, without any symptoms or signs of disease. She is also negative for MPO and PR3 which are more specific for the ANCA associated vasculitides. A gastrointestinal tumour is unlikely given lack of bowel symptoms or anaemia.

Tutorial

While headaches, visual loss, and temporal tenderness are the classic findings in GCA, it can also present with constitutional symptoms like fatigue, weight loss, and pyrexia of unknown origin. In 15% of patients, fevers can exceed 39°C. Around 50% of patients complain of jaw claudication which occurs soon after starting to chew and can be very severe; it is the most strongly correlated symptom with positive temporal artery biopsies. There is also a close association with PMR, as seen in this case, which is characterized by aching and morning stiffness in proximal muscles. Incidence increases with age and there is a female and Caucasian preponderance.

Permanent visual loss is the most feared complication of GCA and is reported in 15–20% of patients; it is often preceded by transient visual symptoms (amaurosis fugax). Once established, it is rarely reversible; loss of vision in one eye is followed by loss of vision in the other eye within one week in 25–50% of untreated patients. It can be caused by anterior ischaemic optic neuropathy, central or branch retinal arterial occlusion, or cerebral ischaemia.

In a study of patients with biopsy-proven GCA, FDG-PET scans showed subclavian arteritis in 74% and thoracic aortitis in 51%. Aortic aneurysms occur in 10–20%; however, aortic dissection is more rare, occurring only in 1–6%. Subclavian artery involvement may lead to bruits, alterations in blood pressure, and diminished pulses. Examination should thus focus on pulses, bruits, any signs of aortic regurgitation, and should include fundoscopy. Laboratory findings include a normochromic anaemia, reactive thrombocytosis, and raised ESR and CRP. ALP can be elevated in 25–35% of patients.

Treatment is with high-dose steroids for 2–4 weeks and then the dose should be tapered slowly. If there is a suspicion of the diagnosis, then treatment should be started promptly before waiting for definitive diagnosis with a temporal artery biopsy. Low-dose aspirin is also recommended to reduce the risk of strokes, TIAs, or visual loss, especially in patients who have already experienced visual loss. Relapses are not common; ESR and CRP can be used as markers but are not uniformly helpful. In the event of steroid-resistant disease, methotrexate and cyclophosphamide have been suggested. There is limited evidence for the use of either agent and this should not be routinely recommended as an additional treatment agent.

Surveillance imaging for the development of thoracic aortic aneurysms should be undertaken with annual chest X-rays.

Further Reading

Buttgereit F, Dejaco C, Matteson E, Dasgupta B (2016). Polymyalgia rheumatica and giant cell arteritis: a systematic review. *Journal of American Medical Association* 315(22): 2442–2458.

Villa-Forte A (2011). Giant cell arteritis: suspect it, treat it promptly. *Cleveland Clinical Journal of Medicine* 78(4): 265–270.

270. A) Adult-onset Still's disease

The patient presents with fevers, arthralgias, and weight loss, and has features of lymphadenopathy and a salmon-coloured rash. These features are classic for adult-onset Still's disease. This patient had no family history of similar problems and no urticarial symptoms, making periodic fever syndrome, which is discussed further in the tutorial, unlikely. Whilst sarcoidosis, TB, and Hodgkin's lymphoma could all present in this manner, this would have resulted in abnormal lymph node biopsy.

Tutorial

Adult-onset Still's disease is a rare inflammatory arthritis of adults that occurs worldwide. The diagnosis is used in adults who have symptoms that closely resemble juvenile idiopathic arthritis more than RA. The underlying cause is unknown but it is likely that it is a disorder of innate immunity. Different viruses and bacteria have been suggested as possible triggers.

It usually presents with fevers, rash, and arthralgias or arthritis (each occurs in 75–90% of patients). Very high fevers occur once or twice a day (quotidian or double-quotidian) associated with a severe myalgia; symptoms can completely resolve between episodes. A salmon-coloured non-pruritic macular or maculopapular rash is present over the trunk and extremities during febrile periods. The arthritis worsens over months from being transitory and oligoarticular to a more severe polyarthritis, which occurs in a similar distribution to RA. Patients often describe a sore throat at or shortly before the onset of illness. Lymphadenopathy is found in up to 60% of patients; splenomegaly in 30–50%; and hepatomegaly in 12–45%.

The diagnosis is clinical: laboratory tests are non-specific, with raised acute phase proteins and a granulocytic leukocytosis. Rheumatoid factor and anti-nuclear antibody should be negative. To fulfil the Yamaguchi diagnostic criteria at least five features, including at least two major diagnostic criteria, should be present.

Muckle-Wells syndrome (MWS) is an autoinflammatory disorder and one of the periodic fever syndromes. It is a rare autosomal dominant disease that causes progressive sensorineural deafness, recurrent urticaria, and AA amyloidosis. Individuals with MWS often have episodic fevers, headaches, and arthritis. MWS is closely related to two other syndromes: familial cold autoinflammatory syndrome and neonatal onset multisystem inflammatory disease. All three are caused by mutations in cryopyrin, which is part of the NALP3 inflammasome complex, and are known as cryopyrin-associated periodic syndromes (CAPS).

Further Reading

Fautrel B (2008) Adult-onset Still disease. *Best Practice and Research: Clinical Rheumatology* 22(5): 773–792.

Riera E, Olivé A, Narváez J, et al. (2011). Adult onset Still's disease: review of 41 cases. *Clinical and Experimental Rheumatology* 29(2): 331–336.

Yamaguchi M, Ohta A, Tsunematsu T, et al. (1992). Preliminary criteria for classification of adult Still's disease. *Journal of Rheumatology* 19: 424–430.

INDEX

Notes: Page numbers in *q* refer to Question and *a* refer to Answer.